THE FINAL FRCR

THE FINAL FRCR
Self-Assessment

Dr Amanda Rabone, FRCR
Consultant Radiologist, Radiology Department, Maidstone and Tunbridge Wells NHS Trust, Kent, United Kingdom

Dr Benedict Thomson, MRCP, FRCR
Interventional Radiology Fellow, Radiology Department, Guy's and St Thomas' NHS Foundation Trust, London, United Kingdom

Dr Nicky Dineen, FRCR
Consultant Radiologist, Radiology Department, Maidstone and Tunbridge Wells NHS Trust, Kent, United Kingdom

Dr Vincent Helyar, FRCR, EBIR
Consultant Interventional Radiologist, Radiology Department, Hampshire Hospitals NHS Foundation Trust, Hampshire, United Kingdom

Dr Aidan Shaw, MRCS, FRCR
Consultant Interventional Radiologist, Radiology Department, Maidstone and Tunbridge Wells NHS Trust, Kent, United Kingdom

CRC Press
Taylor & Francis Group
Boca Raton London New York

CRC Press is an imprint of the
Taylor & Francis Group, an **informa** business

First edition published 2021
by CRC Press
6000 Broken Sound Parkway NW, Suite 300, Boca Raton, FL 33487-2742

and by CRC Press
2 Park Square, Milton Park, Abingdon, Oxon, OX14 4RN

CRC Press is an imprint of Taylor & Francis Group, LLC

Library of Congress Cataloging-in-Publication Data
Names: Rabone, Amanda, author. | Thomson, Benedict, author. | Dineen, Nicky, author. | Helyar, Vincent, author. | Shaw, Aidan, author.
Title: The final FRCR : self-assessment / by Dr. Amanda Rabone, Dr. Benedict Thomson, Dr. Nicky Dineen, Dr. Vincent Helyar, Dr. Aidan Shaw.
Description: First edition. | Boca Raton, FL : CRC Press, 2021. | Includes bibliographical references and index. | Summary: "This is an SBA question book aimed at the post-graduate radiology market, specifically those taking the Fellowship of the Royal College of Radiology (FRCR) part 2 ('final') exams. This is a complementary title to The Final FRCR: Complete Revision Notes, which published in 2018"– Provided by publisher.
Identifiers: LCCN 2020043939 (print) | LCCN 2020043940 (ebook) | ISBN 9781482259742 (paperback) | ISBN 9780367637187 (hardback) | ISBN 9780429195327 (ebook)
Subjects: MESH: Diagnostic Imaging–methods | Radiology | United Kingdom | Examination Questions
Classification: LCC RC78.7.D53 (print) | LCC RC78.7.D53 (ebook) | NLM WN 18.2 | DDC 616.07/54–dc23
LC record available at https://lccn.loc.gov/2020043939
LC ebook record available at https://lccn.loc.gov/2020043940

ISBN: 9780367637187 (hbk)
ISBN: 9781482259742 (pbk)
ISBN: 9780429195327 (ebk)

Typeset in Palatino
by MPS Limited, Dehradun

I dedicate this book to all my family; my parents, Richard and Gill, to whom I owe so much. My husband Bruce and our son Magnus. Thank you for the love, support and happiness that you ceaselessly provide. And finally, to Melanie – never forgotten.

Amanda Rabone

I would like to dedicate this book to my family for their love and support.

Benedict Thomson

To my wonderful family who have been a constant source of joy, love and support.

Nicky Dineen

To my family, my wife Sinéad and my daughters Clara, Elizabeth and Frances for their love and support. I am very grateful to my parents for giving me my love of words and to my mother for the inspiration to write.

Vincent Helyar

I would like to dedicate this book to my incredible wife Juliette and my two wonderful boys, Edward and George, and for their continuing love and support throughout my career. I am also ever grateful to my amazing parents, Bryn and Ozden, who have always been there for me and my family, and without whom I would not be where I am today.

Aidan Shaw

Contents

Foreword

This book provides four papers, each containing 120 FRCR Part 2A examination mock single best answer questions, with answers in a separate section. The questions are well constructed and comprehensive, and closely simulate the style, standard and content of the current FRCR Part 2A questions which cover all body systems in a single examination.

A very valuable feature of the book is the extremely helpful, clear and pertinent explanations of why the best answer is the correct answer, and why the other possible answers are less likely or incorrect. The subject matter of each question is referenced (where relevant) for further revision and reading to the previously published companion book *The Final FRCR: Complete Revision Notes.*

There is no doubt that this book will appeal greatly to radiology candidates preparing for their FRCR examinations, making their personal revision programme much more interesting, focused, and also fun. I only wish I had had the benefit of this book myself when preparing for the examination! Nevertheless, I have hugely enjoyed reading the book and testing myself on the questions. Post-FRCR radiologists will also find this book invaluable as a quick and stimulating way of bringing them 'up to speed' with radiological knowledge across the whole spectrum of modern imaging.

I congratulate the authors on compiling such an excellent revision text, and I have no hesitation in highly recommending this book (and its companion *Revision Notes* book) to all radiologists.

Professor Nicola H Strickland,
BM, BCh, MA Hons (Oxon), FRCP, FRCR,
Immediate Past President of The Royal College of Radiologists

Acknowledgement

We would like to acknowledge all the teachers, supervisors and mentors over the years who have guided and encouraged us throughout our medical and radiology training.

Authors

Dr Amanda Rabone, FRCR is a recently appointed Consultant Radiologist at Maidstone and Tunbridge Wells NHS Trust. Dr Rabone graduated with Distinctions from Guy's, King's and St Thomas' School of Medicine in London. Following 2 years of Foundation training in the South East of England, she completed speciality training at Kent, Surrey and Sussex School of Radiology working in a variety of Kent district general hospitals and tertiary London centres.

Dr Rabone has subspecialist interests in breast and gynaecology imaging, whilst maintaining a broad interest in general radiology. She has won a number of prizes, published in peer-reviewed journals and has presented both nationally and internationally.

Dr Benedict Thomson, MRCP FRCR is a speciality Registrar in clinical radiology at Guy's and St Thomas' NHS Foundation Trust. He undertook his medical and radiological training in London and the South East. He is currently completing a sub-speciality fellowship in interventional radiology. Dr Thomson has a keen interest in teaching and has published research in international peer-reviewed journals and presented at national and international conferences in the field of diagnostic and interventional radiology. He is a member of the Royal College of Radiologists, British Society of Interventional Radiology, Cardiovascular and Interventional Radiology Society of Europe, European Society of Radiology and Radiological Society of North America.

Dr Nicky Dineen, FRCR qualified from Leicester University Medical School in 2011 and completed specialist radiology training in Kent, Surrey and Sussex School of Radiology, rotating across hospitals in Kent and London. She was appointed as a radiology Consultant Radiologist at Maidstone and Tunbridge Wells NHS Trust in 2018. Dr Dineen has particular interest in breast and thoracic imaging. She is a member of the Royal College of Radiologists and the British Society of Breast Radiology.

Dr Vincent Helyar, FRCR EBIR is a Consultant Interventional Radiologist at Hampshire Hospitals NHS Foundation Trust. He trained as a radiologist at Guy's and St Thomas' Hospitals including a 1-year fellowship in Interventional Radiology. His practice includes a broad range of both vascular and non-vascular intervention. Dr Helyar has a keen interest in teaching and has authored several book chapters, numerous articles and has presented widely at national and international conferences. He is a member of the Royal College of Radiologists, the British Society of Interventional Radiology, the European Society of Radiology and the Cardiovascular and Interventional Radiological Society of Europe.

Dr Aidan Shaw, MRCS FRCR is a Consultant Interventional Radiologist at Maidstone and Tunbridge Wells NHS Trust. He completed his speciality training at Guy's and St Thomas' NHS Foundation Trust including a 2-year Interventional Radiology fellowship. He has particular interests in gastrointestinal stenting and embolisation techniques, including uterine artery embolisation and ovarian vein embolisation.

Dr Shaw has authored several books as well as book chapters and has presented widely at national and international meetings. He has been published extensively in a number of international peer-reviewed journals, winning awards and fellowships in the fields of surgery and radiology. He is a member of the Royal College of Radiologists, the Royal College of Surgeons, the British Society of Interventional Radiology and the Cardiovascular and Interventional Radiological Society of Europe.

Introduction

This book was created with the aim of helping candidates to prepare for the new format of the Final Fellowship of the Royal College of Radiologists (FRCR) Part A examinations. It is the perfect accompaniment to the first book from this series, *The Final FRCR: Complete Revision Notes*.

The old style of the Final FRCR Part A examination consisted of six separate papers spread over the initial years of radiology subspecialist training – one for each curriculum module. Candidates now sit one large exam later in their training, consisting of two papers comprising 120 single best answer questions, encompassing all six modules. This is challenging to prepare for, both in terms of the vast amount of knowledge required and the stamina for sitting both papers on the same day.

This book comprises four full length papers, followed by detailed answer explanations. It aims to help candidates improve their radiology knowledge and their examination technique. Both of these attributes are vital for acquiring the Fellowship of the Royal College of Radiologists, not only for all of the written examinations but also for the Final FRCR Part B examination.

We hope you find this book helpful. Unlike the majority of question books available, which follow the old modular examination style, this book provides papers which are comparable to the new format of the Final FRCR Part A. We want candidates to be able to put their knowledge and timing to the test. Each paper has a selection of questions, of varying difficulty, from each curriculum module. Each answer has a page reference for *The Final FRCR: Complete Revision Notes*, so you can easily access extra reading on a topic if required.

The key to passing the Final FRCR is preparation. The volume and depth of knowledge required is quite overwhelming at the start of your revision journey so start reading early.

- Use everyday clinical experiences at work as an opportunity to familiarise yourself with subjects. You will remember the key features of a diagnosis far more easily if you can pin them to a clinical encounter.
- Attend multidisciplinary team meetings; the Final FRCR Part A not only tests diagnostic knowledge but management too.
- Once you have a good knowledge base, test yourself with as many questions as you can.
- Take the opportunity after marking your answers to read around the subject and ensure you are familiar with the imaging characteristics and factors that help distinguish between key differential diagnoses.

The more thoroughly you can prepare for the Final FRCR Part A examination, the easier you will find the preparation for the Final FRCR Part B, because you will already have acquired a strong foundation of radiology knowledge to build upon. We wish you the best of luck!

PAPER 1

1. A 57 year old man had an abdominal aortic aneurysm endovascular repair 6 months ago. The stent graft extends from the infrarenal region to hyperintense and enhance the common iliac arteries bilaterally. A recent CT abdomen and pelvis demonstrates that the aneurysm sac has enlarged following the repair with a blush of contrast within the sac at the origin of the inferior mesenteric artery from the abdominal aorta.

   What is the most likely diagnosis?

   a. Type 1a endoleak
   b. Type 1b endoleak
   c. Type 2 endoleak
   d. Type 3 endoleak
   e. Type 5 endoleak

2. A 46 year old man has an MRI head for persistent headache which demonstrates a 5-mm area in the pituitary with reduced enhancement compared to the rest of the gland. This is isointense on T1 weighted sequences and mildly hyperintense on T2 weighted sequences. Other recent plain films requested by the GP for joint pain demonstrate generalised osteopenia, chondrocalcinosis at the knees and joint space widening at the ankle.

   What other radiological finding would support the diagnosis?

   a. Eleven pairs of ribs
   b. Heel pad thickness of 30 mm
   c. Increased interpedicular distance
   d. Madelung deformity
   e. Sclerosis of the vertebral end plates

3. A 36 year old female patient originally presented to her GP with difficulty swallowing solids and liquids, associated chest discomfort and occasional episodes of regurgitation. Barium swallow helps to obtain the diagnosis. There is smooth distal oesophageal tapering with proximal oesophageal dilatation and tertiary contractions. This is successfully treated at the time but 19 years later the same patient presents with dysphagia again. The barium swallow now demonstrates an irregular, shouldered narrowing with proximal oesophageal dilatation. Endoscopy confirms malignancy.

   Where is the new narrowing most likely to be sited?

   a. Cervical oesophagus
   b. Distal oesophagus
   c. Mid-oesophagus
   d. Mid and distal oesophagus
   e. Proximal stomach

4. A 42 year old female patient, undergoing long-term peritoneal dialysis, has an abdominal ultrasound for left-sided flank pain with haematuria. The kidneys measure up to 5.5 cm in bipolar length with cortical thinning. There is no hydronephrosis or renal calculi. There are several bilateral renal lesions. These are small, exophytic, anechoic and well defined. One lesion on the left side has internal echoes and dependent debris. There is a moderate amount of free fluid in the abdomen and pelvis.

   What is the most likely underlying diagnosis causing the renal lesions?

   a. Acquired cystic kidney disease
   b. Autosomal dominant polycystic kidney disease
   c. Autosomal recessive polycystic kidney disease
   d. Idiopathic bilateral renal cysts
   e. Tuberous sclerosis

5. A CT head is performed on a toddler who has tripped at home, hitting his head. The paediatric team are concerned about a possible seizure following the event and a couple of episodes of vomiting. The scan shows no intracranial haemorrhage. However, there is a hypodense posterior fossa lesion. An MRI more clearly demonstrates that this is in the posterior midline of the posterior fossa displacing the cerebellum anteriorly. The tentorium

cerebelli and cerebellar vermis appear intact and have normal appearances. There is no hydrocephalus and the fourth ventricle is within normal limits. There is no significant enhancement following contrast administration. There is no restricted diffusion. On a FLAIR sequence the lesion is isointense to cerebrospinal fluid.

Which diagnosis is most likely?

a. Dermoid cyst
b. Epidermoid cyst
c. Ependymal cyst
d. Pilocytic astrocytoma
e. Mega cisterna magna

6. An MRI of the spine is performed in a 43 year old patient with no significant medical history complaining of cervical pain. This reveals a solitary, oval, intradural extramedullary lesion extending from C5 to C6. It is sited anteriorly within the spinal canal and is isointense to the cord on T1, hyperintense on T2 sequences with heterogenous enhancement following contrast. It is displacing the spinal cord and right C5 nerve root and mildly widening the neural foramen.

What is the most likely underlying cause?

a. Epidermoid
b. Meningioma
c. Metastasis
d. Paraganglioma
e. Schwannoma

7. A 44 year old male presents to the emergency department with left side renal colic; he has an unenhanced CT urinary tract to investigate. There is no renal calculus and no other significant finding in the abdomen or pelvis. There is an incidental finding of a partially visualised 2-cm subpleural nodule in the right lower lobe. He is discharged back to the care of the GP, with advice to further investigate the nodule. An unenhanced outpatient CT chest demonstrates that the nodule is solitary and slightly lobulated with punctate calcification. There are low density foci within the nodule that have a density of negative Hounsfield units. No other abnormality is seen on the CT chest.

What is the most appropriate next course of action?

a. Staging CT scan to look for a primary malignancy
b. Investigation of the nodule with CT angiogram
c. FDG PET scan to assess whether the nodule is avid
d. Discharge the patient
e. Investigation with a Gallium 68 PET scan

8. A 53 year old diabetic patient presents with right shoulder pain and reduced range of movement which does not improve despite community physiotherapy. The patient is reviewed in the orthopaedic outpatient clinic and an MRI shoulder arthrogram is requested.

Which of the options below is most consistent with adhesive capsulitis?

Table 1.1:

	Joint Capsule	Subscapularis Bursa	Coracohumeral Ligament	Lymphatic Filling
a	Thickened	Small	Thickened	Present
b	Thickened	Enlarged	Thinned	Present
c	Thinned	Enlarged	Thinned	Absent
d	Thinned	Small	Thickened	Present
e	Normal	Enlarged	Thinned	Absent

9. A 56 year old male presents with gradual onset right upper quadrant pain. An ultrasound examination is performed which demonstrates absence of Doppler flow in the hepatic veins. Budd-Chiari syndrome is suspected.

   Which of the following imaging features differentiates chronic from acute Budd-Chiari?

   a. Hepatomegaly
   b. Hypertrophied caudate lobe
   c. Heterogeneous hepatic echotexture
   d. Splenomegaly
   e. Ascites

10. A 5 year old girl has an obvious deformity affecting the right side of her upper back and shoulder with a visible 'bump'. She has spinal imaging which detects fusion of the C2-C4 vertebrae. The patient has also had an MRI brain and spine.

    Given the other findings, which of the following is most likely to be found on the MRI brain?

    a. Chiari I malformation
    b. Haemangioblastoma
    c. Holoprosencephaly
    d. Optic glioma
    e. Polymicrogyria

11. An oncology patient has an MRI spine due to increasing back pain. Apart from mild generalised motor weakness he has no significant neurology. The MRI identifies multiple areas of abnormal T1 and T2 signal which are hypointense compared to the adjacent disc. There is heterogenous high STIR signal in these regions and restricted diffusion. There is no significant narrowing of the canal or neural foramina. The cord returns normal signal.

    What is the most likely underlying primary site of malignancy?

    a. Colorectal carcinoma
    b. Melanoma
    c. Non-small cell lung carcinoma
    d. Prostate carcinoma
    e. Renal cell carcinoma

12. A 47 year old man complains of progressive discomfort and swelling of his right knee over a couple of years which is now causing difficulty walking. An MRI shows no significant degenerative change but there is synovial proliferation. There is some erosion of the bones on both sides of the joint and multiple small, lobulated intra-articular foci which are intermediate signal on T1 and T2 hyperintense. An earlier radiograph confirms some of these intra-articular bodies are calcified.

    What is the most likely diagnosis?

    a. Pigmented villonodular synovitis
    b. Primary osteochondromatosis
    c. Secondary osteochondromatosis
    d. Synovial chondrosarcoma
    e. Synovial haemangioma

13. A 36 year old man is referred by his GP following a diagnosis of hypertension and has a chest radiograph. The lungs and pleural spaces are clear. The mediastinum is abnormal and the aorta has a 'reverse 3' sign with bilateral inferior rib notching.

    What other finding is magnetic resonance angiography most likely to reveal?

    a. Aortic root dilatation
    b. Pulmonary arterial aneurysm
    c. Scoliosis
    d. Truncus arteriosus
    e. Ventricular septal defect

14. A 35 year old male patient presents to the emergency department with atraumatic right hip pain for 10 days; he is otherwise systemically well. A radiograph shows mild osteopenia in the right femoral head. A previous abdominal radiograph from 2 years ago included the right hip, which looked normal at that time, but you notice foci of calcification projected over the upper abdominal quadrants bilaterally and generalised osteosclerosis.

    What MRI finding in the proximal femur would be most specific for the correct diagnosis?

    a. Adjacent subchondral hypo and hyperintense T2 linear signal
    b. Low T1 signal at the medial aspect of the femoral neck
    c. Low T1 signal line parallel to the subarticular cortex
    d. Synovial enhancement with gadolinium
    e. Subchondral high STIR signal

15. You report an outpatient portal venous phase CT abdomen pelvis which has been performed 3 days earlier for a 67 year old male GP patient with a 1-month history of abdominal pain, weight loss and anaemia. There is no discernible abnormality of the solid abdominal viscera. You notice a small amount of pelvic free fluid. There is evidence of previous endovascular repair of an abdominal aortic aneurysm with a fenestrated suprarenal graft. There are a couple of small gas locules adjacent to the proximal aortic graft and the aortic wall appears thickened, with a loop of small bowel in contact with the aorta.

    What is the most appropriate course of action?

    a. Ask radiology secretaries to email report to GP for their attention
    b. Arrange triple phase CT abdomen and pelvis
    c. Inform on-call vascular specialist registrar of findings
    d. No further action required and suggest endoscopy to exclude gastrointestinal malignancy
    e. Suggest 18F-FDG PET/CT to further evaluate

16. A 28 year old female patient is admitted with right flank pain and a temperature of 37.8 °C. Urine dip is positive for blood and leukocytes. The patient is haemodynamically stable. Inflammatory markers are elevated but liver and renal function tests are normal.

    What would be the most appropriate immediate course of action?

    a. Antibiotics followed by blood culture
    b. Antibiotics followed by blood culture and urinary tract ultrasound
    c. Antibiotics followed by blood culture and CT urinary tract
    d. Blood culture followed by antibiotics
    e. Blood culture followed by antibiotics and urinary tract ultrasound

17. A 6 week old baby is undergoing investigation for ongoing jaundice associated with dark urine and pale stools. An ultrasound abdomen demonstrates an enlarged liver with a normal contour. There is an echogenic region just anterior to the portal vein in the region of the porta hepatis. There is no intrahepatic duct dilatation. The spleen and kidneys have normal appearances. The gallbladder is not visualised. The head and body of the pancreas have normal appearances but the tail is obscured by overlying bowel gas. There is no free fluid.

    What is the most appropriate next investigation to aid diagnosis?

    a. CT abdomen
    b. Hepatic iminodiacetic acid (HIDA) scan
    c. Hepatic ultrasound with contrast
    d. MRCP
    e. Ultrasound guided liver biopsy

18. You have an ultrasound list with a thyroid ultrasound booked for a middle-aged male patient referred by the GP for possible thyroid goitre. You complete the scan and are writing the report.

    Which nodule characteristic is most concerning for malignancy?

    a. Hyperechoic echotexture
    b. Greater than 1.5 cm in size

c. Hypoechoic halo
d. Internal vascularity
e. Microcalcification

19. A 22 year old male medical student reports to his GP with recurrent spontaneous epistaxis as well as fatigue and increasing dyspnoea. The patient is found to be tachycardic and tachypnoeic. The GP is concerned and in view of the patient's significant family history refers him to be seen by the on-call medical team at hospital. The medical team organise an urgent chest radiograph and perform an arterial blood gas which demonstrates hypoxia. They refer the patient to you for a CT pulmonary angiogram to exclude a pulmonary embolus.
On review of the plain film, you confirm the presence of multiple pulmonary nodules and the heart appears large. There is no other significant abnormality.

What is the most likely underlying diagnosis?

a. Caplan syndrome
b. Goodpasture's syndrome
c. Granulomatosis with polyangiitis
d. Multiple metastases
e. Osler-Weber-Rendu syndrome

20. A 55 year old female patient has a lateral cervical spine radiograph requested by the rheumatology clinic. On the lateral view, the tip of the odontoid process of C2 sits at the basion-opisthion line.

Which of the conditions below is NOT associated with this appearance?

a. Achondroplasia
b. Fibrous dysplasia
c. Osteopetrosis
d. Paget disease
e. Rheumatoid arthritis

21. An 18 year old girl with a previous history of intussusception as a child presents with abdominal pain. She is noted to have peri-oral pigmentation. A barium meal and follow-through examination demonstrate multiple polyps within the stomach and small bowel. The patient is known to have a congenital syndrome.

What is the most likely underlying diagnosis?

a. Cronkhite-Canada syndrome
b. Cowden syndrome
c. Peutz-Jegher syndrome
d. Familial adenomatous polyposis syndrome
e. Juvenile polyposis syndrome

22. A GP registrar calls for advice regarding an 11 month old girl following the diagnosis of her first urinary tract infection. This has been confirmed on urine culture as positive for *Escherichia coli* which is sensitive to trimethroprim. The patient has had 2 days of oral antibiotics at home and on review again today at the surgery she is improving. The GP registrar asks for your advice regarding further management.

What is the most appropriate advice?

a. Paediatric referral
b. Ultrasound within 6 weeks
c. Ultrasound and DMSA within 6 weeks
d. Ultrasound and DMSA if recurrent infection
e. Urgent ultrasound

23. An MRI lumbar spine performed for back pain is described as having abnormal signal consistent with Modic type I end plate changes at the L1/2 level.

Which of the following signal characteristics would be most consistent with this?

Table 1.2:

	Endplate T1 Signal	Endplate T2 Signal	Endplate Enhancement	Disc T2 Signal
a	Low	High	Yes	Low
b	Low	High	Yes	High
c	High	Low	No	Low
d	High	High	Yes	Low
e	Low	Low	No	High

24. A 43 year old male patient has a barium swallow and meal study. You are asked to review the images by a junior colleague. There is swift passage of contrast to the stomach with normal oesophageal outline and no gastro-oesophageal reflux. The stomach distends well. Gastric folds at the fundus measure 15 mm in thickness and 6 mm in the prepyloric region of the stomach. No gastric wall irregularity is identified and there is evidence of rapid gastric emptying.

    What is the most likely cause of the thickened gastric folds?

    a. Atrophic gastritis
    b. Alcoholic gastritis
    c. Crohn's disease
    d. Lymphoma
    e. Zollinger-Ellison syndrome

25. A 45 year old motorcyclist involved in a high speed road traffic collision is brought into the emergency department intubated and ventilated and has a portable chest radiograph in the resus bay. This demonstrates the endotracheal tube tip projected over the right main bronchus, multiple right rib fractures, large right pneumothorax, right lung consolidation, a left apical cap and bilateral pleural effusions.

    Which finding most urgently needs to be conveyed to the trauma team?

    a. Bilateral pleural effusions
    b. Endotracheal tube tip position
    c. Left apical cap
    d. Right lung consolidation
    e. Right pneumothorax

26. A 60 year old male patient is referred from his GP with 6 weeks of increased right knee pain. The GP palpated a mass at the posterior aspect of the knee. Radiograph of the right knee demonstrates spiking of the intercondylar eminence and reduction in patellofemoral and medial tibiofemoral joint space. There has been no significant interval change since a radiograph 2 years previously. The patient has an MRI knee which reveals a well-defined high T2 and low T1 signal lesion at the posterior aspect of the knee arising, and extending, from the joint space into the soft tissues posteriorly. This is separate to the neurovascular bundle. There is no associated increased STIR signal in the marrow or soft tissues.

    Which anatomical structures would this lesion arise between?

    a. Biceps femoris muscle and medial head of gastrocnemius
    b. Gracilis tendon and semimembranosus tendon
    c. Iliotibial tract and biceps femoris muscle
    d. Semimembranosus tendon and medial head of gastrocnemius
    e. Semitendinosus tendon and medial head of gastrocnemius

27. A 23 year old male presents with fever, loose stools and watery diarrhoea for the last 2 weeks. He has recently returned from a trip to southeast Asia. Blood tests show raised inflammatory markers. An abdominal radiograph is performed which shows mucosal oedema and thumb printing affecting the ascending colon. Stool cultures are sent.

Given the distribution of the abnormality, what is the most likely organism responsible for the appearances?

a. *Salmonella*
b. *Shigella*
c. Cytomegalovirus
d. Herpes simplex virus
e. *Clostridioides difficile*

28. A 54 year old female patient has an abdominal ultrasound for right upper quadrant pain. This demonstrates a homogenous, echogenic lesion in the upper pole of the left kidney. It is well defined, exophytic and measures 46 mm with posterior acoustic shadowing. There is no hydronephrosis and the kidney otherwise has normal appearances. Appearances of the right kidney are within normal limits.

    What would be the next most appropriate step?

    a. CT chest, abdomen and pelvis
    b. CT abdomen as next available outpatient appointment
    c. CT abdomen in 3–6 months
    d. Discussion at the urology multidisciplinary team meeting
    e. Repeat ultrasound in 3–6 months

29. The urology team request an urgent testicular ultrasound on a teenager with left sided scrotal pain and swelling. The ultrasound demonstrates scrotal wall thickening with associated increased Doppler flow. The testicles have a homogenous echotexture with symmetrical vascularity. The left testicle is marginally bigger than the right testicle. There is a trace amount of fluid around the left testicle. There is a 3-mm thin-walled, avascular, anechoic structure with posterior acoustic enhancement at the left epididymal head adjacent to the upper pole of the testicle. The left epididymal tail is swollen with a heterogenous echotexture and diffusely increased vascularity compared to the right side. The right epididymis has a homogenous echotexture. There is no evidence of varicocele. The urology registrar comes to discuss the findings after the scan.

    What is the most appropriate report conclusion?

    a. Epididymitis
    b. Epididymo-orchitis
    c. Orchitis
    d. Testicular torsion
    e. Torsion of the appendix testis

30. You are the radiology registrar in a major trauma centre. An intubated and ventilated 35 year old motorcyclist has an MRI whole spine following a road traffic collision earlier the same day. The initial trauma CT identified intracranial haemorrhage and fractures of the T4, T5 and L1 vertebrae. The MRI reveals a thoracic epidural collection which is isointense on T1 sequences and mildly hyperintense on T2 sequences. The radiology consultant agrees with your observations.

    What is the most appropriate next step in management?

    a. Inform neurosurgical team
    b. Request immediate T2* MRI sequence
    c. Request immediate additional contrast enhanced MRI sequences
    d. Repeat MRI in 24 hours
    e. Urgent discussion with microbiology

31. A 59 year old male patient is referred to radiology from the GP for investigation of a chronic cough. No other history is provided. He has a chest radiograph. The performing radiographer notices an abnormality and asks you to review the image before the patient is sent away. There are scattered tiny nodules seen in both lungs; there is also eggshell calcification of the nodes in the hilar regions bilaterally and the mediastinum. No other finding is seen on the plain film. You reassure the radiographer that the patient can go home. You report the imaging, suggesting further investigation with non-contrast CT chest.

    Which diagnosis is LEAST likely?

a. Amyloidosis
b. Histoplasmosis
c. Sarcoidosis
d. Silicosis
e. Treated lymphoma

32. A 67 year old diabetic male patient presents to hospital with a 4-day history of erythema and swelling of his left elbow which has not improved despite 2 days of antibiotics from his GP. There is no history of preceding trauma. Inflammatory markers are raised and he has a temperature of 38.5 °C. A blood culture is negative. A radiograph of the left elbow demonstrates soft tissue swelling but the bones are normal in appearance. The MRI scanner is undergoing maintenance; therefore a nuclear medicine triple phase bone scan is performed.

    Which of the below patterns of tracer uptake would be most consistent with osteomyelitis?

Table 1.3:

	Angiographic Phase	Tissue Phase	Osseous Phase
a	Normal	Normal	Increased
b	Normal	Increased	Increased
c	Increased	Increased	Increased
d	Increased	Increased	Normal
e	Increased	Increased	Decreased

33. A 58 year old male patient has a barium swallow and meal study for heartburn and symptoms of gastritis which have not responded to treatment. This demonstrates a malignant appearing gastric ulcer and the patient subsequently has an endoscopy that confirms malignancy. CT chest, abdomen and pelvis confirms no distant spread of the disease.

    With regard to the ulcer, what imaging finding on barium meal best correlates with this diagnosis?

    a. Carmen meniscus
    b. Hampton's line
    c. Location on the lesser curve
    d. Extending beyond the gastric wall
    e. Gastric folds reach the edge of the ulcer

34. A 2 month old boy has an abdominal ultrasound scan which identifies small kidneys bilaterally with bilateral hydronephrosis and hydroureter. The urinary bladder is thickened and trabeculated. On micturating cystourethrogram there is bilateral vesicoureteral reflux and dilatation of the posterior urethra. Contrast also fills a small diverticulum, continuous with the bladder dome, at the bladder's anterosuperior aspect. Assessment of the scrotum finds that the testicles are undescended.

    Which one of the following conditions is most consistent with these radiological findings?

    a. Bladder exstrophy
    b. Eagle-Barrett syndrome
    c. Edwards syndrome
    d. Patau syndrome
    e. Posterior urethral valve

35. A 70 year woman falls on the pavement whilst walking, hits her head and loses consciousness. She is assessed in the emergency department.

    Which of the following findings is an indication to perform an immediate CT according to NICE guidelines?

    a. 30 minutes of antegrade amnesia
    b. High energy trauma
    c. Age >65

d. One episode of vomiting since head injury
e. GCS <15 at 2 hours post injury

36. The abdominal radiograph of an 18 month old child reveals a large soft tissue density mass in the left upper quadrant displacing the adjacent bowel loops. An abdominal ultrasound confirms a vascular, heterogenous, solid and cystic left upper quadrant mass. There are highly reflective foci which exhibit posterior acoustic shadowing. The left kidney is displaced anteroinferiorly and the mass extends posteriorly and is seen adjacent to the vertebral column, with the aorta seen pulsating within the mass. The liver and spleen have normal appearances. The case is discussed at the paediatric oncology multidisciplinary team meeting with the paediatric surgeons.

Which imaging test would be most appropriate for assessing the local disease extent?

a. CT chest, abdomen and pelvis
b. MIBG
c. MRI abdomen
d. Technetium 99-m bone scan
e. 18F-FDG PET/CT

37. A CT pulmonary angiogram of a 42 year old female patient demonstrates a well-defined, round filling defect in the left atrium. This is confirmed with echocardiogram and the lesion can be seen protruding through the mitral valve. MRI demonstrates low T1 signal and heterogenous T2 signal with enhancement on post contrast sequences.

What is the most likely diagnosis?

a. Fibroma
b. Metastasis
c. Myxoma
d. Rhabdomyoma
e. Thrombus

38. A 55 year old male patient is referred by his GP due to pain in his non-dominant left wrist, particularly at night, and associated pins and needles in his thumb, index and middle fingers. Carpal tunnel syndrome is suspected and the patient has an MRI of the left wrist.

What is the most specific sign on MRI?

a. Abrupt change in median nerve diameter
b. Bowing of the flexor retinaculum
c. Enhancement of the median nerve
d. Flattening of the median nerve
e. Oedema within the carpal tunnel

39. A 34 year old male presents to the emergency department with generalised abdominal pain, weight loss and diarrhoea. He is seen by the general surgeons who request a CT abdomen and pelvis. This shows mucosal thickening mainly involving the caecum, and to a lesser extent the terminal ileum. There are several enlarged ileo-colic lymph nodes that are hypoattenuating. Small volume hyperattenuating ascites is also seen.

What is the most likely diagnosis?

a. Small bowel lymphoma
b. Small bowel tuberculosis
c. Yersiniosis
d. Crohn's disease
e. Actinomycosis

40. You are attending the urology multidisciplinary team meeting and have reviewed a CT urogram for a 53 year old male patient with a performance status of 0. The patient was seen in clinic with repeated haematuria. The CT shows unobstructed kidneys with no renal calculi and no filling defects in the pelvicalyceal system or ureters. There is an exophytic 15-mm right renal lesion which has a Hounsfield unit (HU) of 42 on the unenhanced study and 50HU on the delayed phase split bolus sequence. The bladder is partially filled and there is no differentially enhancing bladder lesion visible. There are no enlarged retroperitoneal or pelvic

lymph nodes. No further abnormalities are seen on the CT.

What would be the most appropriate recommendation to the multidisciplinary team?

a. Cystoscopy
b. No further action
c. Repeat CT in 3–6 months
d. Staging CT chest
e. Ultrasound guided right renal biopsy

41. An 11 month old baby has an abdominal ultrasound for possible intussusception following an episode of abdominal pain and haematochezia. This does not identify any evidence of intussusception and the child's symptoms resolve after treatment for constipation. During this scan the right kidney was noted to have a 20-mm hypoechoic, peripherally sited, right renal lesion distant to the renal sinus. The left kidney has normal appearances. An MRI abdomen confirmed the presence of the lesion, which was limited to the kidney and demonstrated homogenously low signal on T1 and T2 weighted imaging. Following contrast there was minimal homogenous enhancement compared to the adjacent renal cortex.

    Which of the following does this renal lesion most likely represent?

    a. Mesoblastic nephroma
    b. Multilocular cystic nephroma
    c. Nephroblastoma
    d. Nephroblastomatosis
    e. Prominent column of Bertin

42. A 30 year old male driver is involved in a high-speed road traffic collision. At the scene of the accident his GCS is 7. On arrival in hospital his initial CT scan is normal. Following 48 hours on intensive care, his GCS remains inappropriately low and he undergoes an MRI brain which demonstrates multiple FLAIR hyperintensities at the grey–white matter junction in the frontotemporal regions and the periventricular temporal lobes.

    What is the most likely diagnosis?

    a. Diffuse axonal injury
    b. Cerebral contusions
    c. Subdural haematoma
    d. Intraparenchymal haematoma
    e. Cavernomas

43. A 56 year old female is on intensive care for the second day after presenting with severe community acquired pneumonia and acute kidney injury. She has no previous history of renal impairment or other significant medical history. On admission the radiograph demonstrates density overlying the cardiac silhouette in keeping with left lower lobe pneumonia. She develops respiratory failure which is not improving with oxygen administration. She has a chest radiograph every day, and on subsequent plain films there are increasing ill-defined airspace opacities bilaterally.

    Which of the following is LEAST likely to be a feature of acute respiratory distress syndrome?

    a. Anterior airway dilatation
    b. Patchy airspace opacification
    c. Peripheral airspace opacification
    d. Pleural effusion
    e. Reticular opacities

44. A patient presents with a 6-month history of a painless swollen right shoulder with no known preceding history of trauma. Inflammatory markers are normal and the patient is systemically well with no fever. Radiograph of the shoulder reveals normal bone density; however there is fragmentation of the right humeral head with glenohumeral dislocation and loose bodies in the joint space.

    What is the most likely underlying diagnosis?

a. Chronic alcohol excess
b. Diabetes
c. Multiple sclerosis
d. Previous spinal cord trauma
e. Syringomyelia

45. An abdominal ultrasound of a 52 year old febrile woman with right upper quadrant discomfort and a history of gallstones, raised body mass index, type 2 diabetes and previous alcohol excess identifies a 6-mm mobile gallstone at the neck of the gallbladder. The gallbladder wall measures 4 mm in thickness. There is a more focal area of wall thickening at the fundus. There is no intra- or extrahepatic biliary dilatation. This focal fundal thickening does not alter with patient movement. There is a small amount of pericholecystic fluid. The patient is discharged and an outpatient MRCP confirms a solitary non-obstructing gallstone and also better visualises the area of focal fundal mural thickening which demonstrates multiple small curvilinear foci of T2 weighted hyperintensity within the wall.

What is the most likely diagnosis?

a. Adenomyomatosis
b. Gangrenous cholecystitis
c. Gallbladder carcinoma
d. Gallbladder polyp
e. Phrygian cap

46. An MRI spine for a patient with back pain radiating down the left leg has a report which states that there is a broad-based disc protrusion at L2/3 causing significant stenosis of the left exit foramen and impingement of the exiting nerve at this level.

Which of the following descriptions fits this observation most accurately?

a. Disc material extending >90° circumference and >3 mm beyond the vertebral body margin impinging the left L2 nerve
b. Disc material extending >90° circumference and >3 mm beyond the vertebral body margin impinging the left L3 nerve
c. Disc material extending >90° circumference and >3 mm beyond the vertebral body margin impinging the right L3 nerve
d. Disc material extending >180° circumference and >3 mm beyond the vertebral body margin impinging the left L2 nerve
e. Disc material extending >180° circumference and >3 mm beyond the vertebral body margin impinging the left L3 nerve

47. A renal ultrasound on a 1 year old girl being followed up following an abnormal antenatal scan finds an enlarged right kidney. There are several thin-walled, large anechoic lesions which are variable in size but demonstrate posterior acoustic enhancement. The morphology of the kidney is distorted with no visible normal renal parenchyma. It is difficult to assess if these lesions are continuous with the renal pelvis. There is no associated increased Doppler vascularity. There is no uptake in this kidney on a MAG3 study. The left kidney has normal appearances.

What is the most likely diagnosis?

a. Autosomal recessive polycystic kidney disease
b. Congenital mesoblastic nephroma
c. Hydronephrotic right kidney
d. Multicystic dysplastic kidney
e. Multilocular cystic nephroma

48. A 25 year old male boxer loses consciousness during a fight. He is brought to the emergency department where a CT shows an extra-axial haemorrhage at the vertex. This crosses the midline and also displaces the superior sagittal sinus inferiorly.

What is the most likely diagnosis?

a. Subdural haematoma
b. Mixed extradural and subdural haematoma

c. Extradural haematoma
d. Intraparenchymal haematoma
e. Subarachnoid haemorrhage

49. A 31 year old football player with a family history of heart disease has a cardiac MRI following syncopal episodes during exertion. This demonstrates an overall ejection fraction of 60% (normal 50–70%), segmental right ventricular dilatation and wall motion abnormality with T1 hyperintensity in the right free wall basally and apically. There is normal left wall motion.

    What is the most likely diagnosis?

    a. Arrhythmogenic right ventricular dysplasia
    b. Dilated cardiomyopathy
    c. Established myocardial infarct
    d. Hypertrophic cardiomyopathy
    e. Restrictive cardiomyopathy

50. A 52 year old female patient presents to hospital feeling unwell with fever, fatigue and generalised aches and pains causing difficulty mobilising. There is a rash on her back and upper arms. The emergency department team request blood tests and chest and abdominal radiographs. The chest radiograph shows some air space opacification and bibasal atelectasis. The abdominal radiograph demonstrates a normal bowel gas pattern with subcutaneous calcification in a linear distribution projected over the soft tissues of the pelvis and upper thigh.

    What is the most appropriate next investigation?

    a. Barium swallow
    b. CT chest
    c. Oesophageal endoscopy
    d. Nuclear medicine cardiac perfusion study
    e. Ultrasound Doppler lower limbs

51. A 30 year old female is referred to the gastroenterologists by her GP with intermittent abdominal pain. She has recently undergone significant weight loss through intense dieting and exercise. She describes an intermittent cramping abdominal pain that is relieved by lying prone in bed. The gastroenterology team request a CT abdomen and pelvis. This shows a paucity of intrabdominal fat. The proximal duodenum is noted to be dilated and there is an abrupt transition point as the D3 segment passes between the duodenum and aorta.

    What is the most likely diagnosis?

    a. Nutcracker syndrome
    b. Mesenteric ischaemia
    c. Irritable bowel syndrome
    d. Superior mesenteric artery syndrome
    e. Duodenal ulcer

52. A 31 year old male patient falls off a horse and is brought into the emergency department with generalised abdominopelvic pain and haematuria upon catheterisation. Following initial review the team request a CT abdomen and pelvis. A portal venous phase scan is performed. This demonstrates a fracture of the L2–4 left transverse processes and comminuted, displaced fractures of the left superior and inferior pubic rami. The solid organs appear intact. The urinary catheter is appropriately sited. There is a moderate volume of free fluid in the pelvis with a density of approximately 5HU but no free gas. No focal bowel wall thickening or mesenteric fat stranding is evident.

    What would be the most appropriate next step?

    a. CT cystogram
    b. Cystoscopy
    c. Repeat CT abdomen and pelvis in 20 minutes
    d. Repeat CT in 24 hours
    e. Immediate triple phase CT abdomen and pelvis

53. An abdominal radiograph is performed for a 51 year old patient with abdominal pain presenting to hospital. Bilateral renal calcification is evident in a medullary distribution.

    Which of the following is unlikely to be a cause for this appearance?

    a. Hyperparathyroidism
    b. Hypothyroidism
    c. Multiple myeloma
    d. Sarcoidosis
    e. Tuberculosis

54. A 20 year old man is assaulted sustaining several heavy blows to the face. Facial bone radiographs are performed in the emergency department followed by CT facial bones. There are bilateral complex facial bone fractures.

    Which structure needs to be involved to classify the injury as a Le Fort fracture?

    a. Zygomatic arch
    b. Inferior orbital rim
    c. Pterygoid plates
    d. Nasal septum
    e. Lateral walls of maxillary sinuses

55. A 68 year old female with known HIV infection presents to the emergency department with insidious onset exertional dyspnoea. Her CD4 count is 120 cells/mm^3 (500–1400 cells/mm^3) and her chest radiograph demonstrates bilateral perihilar ground glass opacification. *Pneumocystis jiroveci* is suspected and the clinical team refer her for a CT chest prior to bronchoscopy.

    Which of the following imaging features are LEAST likely to be seen on CT chest?

    a. Perihilar ground glass opacification
    b. Pleural effusion
    c. Pneumatoceles
    d. Pneumothorax
    e. Septal thickening

56. A 69 year old male patient has a radiograph of the spine following a fall from standing which shows an incidental finding of diffuse idiopathic skeletal hyperostosis.

    Which feature is NOT associated with this condition?

    a. Calcaneal spur
    b. Dysphagia
    c. Facet joint ankylosis
    d. Ossification of the patella tendon
    e. Posterior longitudinal ligament calcification

57. A CT abdomen pelvis is performed for a 51 year old female patient with abdominal discomfort, change in bowel habit and generalised fatigue. This demonstrates a small, hyper-enhancing polypoid lesion in the distal small bowel measuring 15 mm with adjacent mural thickening. The small bowel loops proximal to this are prominent with faecalisation of small bowel contents. There is a 2-mm focus within the lesion with a density of 956HU and there are a couple of adjacent 10-mm short axis low density mesenteric lymph nodes.

    What is the most appropriate next step in the management of this patient to aid diagnosis and treatment planning?

    a. Arterial phase CT chest and abdomen
    b. MIBG scan
    c. 5-HIAA serum levels
    d. 111In-octreotide study
    e. 18F-FDG PET/CT

58. An athletic 45 year old man is seen in a follow-up orthopaedic clinic following surgery for a prolapsed L3/4 disc 12 months ago as an emergency case for cauda equina. He recovered well immediately postoperatively but is concerned because he has been suffering from increasing

back pain for 3 months radiating down his left leg. The patient has no neurological symptoms on examination. The orthopaedic team request an MRI of the lumbar spine. At the L3/4 disc space there is moderate low T1 signal narrowing the left subarticular zone.

Which finding in the left subarticular zone is most in keeping with post-surgical fibrosis versus recurrent disc prolapse?

a. Early enhancement following gadolinium
b. High T2 signal
c. Smooth border
d. Late enhancement following gadolinium
e. Restricted diffusion

59. A 7 year old girl with urinary incontinence is referred for a micturating cystourethrogram. The patient has an ultrasound followed by an intravenous urogram. Both kidneys have a normal position and size. The left kidney has two ureters draining it and one of the ureters drains into the vagina with the other ureter draining into the urinary bladder.

Which of the following is the most accurate statement?

a. The anatomy in this case represents a bifid ureter
b. The lower pole moiety is frequently obstructed by a ureterocoele
c. The upper pole moiety can have a 'drooping lily' appearance
d. The ureter draining into the vagina is associated with the upper pole moiety
e. Vesicoureteral reflux is associated with the ureter draining into the vagina

60. A 60 year old woman presents following a traumatic head injury. She is noted to have haemotympanum. A CT head is performed which shows a transverse fracture extending through the left petrous temporal bone.

What likely complication is most associated with this type of fracture?

a. Tympanic membrane disruption
b. Sensorineural hearing loss
c. Conductive hearing loss
d. Carotid artery dissection
e. Sigmoid sinus injury

61. A 37 year old male presents to his GP with a long-standing cough. A plain film demonstrates a large, smoothly marginated opacity in the right lower zone abutting the right heart border. A second similar density is seen in the periphery of the left lower zone. A contrast-enhanced CT helps investigate further. This confirms the presence of two well circumscribed, rounded, slightly lobulated densities with thin walls and low density contents (10HU). Within left lower zone lesion there is the presence of a serpiginous structure; the surrounding lung is normal.

What is the most likely diagnosis?

a. Bronchogenic cysts
b. Diaphragmatic hernias
c. Hydatid cysts
d. Pericardial cysts
e. Pulmonary abscesses

62. A 31 year old patient comes to the emergency department with worsening lower lumbar back pain over the past 7 weeks. The patient has no fixed abode and has a recent history of intravenous drug use. Inflammatory markers are raised and the patient has a temperature of 37.5 °C. Chest radiograph is normal and urine dip is negative. Blood cultures are sent to the laboratory. Radiograph of the spine shows reduction in disc space at L3/4. MRI reveals high T2 signal and post contrast enhancement in the L3/4 disc with low T1 and high T2 signal in the adjacent vertebral bodies. There is also an enhancing paravertebral collection which is inseparable from the left psoas muscle.

What is the most likely causative organism?

a. *Burkholderia pseudomallei*
b. *Candida*

c. *Mycobacterium tuberculosis*
d. *Salmonella*
e. *Streptococcus viridans*

63. A 75 year old male patient is admitted with fever, reduced appetite, shortness of breath and chest pain. Contrast enhanced CT chest, abdomen and pelvis identifies no consolidation or intrabdominal collections however there are multiple low attenuation hepatic lesions consistent with metastases and subsegmental bilateral lower lobe pulmonary emboli. An echocardiogram reveals tricuspid valve vegetations. Blood cultures obtained upon presentation to hospital have grown *Streptococcus bovis*.

    Which is the most likely primary site of malignancy?

    a. Biliary tree
    b. Colon
    c. Oesophagus
    d. Pancreas
    e. Prostate

64. A 57 year old woman has a breast assessment following a positive CT pulmonary angiogram which reported a small, enhancing, solid mass in the right breast and two similar lesions in the left breast. The lesions are assessed in the clinic and biopsied. The pathology reports they are metastatic lesions rather than primary breast carcinoma.

    Which of the following is the most likely underlying malignancy?

    a. Colonic carcinoma
    b. Lung carcinoma
    c. Lymphoma
    d. Ovarian carcinoma
    e. Renal cell carcinoma

65. You are telephoned to review a paediatric emergency department chest radiograph for a 3 year old boy brought in by his parents with a short history of a cough and wheeze. An inspiratory chest film demonstrates a mildly lucent right lung with increased right rib spacing. The lungs are clear with no consolidation and no pleural effusion. The mediastinum, imaged skeleton and soft tissues have normal appearances.

    What is the most appropriate next step to help obtain the diagnosis?

    a. Arterial phase low dose CT chest
    b. Expiratory chest radiograph
    c. Spirometry
    d. Sputum sample
    e. Ventilation-perfusion nuclear medicine study

66. An 80 year old women is admitted from a nursing home with acute onset right hemiparesis. A CT is performed which shows an acute intraparenchymal haemorrhage in the subcortical white matter of the left frontal lobe. There is a small amount of surrounding oedema. Small foci of blooming artefact are evident on gradient echo sequences at the grey–white matter junction in both cerebral hemispheres and in the cerebellum. Generalised parenchymal volume loss and moderate small vessel ischaemia are also present.

    What is the most likely diagnosis?

    a. Hypertensive bleed
    b. Arteriovenous malformation
    c. Haemorrhagic metastases
    d. Amyloid angiopathy
    e. Herpes encephalitis

67. A 44 year old female patient presents with a couple of months' history of feeling generally unwell and more recently with headaches. On admission the patient is hypertensive with a blood pressure of 180/110. Following further workup the patient has an arterial and portal venous phase CT chest and abdomen. On the arterial phase there is bilateral renal artery

stenosis with wall thickening but no associated vascular calcification. The appearance of the kidneys on the portal venous phase imaging are symmetrical with no focal abnormality identified. The renal artery walls mildly enhance. Similar stenosis, arterial wall thickening and enhancement is also noted at the proximal left subclavian artery and descending thoracic aorta.

Which other investigation would be most appropriate in this patient?

a. Carotid Doppler ultrasound
b. Circle of Willis CT
c. CT pelvis with contrast
d. Lower limb Doppler ultrasound
e. MRA renal arteries

68. A 67 year old female patient has a chest radiograph following presentation to hospital with chest pain. The lungs and pleural spaces are clear and appearances of the mediastinum are within normal limits; however, there are multiple osseous lytic lesions. The patient is investigated further with a CT chest, abdomen and pelvis and a nuclear medicine bone scan. The CT scanner is currently undergoing maintenance awaiting a new part and therefore the nuclear medicine bone scan occurs first and is reported as normal osseous uptake.

What is the next best available test to confirm the diagnosis?

a. Breast clinic triple assessment
b. Bone marrow biopsy
c. Blood culture
d. Serum alkaline phosphatase levels
e. Serum parathyroid hormone levels

69. A 40 year old man with known HIV presents with night sweats, abdominal pain and weight loss. His CD4 count is <200 cells/mm^3 (500–1400 cells/mm^3). He is noted to have multiple purple, painless plaques on both legs. A CT abdomen and pelvis demonstrates multiple enlarged and enhancing periportal lymph nodes around the liver. Multiple submucosal duodenal nodules are also seen.

What is the most likely diagnosis?

a. Lymphoma
b. Mycobacterial disease
c. Histoplasmosis
d. Kaposi sarcoma
e. Candidiasis

70. An abdominal ultrasound in a 5 year old girl finds hepatomegaly with increased periportal echogenicity and reversal of hepatic venous flow. There are dilated intrahepatic bile ducts. The gallbladder and pancreas have normal appearances. The spleen is enlarged. The kidneys are enlarged bilaterally and echogenic with reduction in corticomedullary differentiation.

Which inheritance pattern does the condition associated with this constellation of radiological findings have?

a. Autosomal dominant
b. Autosomal recessive
c. Spontaneous mutation
d. X-linked dominant
e. X-linked recessive

71. A 23 year old gastroenterology clinic patient is being investigated for iron deficiency anaemia and abdominal pain. A small bowel meal and follow-through are performed.

Regarding the findings of coeliac disease on fluoroscopic imaging, which feature is the most likely to be associated with the diagnosis?

a. Crowding of the valvulae conniventes
b. Jejunoileal fold pattern reversal

c. Luminal dilatation
d. Reduced peristalsis
e. Small bowel sacculation

72. A 22 year old student develops cognitive decline and then worsening ataxia and spasticity over a period of a few weeks. Following admission she has an MRI head which demonstrates subcortical and deep white matter T2 hyperintensity affecting the majority of the right parietal lobe, the left temporoparietal region and minimal signal changes in the left putamen and globus pallidus. There is evidence of adjacent oedema and patchy white matter enhancement. There is also mild volume loss in the frontotemporal region.

Past medical history is unremarkable apart from appendicectomy as a child. Upon further questioning she recalls an episode of feeling unwell about 6 months ago with fever and flu-like symptoms before developing white spots on the inside of her cheeks and then a more generalised rash.

What is the most likely diagnosis?

a. Acute demyelinating encephalomyelitis
b. Acute haemorrhagic leukoencephalopathy
c. Herpes simplex encephalitis
d. Japanese encephalitis
e. Subacute sclerosing panencephalitis

73. A 34 year old male is under investigation for a newly diagnosed malignancy. Lymph node biopsy demonstrates Reed-Sternberg cells.

Where is the most likely site of thoracic lymph node enlargement on the CT chest?

a. Hilar
b. Internal mammary
c. Paratracheal
d. Peri-oesophageal
e. Subcarinal

74. A 37 year old semi-professional footballer attends the orthopaedic clinic due to left hip pain which is causing him difficulty when playing. Following clinical review, radiographs and subsequent MRI, a diagnosis of cam femoroacetabular impingement is made.

Which radiological findings are most consistent with this diagnosis?

Table 1.4:

	Radiographic Feature	α Angle	MRI Feature
a	Deep acetabulum	65°	Labral tear
b	Degenerative change	45°	Circumferential cartilage lesion
c	Flattening of the femoral head/neck junction	50°	Antero-superior cartilage lesion
d	Lateral osseous bump	65°	Labral tear
e	Deep acetabulum	50°	Labral tear

75. A 52 year old male patient with anaemia has a CT staging study following a colonoscopic biopsy confirming colorectal malignancy. The CT demonstrates some mild bowel wall thickening correlating with the area biopsied. There are a couple of small low attenuation areas in the liver which are unchanged from a CT study following trauma 2 years ago. However, there are multiple new bilateral sub-centimetre lung nodules.

In which venous drainage distribution is the primary tumour likely located?

a. Inferior mesenteric vein
b. Middle rectal vein
c. Sigmoid vein

d. Superior mesenteric vein
e. Superior rectal vein

76. A 54 year old male patient with no significant past medical history has an enhanced CT abdomen pelvis requested by the emergency department for right sided abdominal pain which confirms appendicitis. There is an incidental finding of a 23 mm exophytic right renal lesion which has a density of 2HU, multiple thin septae and nodular calcifications. On the left kidney there is another exophytic lesion which is 15 mm, homogenous and has a density of 72HU; there is thin wall calcification but no septations. Both lesions are classified as per the Bosniak classification system. The CT report is forwarded to the urology multidisciplinary team meeting co-ordinator.

What is the most appropriate management for this patient?

a. CT chest
b. Follow-up CT in 3–6 months
c. No further follow-up required
d. Surgical excision of the right renal lesion
e. Unenhanced CT abdomen

77. A 7 year old boy with no significant past medical history is being investigated for increased thirst. An MRI head demonstrates mild exophthalmos but no intracranial abnormality. A chest radiograph shows that the lungs are clear. Hepatosplenomegaly is reported on an ultrasound abdomen. Imaging 1 month previously for a painful right leg identified a lucent lesion in the distal right femoral metadiaphysis with a narrow zone of transition and a fine sclerotic border. There is minimal adjacent periosteal reaction but no matrix calcification and no soft tissue component evident.

What is the most likely underlying diagnosis?

a. Diabetes mellitus
b. Graves disease
c. Langerhans cell histiocytosis
d. Sarcoidosis
e. Tuberculosis

78. A 40 year old woman is referred for an MRI by the endocrinologists for investigation of hyperprolactinaemia.

Which of the following sequences would be most useful in an MRI protocol for the pituitary gland?

a. T1 axial and coronal, T1 post contrast axial and coronal, T1 coronal with dynamic contrast
b. T1 axial and coronal, T1 post contrast axial and coronal, T2 coronal with dynamic contrast
c. T1 sagittal and axial, T1 post contrast sagittal and axial, T1 coronal with dynamic contrast
d. T1 sagittal and coronal, T1 post contrast sagittal and coronal, T1 coronal with dynamic contrast
e. T1 sagittal and coronal, T1 post contrast sagittal and coronal, T2 coronal with dynamic contrast

79. A 63 year old man presents to the emergency department with an episode of slurred speech and right facial droop. The symptoms last for approximately 40 minutes. CT head demonstrates no acute abnormality. MRI head the following day reveals evidence of periventricular small vessel ischaemic change but no foci of restricted diffusion. The patient is referred for a carotid artery ultrasound Doppler which is reported as normal.

Which values are most compatible with this diagnosis?

Table 1.5:

	ICA PSV (cm/sec)	ICA/CCA PSV ratio	ICA EDV (cm/sec)
a	<125	<2.0	<40
b	<125	>4.0	<40
c	<125	<2.0	40–100
d	<125	>4.0	40–100
e	<125	2.0–4.0	40–100

80. A 6 year old patient has a chest radiograph for cough which is not responding to antibiotics. There is hyperinflation of the lungs and mild bronchial wall thickening suggestive of asthma. Incidental note is made of complete collapse of the T8 vertebral body.

What other finding would best correlate with the most common paediatric cause of this vertebral appearance?

a. Abdominal mass on ultrasound abdomen arising adjacent to aorta
b. Enlarged rounded lymph nodes on ultrasound neck and axilla
c. Multiple lytic skull lesions
d. Permeative lytic lesion with laminated periosteal reaction in the right femur
e. Raised inflammatory markers

81. A 24 year old motorcyclist is admitted following a road traffic collision. He has sustained significant blunt force trauma, falling off his motorbike at around 20 mph and hitting a tree. On arrival at hospital he is cardiovascularly compromised. Following stabilisation he is brought for a trauma CT. Internal haemorrhage is suspected and his abdomen is acutely tender.

Which of the following organs is he most likely to have injured?

a. Kidney
b. Liver
c. Pancreas
d. Spleen
e. Small bowel and mesentery

82. A 6 year old boy has a chest radiograph requested by his GP following a week of fever and productive cough. There is a small region of air space opacification in the right lower zone. Asymmetry is noted between both sides of the chest; the left hemithorax is smaller and more lucent compared to the right with reduced vascular markings. There is no significant mediastinal shift. The heart size is normal.

What is the most likely cause?

a. Congenital lobar over inflation
b. MacLeod syndrome
c. Poland syndrome
d. Pulmonary agenesis
e. Scimitar syndrome

83. A 40 year old male had an incidental finding of a low density sella mass on a CT head which was performed for trauma. The report states that a Rathke cleft cyst is the most likely differential and an MRI brain is recommended.

Which of the following statements regarding Rathke cleft cysts is correct?

a. They commonly calcify
b. They frequently show diffusion restriction
c. They sometimes contain an intracystic nodule
d. They often extend beyond the boundaries of the sella
e. Uniform enhancement is typical

84. A neonate has an abdominal ultrasound for a right sided abdominal mass. The patient is 3 days old and was born by emergency caesarean section following an unsuccessful induction of labour. The pregnancy was uncomplicated and antenatal scans unremarkable.

The ultrasound finds there is a hypoechoic mass in the right upper quadrant containing internal echoes without Doppler vascularity. This is posterior to the liver and the right kidney is seen inferiorly.

What is the most appropriate next step in management?

a. MIBG study
b. MRI abdomen
c. No further management required
d. Repeat ultrasound in 3 weeks
e. Ultrasound-guided biopsy

85. A 56 year old male presents with increasing shortness of breath and persistent cough. He has never smoked and has a medical history of rheumatoid arthritis. His GP requests a plain film of the chest which is abnormal. Therefore, a non-contrast CT chest is suggested to assess further. The CT chest reveals volume loss in the lower zones. There is diffuse ground glass opacification seen in the mid and lower zones which demonstrates immediate subpleural sparing with fine subpleural reticulation and traction dilatation of the small airways.

    What is the most likely diagnosis?

    a. Cryptogenic organising pneumonia
    b. Hypersensitivity pneumonitis
    c. Lymphocytic interstitial pneumonitis
    d. Non-specific interstitial pneumonia
    e. Usual interstitial pneumonia pattern of disease

86. A 25 year old male patient has a CT head and sinuses after review in the Ear, Nose and Throat clinic for symptoms of recurrent sinusitis. The CT shows the paranasal sinuses are lacking normal aeration and obliterated due to medullary expansion of the adjacent bones. An abdominal ultrasound from the previous year described the spleen as measuring 17 cm in craniocaudal extent and the inferior border of the liver extending to 6 cm below the lower pole of the right kidney. A recent radiograph of the left shoulder demonstrates normal bone density with metaphyseal flaring at the proximal humerus.

    What is the most likely diagnosis?

    a. Gaucher disease
    b. Osteopetrosis
    c. Sarcoidosis
    d. Thalassaemia
    e. Granulomatosis with polyangiitis (previously known as Wegener granulomatosis)

87. One of the gastroenterology consultants discusses a case with you of a patient with weight loss and suspicious gastric findings on a recent CT abdomen pelvis. The patient has declined endoscopy. Based on imaging findings, the differential lies between gastric lymphoma and primary gastric carcinoma.

    Which of the following is more consistent with gastric lymphoma than carcinoma?

    a. Associated with a history of atrophic gastritis
    b. Duodenal involvement
    c. Large polypoid mass
    d. Gastric outlet obstruction
    e. Perigastric fat invasion

88. A 49 year old woman has an MRI of her pelvis to assess her uterus. The patient has been having heavy, painful periods. A pelvic ultrasound identified a heterogenous area of uterine wall thickening. This area is evident on the MRI as a focal but ill-defined, thickened area of the posterior uterine wall with T2 hyperintensities. Enhancement is similar to the adjacent uterus. The endometrium measures up to 7 mm. The junctional zone measures 15 mm. There is a right ovarian corpus luteum. The left ovary has normal appearances. There are a couple of cervical Nabothian cysts.

    What is the most likely diagnosis?

    a. Adenomyosis
    b. Endometrial carcinoma
    c. Endometriosis
    d. Leiomyoma
    e. Leiomyosarcoma

89. The radiology department performs a skeletal survey for a 4 month old child with injuries suspicious for non-accidental injury (NAI).

    Which of the following injuries is most specific for NAI?

    a. Diaphyseal metacarpal fracture
    b. Fractures of different ages

c. Fracture of the acromion of the scapula
d. Parietal skull fracture
e. Spiral humeral fracture

90. A 35 year old woman presents with recurrent episodes of transient left sided weakness and dysphagia. An MRI brain shows multiple, bilateral white matter lesions predominantly within both anterior temporal lobes and external capsules. These lesions do not show restricted diffusion. There is a family history of strokes occurring at a young age.

    What is the most likely diagnosis?

    a. Susac syndrome
    b. MELAS
    c. CADASIL
    d. Acute demyelinating encephalomyelitis
    e. Amyloid angiopathy

91. A 52 year old patient who received a heart transplant 12 months ago secondary to viral myocarditis has a chest radiograph for increasing shortness of breath and fever. This shows several densities projected over both lungs and a widened right paratracheal stripe. CT chest confirms multiple small medium sized nodules throughout both lungs with mediastinal and hila lymph node enlargement.

    What is the most likely diagnosis?

    a. Aspergillus infection
    b. Drug reaction
    c. Lymphoid interstitial pneumonia
    d. Metastatic malignancy
    e. Post-transplant lymphoproliferative disease

92. You are on-call overnight and a 10 year old rear seat passenger is brought in following a road traffic collision at 30 mph. The child was wearing a seatbelt. Glasgow Coma Scale is 15/15 at the scene and the patient is haemodynamically stable. There is a 2-cm bruise on the forehead but there is no focal neurology and the patient has not vomited. The patient is complaining of neck pain and is immobilised. The chest is clear on auscultation and the abdomen is soft. There is no thoracic or lumbar spine pain on secondary survey. The trauma team discuss with you regarding imaging the child.

    Based on the available information what is the most appropriate form of initial imaging for this child?

    a. CT head and cervical spine
    b. CT head, cervical spine, chest, abdomen and pelvis
    c. CT cervical spine
    d. MRI head, cervical spine and chest radiograph
    e. Radiographs of the cervical spine

93. A 15 year old boy is undergoing chemotherapy for Hodgkin's lymphoma. He is admitted with severe right iliac fossa pain and fevers. A CT abdomen and pelvis shows mucosal thickening affecting the caecum. It also involves the appendix and terminal ileum, with surrounding inflammatory fat stranding.

    What is the most likely diagnosis?

    a. Acute appendicitis
    b. Typhlitis
    c. Lymphoma of the bowel
    d. Crohn's disease
    e. Necrotising enterocolitis

94. An emergency department patient has a mandibular radiograph due to jaw pain following a fight. There is no fracture; however there is a lucency in the posterior left mandible adjacent to an unerupted wisdom tooth. The lucent area is unilocular and appears well

corticated with a narrow zone of transition. There is no evidence of root resorption or periodontal ligament widening.

What is the most likely diagnosis?

a. Ameloblastoma
b. Dentigerous cyst
c. Odontogenic keratocyst
d. Radicular cyst
e. Solitary bone cyst

95. You are asked to review the radiograph of a neonate with an umbilical artery catheter in situ. The clinical team ask you to report the position of the arterial catheter.

Which of the catheters described below is sited appropriately?

a. Catheter passes inferiorly from umbilicus into pelvis, turning cephalad with the tip at the level of T9
b. Catheter passes inferiorly from umbilicus into pelvis, turning cephalad with the tip at the level of T11
c. Catheter passes inferiorly from umbilicus into pelvis, turning cephalad with the tip at the level of L1
d. Catheter passes superiorly from umbilicus with the tip at the level of the diaphragm
e. Catheter passes superiorly from umbilicus with the tip at the level of T8

96. A 40 year old male undergoes an MRI brain. This shows a durally based, extra-axial lesion in the left anterior cranial fossa. It is T1/T2 isointense to grey matter. It shows avid contrast enhancement.

Which of the following features help distinguish a haemangiopericytoma from a meningioma?

a. Absence of a dural tail
b. Alanine peak on MR spectroscopy
c. Bone erosion
d. Multiple lesions
e. Older patient

97. A 39 year old man is seen in the emergency department feeling generally unwell, intoxicated and has right sided chest pain. He has no fixed abode and a history of chronic alcohol excess and pulmonary tuberculosis. He is a frequent attender to the department. A chest radiograph demonstrates persistent opacification in the right lower lobe. In view of the persistence of this finding, as well as chest pain, the team organise a CT pulmonary angiogram. The timing of the scan is suboptimal; however it does demonstrate a focus of mass-like consolidation in the right lower lobe, which has several low attenuation foci centrally and peripheral enhancement. There is also pleural thickening with periostitis of the adjacent ribs and probable chest wall involvement. Biopsy of the lesion demonstrates 'sulphur granules' within the histopathologic specimen.

What is the most likely causative organism?

a. Actinomycosis
b. *Haemophilus influenzae*
c. *Klebsiella pneumoniae*
d. *Legionella pneumophila*
e. *Streptococcus pneumoniae*

98. A 70 year old male patient has pain in his right knee following a skiing injury. Numerous skeletal radiographs over the past 10 years demonstrate signs of an asymmetrical, polyarticular arthropathy not previously investigated. The patient has an MRI of the knee which reveals a horizontal medial meniscus tear. Other findings include marginal erosions and several lesions around the joint. These lesions are isointense to muscle on T1 weighted imaging, heterogeneously low signal on T2 sequences and enhance following gadolinium administration. One of these lesions is minimally infiltrating the patellar tendon.

What would be the most appropriate test to help confirm the underlying diagnosis?

a. 24-hour urine collection
b. CT chest abdomen pelvis

c. Joint aspiration
d. 18F-FDG PET/CT
e. Serum parathyroid hormone levels

99. The colorectal nurse specialist calls for advice regarding a 48 year old male patient who underwent total mesorectal excision 23 months ago for T3 N1b M0 rectal carcinoma. More recently he has had a stoma reversal and anastomosis. The patient's serum carcinoembryonic antigen (CEA) level has increased over the past 3 months.

    What would be the most appropriate course of action?

    a. CT cologram and CT chest
    b. Ultrasound abdomen
    c. FDG-PET/CT study
    d. MRI liver with liver specific contrast agent
    e. Re-check serum CEA in 3 months

100. A 43 year old male patient is brought in as a trauma call following a fight where he was stabbed multiple times in the posterior chest and abdomen. Arterial and portal venous phase CT chest abdomen pelvis are performed which demonstrate a couple of subcutaneous gas bubbles and a skin defect in the posterior left abdomen. There is adjacent subcutaneous fat stranding and left perinephric fat stranding with a thin rim of fluid with a density of 2HU around the left kidney. There is a 16-mm laceration of the right kidney extending to the renal pelvis. There is no evidence of contrast extravasation on the arterial or portal venous phase sequence.

    Using the American Association for the Surgery of Trauma (AAST) guidelines, what grade of renal trauma would this be?

    a. Grade I
    b. Grade II
    c. Grade III
    d. Grade IV
    e. Grade V

101. A chest radiograph is performed for a neonate followed repeated episodes of aspiration. The paediatric team feel tracheo-oesophageal fistula ± oesophageal atresia is likely due to cardiac abnormalities detected on antenatal scans. The chest radiograph demonstrates right lower zone air space opacification. The gastric air bubble is visible under the left hemidiaphragm.

    Which of the following is most likely?

    a. Double fistula with intervening oesophageal atresia
    b. Isolated fistula without oesophageal atresia
    c. Isolated oesophageal atresia
    d. Proximal fistula with distal oesophageal atresia
    e. Proximal oesophageal atresia with distal fistula

102. A 43 year old man with a three day history of headache, fever and vomiting is admitted. Neurological assessment finds he has a GCS of 12. The right eyelid is drooping and the eye is deviated outwards and downwards. A non-contrast CT head is normal. The scan acquired following contrast injection shows evidence of leptomeningeal enhancement with thickening and enhancement of the basal meninges extending into the sylvian fissures. The brain parenchyma returns normal signal. The leptomeninges overlying the cerebral convexities are not thickened or enhancing. There is mild dilatation of the temporal horns of the lateral ventricles.

    What is the most likely underlying cause for these changes?

    a. Enterovirus
    b. Group B streptococcus
    c. *Mycobacterium tuberculosis*
    d. Neurosarcoidosis
    e. *Streptococcus pneumoniae*

103. An active 48 year old man presents with a history of fatigue, weight loss and fever with right sided loin pain. The patient is tachycardic, hypotensive and has a low haemoglobin. Urine dip

demonstrates a small amount of blood and protein. Triple phase CT abdomen and pelvis reveals a right perinephric haematoma with a blush of contrast at the right lower pole on arterial phase imaging with pooling on the portal venous phase sequence. The patient undergoes urgent interventional radiology procedure. During the procedure the radiologist reports abnormality of the interlobar and arcuate arteries, with segments of short stenoses and aneurysmal dilatation.

What is the most likely underlying diagnosis?

a. Behçet disease
b. Fibromuscular dysplasia
c. Goodpasture syndrome
d. Polyarteritis nodosa
e. Takayasu disease

104. A young patient has a diagnosis of cleidocranial dysostosis; he is reviewed regularly in the paediatric outpatient clinic. The clinical team are concerned as he has a 1-week history of productive cough and increased shortness of breath. The paediatric junior doctor asks you to review his chest radiograph. There is consolidation in the left mid-lower zone which obscures the left heart border. The clavicles are absent.

What other feature would correlate with the patient's underlying congenital skeletal abnormality?

a. Decreasing interpedicular distance
b. Incompletely ossified sternum
c. Pectus excavatum
d. Platyspondyly
e. Shortened horizontally orientated ribs

105. A 52 year old woman under surveillance following previous colorectal carcinoma resection has a CT chest abdomen and pelvis. This shows a splenic artery aneurysm measuring 2 cm in maximal diameter.

Which of the following statements is most accurate regarding splenic artery aneurysms?

a. Aneurysms below 15 mm do not require follow-up
b. Increased rupture risk is associated with cirrhosis
c. Peripheral calcification is uncommon
d. Splenic artery aneurysms in pregnancy should be treated conservatively
e. The majority represent pseudoaneurysms

106. A 45 year old female patient has been referred to the orthopaedic service with anterior right knee pain, exacerbated by climbing stairs. A radiograph is unremarkable. Chondromalacia patellae is suspected clinically. The patient is mildly claustrophobic and the radiographer from the MRI scanner asks you which sequences you would like to prioritise in case the patient cannot tolerate the whole scan.

What sequence would be most helpful in assessing the cartilage?

a. Axial T1 weighted
b. Axial proton density fat saturation
c. Coronal short tau inversion recovery (STIR)
d. Sagittal T1 post gadolinium
e. Sagittal T1 weighted

107. A baby is born with radial dysplasia and anal atresia. Following further investigation two hemivertebrae are noted. The child has further investigations and is found to have a cardiac anomaly.

What is the most likely cardiac anomaly?

a. Atrial septal defect
b. Coarctation of the aorta
c. Patient ductus arteriosus
d. Tetralogy of Fallot
e. Ventricular septal defect

108. A 25 year old woman has a simple, partial seizure and goes on to have a CT head. This shows a focal, 9-mm hyperdense mass in the left centrum semiovale. There is speckled calcification within the lesion. The patient is suspected to have a cerebral cavernoma and a MRI brain is requested.

What is the best MRI sequence to diagnose cerebral cavernomas?

a. T2*
b. T2
c. T1 post contrast
d. Diffusion weighted imaging
e. FLAIR

109. You are asked to review a plain film by a junior doctor working in the emergency department who is concerned about the appearance of the mediastinum. The case is that of a 25 year old male who has presented with a productive cough and a fever. You review the chest radiograph; there is consolidation in the left lower zone which obscures the left hemidiaphragm, the airways appear dilated and abnormally thick walled and there is evidence of dextrocardia. You look back at the patient's previous imaging and see the patient had a CT for investigation of sinusitis.

What is the most likely unifying diagnosis?

a. Cystic fibrosis
b. Hypogammaglobulinaemia
c. Post-infective bronchiectasis
d. Primary ciliary dyskinesia
e. Recurrent aspiration

110. A 12 year old girl presents to the emergency department with pain weight bearing on her right leg after a school hockey tournament. Pelvic radiograph demonstrates a small linear flake of bone adjacent to the right ischial tuberosity.

Which tendinous avulsion is most likely to cause this appearance?

a. Adductor magnus
b. Gracilis
c. Iliopsoas
d. Rectus femoris
e. Tensor fascia lata

111. An 84 year old care home resident is brought into hospital with fever, abdominal pain, distension and vomiting. The patient is referred to the surgeons, made nil by mouth and an attempted nasogastric tube insertion is unsuccessful. Chest radiograph demonstrates right lower lobe consolidation and an air-fluid level projected over the heart extending just to the right of the midline. A chest radiograph taken 1 year previously demonstrates a smaller retrocardiac air-fluid level. A current abdominal radiograph demonstrates no gas-filled dilated small or large bowel loops. Inflammatory markers, lactate and renal function tests are raised. Liver function tests are normal.

Which is the most likely diagnosis?

a. Epiphrenic diverticulum
b. Hiatus hernia with aspiration pneumonia
c. Lung abscess
d. Mesentero-axial gastric volvulus
e. Organo-axial gastric volvulus

112. A 59 year old male patient has an MRI spine for back pain which incidentally identifies an exophytic right sided renal mass. This measures up to 35 mm and is homogenously low signal on both T1 and T2 weighted images. A subsequent unenhanced CT followed by a contrast enhanced scan visualises the renal mass. This has a density of 35HU which increases to 40HU following contrast. Additional MRI sequences are performed which confirm restricted diffusion of the mass and similar enhancement characteristics to the CT.

Based on the imaging characteristics, what is the most likely diagnosis?

a. Clear cell carcinoma
b. Haemorrhagic renal cyst
c. Oncocytoma
d. Papillary carcinoma
e. Renal lymphoma

113. A 4 year old boy presents with vomiting and confusion. A CT head is performed which shows hydrocephalus. There is also a hyperdense mass within the midline of the cerebellum with adjacent mass effect. On MRI the mass has low T1 and heterogenous T2 signal with diffusion restriction.

What is the most appropriate next investigation?

a. CT chest, abdomen and pelvis
b. MRI whole spine
c. MR spectroscopy
d. Thallium SPECT
e. Ultrasound abdomen

114. Ophthalmology refer a 57 year old female patient with a painful left eye, diplopia and proptosis for an MRI orbits. The MRI reveals an abnormality affecting the left orbit. There is a mass at the inferior aspect of the orbit involving the left inferior rectus, inferior oblique and lateral rectus muscles, including the tendons. The abnormality infiltrates the adjacent intraconal fat. The lesion is T1 isointense to the muscle, T2 hypointense and enhances following contrast injection. The adjacent bone returns normal signal.

What is the most likely diagnosis?

a. Lymphoma
b. Metastases
c. Pseudotumour
d. Rhabdomyosarcoma
e. Thyroid ophthalmopathy

115. A 67 year old male patient with a history of hypertension and diabetes is brought to hospital by ambulance with sudden onset chest pain radiating to his back. A CT aorta confirms a Stanford Type B and Debakey Type IIIB aortic dissection. Following the CT scan he develops bladder and bowel dysfunction and bilateral lower limb motor impairment. Neurological assessment reveals bilateral proprioception is intact but pain sensation is absent.

Which of the below is/are most likely to be affected?

a. Artery of Adamkiewicz
b. Artery of Percheron
c. Posterior spinal arteries
d. Recurrent artery of Heubner
e. Vertebral arteries

116. The rheumatology team ask you to review a lumbar spine radiograph of a 42 year old female patient with a significant past medical history. There is symmetrical irregularity of the sacroiliac joints with sclerosis on both sides of the joint. Elsewhere in the lumbar spine, particularly at L1-L3 there are symmetrical marginal paravertebral ossifications which align vertically.

What test would most likely confirm the underlying diagnosis?

a. Faecal calprotectin levels
b. Serum anti-CCP levels
c. Serum HLA B27 levels
d. Serum parathyroid hormone levels
e. Punch biopsy

117. A 60 year old man presents to the emergency department with a 1-day history of absolute constipation and abdominal pain. Clinical examination reveals a distended, tympanic abdomen. An abdominal radiograph shows a grossly distended loop of bowel.

Which of the following radiological features favours a diagnosis of caecal over sigmoid volvulus?

a. Ahaustral bowel wall
b. Coffee bean sign
c. Pelvic overlap sign
d. Long axis of the distended loops arises from the right lower quadrant
e. Extends towards the right upper quadrant

118. An infant is diagnosed with intussusception following an abdominal ultrasound.

Regarding the technique of image guided pneumatic reduction of intussusception, which of the following is correct?

a. >24 hours symptom duration is a contraindication
b. Maximum pressure generated of 120 mmHg within the colon
c. No more than two attempts
d. The procedural risks are failure and recurrence of intussusception
e. One minute should be left between reduction attempts

119. A 43 year old female patient with a history of asthma and rheumatoid arthritis has a barium swallow following GP referral. Symptoms include dysphagia and globus sensation with infrequent regurgitation. The study identifies a pharyngeal pouch.

Which imaging findings are most likely to be present to support this diagnosis?

a. Distal oesophageal diverticulum with tertiary contractions
b. Left sided lateral diverticulum distal to cricopharyngeus
c. Left sided lateral diverticulum proximal to cricopharyngeus
d. Posterior midline diverticulum distal to cricopharyngeus
e. Posterior midline diverticulum proximal to cricopharyngeus

120. A 40 year old female with a background of invasive ductal breast carcinoma and mastectomy presents with headache and diplopia. An MRI brain is performed. The radiologist's report states that the appearances are suggestive of leptomeningeal carcinomatosis.

Which of the following radiological features is most likely to be present?

a. Adjacent skull involvement
b. Multiple nodular durally based lesions
c. Parenchymal brain lesions
d. Contrast enhancement extending into the sulci
e. Normal DWI and ADC signal

ANSWERS 1

1. (c) Type 2 endoleak
(*The Final FRCR Complete Revision Notes*pages 1–3)

Table 1.6: The Classification of Endovascular Stent Graft Endoleaks

Type of Endoleak	Site
Type 1	Leak from the stent/graft attachment due to an inadequate seal
1a	Proximal
1b	Distal
Type 2 (most common 80%)	Filling of the sac from retrograde flow through aortic branches (e.g. lumbar arteries, inferior mesenteric)
Type 3	Structural failure of the stent graft/leak from mid-graft component junction
Type 4	Porosity of the graft (corrects with reversal of anticoagulation)
Type 5	Endotension (i.e. aneurysm sac enlargement without demonstrable leak)

Source: Reprinted with permission from V Helyar and A Shaw, *The Final FRCR: Complete Revision Notes.* CRC Press, Taylor & Francis Group, 2018, p. 3.

2. (b) Heel pad thickness of 30 mm

The case describes a case of acromegaly. Typical features include frontal bossing and enlargement of the sinuses and mastoid air cells. Pituitary adenomas are frequently discovered and microadenomas are identified as small areas of reduced enhancement compared to the surrounding pituitary gland. Musculoskeletal findings include posterior vertebral body scalloping, spade-like terminal phalangeal tufts, calcified intervertebral discs and joint cartilage. Cartilage can also be subject to overgrowth causing joint space widening. Heel pad thickness above 25 mm is considered abnormal, and this can be assessed on lateral ankle radiographs.

Decreased interpedicular distance is a feature of acromegaly and can lead to cord compression. In contrast to this, increased interpedicular distance is associated with dural ectasia which is described in conditions such as neurofibromatosis 1, ankylosing spondylitis, Ehlers-Danlos syndrome and Marfan syndrome.

Eleven paired ribs is linked with various conditions including several skeletal dysplasias and trisomy 18 and 21; however it is not associated with acromegaly.

Madelung deformity is also not a feature of acromegaly but is described in Turner syndrome, Ollier disease, nail-patella syndrome, achondroplasia and Leri Weill syndrome.

Sclerosis of the vertebral end plates, also known as 'sandwich' vertebrae in osteopetrosis and 'rugger jersey spine' in hyperparathyroidism, is not associated with acromegaly.

(The Final FRCR Complete Revision Notes Page 61)

3. (c) Mid-oesophagus

The patient was originally suffering with achalasia leading to dysphagia to both solids and liquids, which can be relieved with warm fluids. Barium swallow typically causes a characteristic 'rat-tail' narrowing of the distal oesophagus with associated oesophageal dilatation, an oesophageal air-fluid level and tertiary contractions. Warm water can be administered during the barium study to demonstrate relaxation of the lower oesophageal sphincter. Complications from achalasia include aspiration, pneumonia, oesophagitis and also malignancy. Approximately 5% of patients with achalasia develop oesophageal carcinoma and these strictures tend to occur in the mid-oesophagus.

Most idiopathic oesophageal carcinomas are squamous cell carcinomas and these similarly arise in the mid-oesophagus. Oesophageal adenocarcinoma is less common but frequently related to Barrett oesophagus and arises distally at the gastro-oesophageal junction, therefore more commonly involving the proximal stomach.

(The Final FRCR Complete Revision Notes Pages 151, 177)

4. (a) Acquired cystic kidney disease

Acquired cystic kidney disease is associated with end stage renal failure and can affect patients having either peritoneal or haemodialysis. The condition becomes much more common the longer a patient has been on dialysis, with 90% of patients estimated to have developed it after a decade. The typical features include small kidneys and >3–5 cysts in each kidney. Unfortunately, there can be complications such as cyst haemorrhage – as has happened to this patient. There is also a risk of renal cell carcinoma; findings such as solid nodules and septations would warrant further assessment and this risk continues in the native kidneys following transplantation.

Autosomal dominant polycystic kidney disease is the most common hereditary cause of end stage renal failure; however the kidneys usually appear enlarged due to the innumerable cysts. The cysts can be variable in size and can become very large rather than the small cysts described in the question.

Autosomal recessive polycystic kidney disease is a paediatric condition which tends to cause enlarged kidneys with a lot of small cysts and is also associated with hepatic fibrosis.

Tuberous sclerosis is associated with renal cysts as well as angiomyolipomas, which can also haemorrhage; however the most likely cause is acquired cystic kidney disease in the context of end stage renal failure.

(The Final FRCR Complete Revision Notes Page 245)

5. (e) Mega cisterna magna

Mega cisterna magna is usually an incidental diagnosis which causes the appearances of a cystic midline posterior fossa lesion located posteriorly and displacing the cerebellum. It follows cerebrospinal fluid (CSF) on all MRI sequences. An arachnoid cyst would be another possible differential as it has the same signal characteristics, although the position is suggestive of mega cisterna magna. This appearance can be detected antenatally and in these cases can be associated with infections such as cytomegalovirus or chromosomal abnormalities.

An epidermoid cyst has similar appearances to an arachnoid cyst on imaging apart from on DWI and FLAIR sequences where there will be restricted diffusion and FLAIR hyperintensity compared to CSF.

Dermoid cysts are usually in the midline but they characteristically contain fat and will therefore have high T1 signal. If they rupture they may cause a chemical meningitis.

Ependymal cysts also have similar imaging features to arachnoid cysts but are usually deep within the parenchyma or associated with the ventricles, being either peri or intraventricular.

Pilocytic astrocytoma is an important differential for midline paediatric posterior fossa lesions. They usually have a large cystic component with an enhancing solid nodule.

(The Final FRCR Complete Revision Notes Page 294)

6. (e) Schwannoma

The intradural, extramedullary location raises the possibility of a variety of lesions. One mnemonic to aid memory is 'MNM': Meningioma, Nerve sheath tumours, Metastases. The lesion described in the case has typical imaging features of a schwannoma. They are most commonly found in the cervical and lumbar spine and cause neural displacement, bone remodelling and can have a dumbbell appearance.

Spinal meningiomas are most commonly found in the thoracic spine. They have a characteristic dural tail and broad based dural attachment. They are usually T1 iso to hypointense, T2 iso to hyperintense and enhance homogenously following contrast. They are unusual in that they can calcify, but less commonly than intracranial meningiomas.

Metastases in the spinal canal can arise from a primary within the brain or via haematogenous seeding from primaries such as breast, lung or melanoma. They can manifest as diffuse dural thickening and nodularity.

Spinal paragangliomas are extramedullary and intradural however they usually involve the cauda equina region and so the location does not fit with this diagnosis. Their imaging characteristics are the same as for paragangliomas elsewhere in the body; they enhance avidly, can have flow voids and are T2 hyperintense. Additionally, they frequently show evidence of haemorrhage.

Epidermoid cysts have a similar appearance to cerebrospinal fluid and would exhibit low T1 signal, high T2 signal and would not demonstrate the enhancement pattern described in this case. DWI and FLAIR imaging is important in the diagnosis of epidermoid cysts.

(The Final FRCR Complete Revision Notes Page 454)

7. (d) Discharge the patient

The presence of fat and description of 'punctate calcification' is typical for a hamartoma, which is a benign entity. Hamartomas are usually asymptomatic and most are detected incidentally. Typically they are peripheral; a minority (10%) are endobronchial. Malignant transformation is very rare. According to the most recent 2015 British Thoracic Society guidelines, nodules with clear benign features can be discharged without further imaging. Hamartomas can demonstrate avidity on FDG PET in 20% of cases but this investigation is not warranted and likely to cause confusion rather than aid diagnosis.

CT angiogram is not an appropriate next investigation; calcification is rare in arteriovenous malformations and there is no description provided of a feeding vessel. A Gallium 68 PET-CT scan can aid diagnosis of carcinoid tumour, however the description provided in the main stem is not suggestive of a carcinoid owing to the presence of fat. Although carcinoid tumours can be peripherally located (atypical 10%), more commonly they are central (typical 90%).

(The Final FRCR Complete Revision Notes Page 32)

8. (a)

Adhesive capsulitis is also known as frozen shoulder and classically presents with restriction in shoulder elevation and external rotation. It is most common in middle-aged women, particularly diabetic patients, and can also be associated with previous trauma. Classical radiological features are a thickened joint capsule and coracohumeral ligament. The subscapularis bursa is small, and lymphatic filling is a feature. The subcoracoid fat triangle between the coracohumeral ligament and coracoid process can be obliterated. The joint volume

is reduced and therefore there is limited filling capacity during arthrogram injection.
(The Final FRCR Complete Revision Notes Page 62)

9. (b) Hypertrophied caudate lobe
In the chronic phase of Budd-Chiari there is compensatory enlargement of the caudate lobe as it drains directly into the inferior vena cava. There is associated atrophy of the peripheral segments, and regenerative nodules may be a feature.
In the acute presentation there is classically hepatosplenomegaly and ascites. CT can demonstrate a 'flip-flop' pattern of enhancement due to hyperenhancement of the central liver segments on early-phase images, with peripheral hypoenhancement. This appearance is reversed on delayed phase images.
(The Final FRCR Complete Revision Notes Page 198)

10. (a) Chiari I malformation
The patient has characteristic features of Klippel-Feil syndrome with Sprengel deformity of the shoulder and cervical vertebral fusion. Chiari I malformation is associated with Klippel-Feil syndrome and is when the cerebellar tonsils descend ≥5 mm below the level of the foramen magnum. It is often asymptomatic and found incidentally in adults. As well as being associated with Klippel-Feil syndrome, it is also associated with craniosynostosis, hydrocephalus, syrinx and a tethered cord.
Haemangioblastomas are a cause of predominantly posterior fossa cystic lesions and are associated with von Hippel-Lindau. They often have an enhancing solid nodule and flow voids.
Optic gliomas are associated with neurofibromatosis type I, along with pilocytic astrocytoma, sphenoid wing dysplasia and focal areas of parenchymal T2 signal hyperintensity.
Holoprosencephaly is a cleavage failure and appearances range from severe (alobar) to less severe (lobar).
Polymicrogyria is associated with a number of infections during pregnancy including toxoplasmosis, rubella and cytomegalovirus.
(The Final FRCR Complete Revision Notes Page 289)

11. (d) Prostate carcinoma
Vertebral metastases, when diffuse, can be difficult to appreciate. It is always important to compare the vertebral body signal to the adjacent disc. The signal of metastases depends on whether they are sclerotic or lytic. STIR signal is usually high and they demonstrate restricted diffusion. Lytic metastases would be low on T1 and high on T2 compared to the disc. However, sclerotic metastases would be low on both sequences.
The metastases in this case are consistent with sclerotic lesions and therefore the most likely primary site is prostate cancer. The other cancers are more commonly associated with lytic metastases. Melanoma is unusual in that it can demonstrate high T1 signal due to melanin.
(The Final FRCR Complete Revision Notes Page 453)

12. (b) Primary osteochondromatosis
The question describes multiple, intra-articular, cartilaginous nodules, with some early calcification. This is in keeping with osteochondromatosis and the relatively young age of the patient and lack of degenerative change is suggestive of the primary, rather than the secondary form of the condition. Radiographic appearances can be variable depending on the degree of ossification of the nodules but the typical calcification is described and 'ring and arc' which fits with a chondral pattern. Erosion on both sides of the joint can occur due to the synovial proliferation and mass effect.
Calcification is rare in pigmented villonodular synovitis and when diffuse it can be more mass-like in appearance. Haemosiderin deposition within the synovial proliferation will demonstrate blooming artefact on gradient echo sequences.
Synovial chondrosarcoma is rare but tends to have much more aggressive appearances extending beyond the joint with cortical erosion, marrow infiltration and potentially metastatic spread.
Synovial haemangioma present as a soft tissue mass which will demonstrate linear areas of flow void on MRI and marked enhancement of the mass.
(The Final FRCR Complete Revision Notes Page 98)

13. (a) Aortic root dilatation
The patient has typical radiographic features of aortic coarctation. The most common association (75–80%) is with a bicuspid aortic valve. A bicuspid aortic valve is predisposed to stenosis and over time can cause aortic root dilatation due to the high pressure jet of blood

through the stenotic valve. A congenital bicuspid aortic valve is one of the most common causes of aortic valve disease in young adults.

Other conditions associated with aortic coarctation include ventricular septal defect, hypoplastic aortic arch, truncus arteriosus, scoliosis and Turner syndrome. Congenital truncus arteriosus and ventricular septal defect would become symptomatic much earlier in the patient's life. Pulmonary artery aneurysms are not associated with aortic coarctation.

(The Final FRCR Complete Revision Notes Page 3)

14. (a) Adjacent subchondral hypo- and hyperintense T2 linear signal

The patient has features of sickle cell disease on abdominal radiograph with osteosclerosis, likely calcified gallstones in his right upper quadrant and a calcified spleen in the left upper quadrant. Therefore, the most likely diagnosis is avascular necrosis of the hip.

Radiographic features are often not visible, or subtle in the early stages, and osteopenia may be present. It is only later in the disease process that sclerosis, lucency, irregularity and flattening of the femoral heads develop.

MRI is the most sensitive test for diagnosis and the most specific sign is the 'double line' sign which is paired high and low T2 linear signal. The low T1 signal parallels the subarticular cortex, also known as the 'crescent' sign – representing a subchrondral fracture. This would likely be associated with subchrondral high STIR signal in the acute phase.

Low signal at the medial aspect of the femoral neck can be seen in stress fractures, which typically affect young patients; however the clinical findings are more in keeping with sickle cell anaemia and subsequent avascular necrosis.

Synovial enhancement with gadolinium is not typical for avascular necrosis but would be seen in septic arthritis, which patients with sickle cell disease are at higher risk of; however you would also expect systemic illness.

(The Final FRCR Complete Revision Notes Pages 65, 348)

15. (c) Inform on-call vascular specialist registrar of findings

The finding of gas locules adjacent to an aortic graft >3 months following surgery, a loop of small bowel in contact with the aorta, and thickening of the aortic wall are all concerning for a possible aorto-enteric fistula. These most commonly occur between the duodenum and aorta. This patient's graft is suprarenal and therefore the position potentially places the patient at risk. Other radiological signs include pseudoaneurysm formation and disruption of the aortic wall. In acute cases there may be extravasation of contrast into the bowel lumen. Often patients present with a herald bleed which can then be followed by massive haemorrhage. This patient is anaemic, which, given the radiological findings, is concerning. Urgent action is required and the most appropriate step is to inform the vascular specialist registrar on-call; their team can review the patient and decide regarding further management.

Another differential diagnosis would be graft infection, also a serious complication. Recent studies have suggested 18F-FDG PET/CT studies can help differentiate cases of infection from non-infected grafts; however, a more appropriate initial step would be to correlate with inflammatory markers and blood cultures.

(The Final FRCR Complete Revision Notes Page 152)

16. (d) Blood culture followed by antibiotics

The patient has typical signs and symptoms of pyelonephritis. If the patient is septic then antibiotics need to be given within an hour as per sepsis protocol; however, from the description there is no indication of sepsis and the patient is haemodynamically stable. Blood cultures should be obtained prior to antibiotics where possible. Urinary tract ultrasound is insensitive for pyelonephritis and the diagnosis should be clinical. Radiology can be helpful if there is concern regarding other diagnoses, such as urinary tract calculi; however, these are uncommon, particularly in young women. In an uncomplicated case of pyelonephritis no imaging may be required. Radiology can be incorporated if there is concern regarding abscess formation, infarction or obstruction. Ultrasound would be preferable over CT in the first instance to reduce radiation exposure in a relatively young patient.

(The Final FRCR Complete Revision Notes Page 246)

17. (b) Hepatic iminodiacetic acid (HIDA) scan

The baby has typical radiological features of biliary atresia with hepatomegaly and the 'triangular cord' sign which is caused by fibrous echogenic tissue anterior to the portal vein.

Intrahepatic biliary duct dilatation may or may not be present. The inability to see the gallbladder is suspicious and the common bile duct may also not be visible. Biliary atresia most commonly presents within the first couple of months of life with jaundice, pale stools and dark urine. Prompt diagnosis and surgical treatment is important to avoid cirrhosis and liver transplant.

A HIDA scan will demonstrate hepatic tracer uptake but absent bowel tracer excretion at 24 hours. In contrast to this, neonatal hepatitis will cause reduced hepatic uptake and maintained excretion.

(The Final FRCR Complete Revision Notes Page 334)

18. (e) Microcalcification

Concerning features in thyroid nodules include microcalcification, irregular margins, a nodule being taller than it is wide, invasion into adjacent structures, an incomplete hypoechoic halo and enlarged or abnormal appearing cervical lymph nodes. A hyperechoic echotexture is reassuring compared to hypoechoic nodules, which are more frequently associated with malignancy. However, some benign nodules can be hypoechoic. No one characteristic is completely diagnostic for malignancy but there are various guidelines to help guide management. Ultrasound follow-up can be undertaken and depending on the level of suspicion if a nodule reaches 1–1.5 cm then fine needle aspiration would be indicated.

(The Final FRCR Complete Revision Notes Page 435)

19. (e) Osler-Weber-Rendu syndrome

The most likely diagnosis is Osler-Weber-Rendu syndrome, or hereditary haemorrhagic telangiectasia. It is characterised by multiple arteriovenous malformations (AVMs) with a triad of telangiectasia, epistaxis (due to nasal telangiectasia) and a positive family history (autosomal dominant). The pulmonary nodules seen on plain film are multiple AVMs. The AVMs cause cyanosis and can cause high output heart failure.

Although multiple pulmonary nodules are seen in granulomatosis with polyangiitis (previously known as Wegener granulomatosis), the associated upper respiratory tract symptom is sinusitis rather than epistaxis, and cyanosis is not usually a feature.

Caplan syndrome is a combination of rheumatoid arthritis and pneumoconiosis. Although lung nodules are seen in this condition, there is no relevant history provided in the main stem, and there is no evidence of interstitial abnormality provided on plain film.

Goodpasture syndrome may present with haemoptysis; however, pulmonary nodules are not a typical feature.

Multiple metastases is a possible answer; however it is not the most likely from the information provided, especially given the patient's age.

(The Final FRCR Complete Revision Notes Page 32)

20. (c) Osteopetrosis

Basilar invagination is where the odontoid process of C2 sits at or above the level of the basion-opthision line which is also known as the McRae line. It should sit >5 mm below this line and it can lead to compression of the brainstem and subsequent hydrocephalus, syringomyelia and neurological symptoms.

Causes can be acquired or congenital, and a common mnemonic is **PF ROACH**:

Paget disease
Fibrous dysplasia
Rheumatoid arthritis, rickets
Osteogenesis imperfecta, osteomalacia
Achondroplaisa
Chiari I/II, cleidocranial dysostosis
Hyperparathyroidism

Osteopetrosis is not associated with basilar invagination.

(The Final FRCR Complete Revision Notes Page 67)

21. (c) Peutz-Jegher syndrome

The vignette alludes to a history of Peutz-Jegher syndrome. This is an autosomal dominant syndrome that causes multiple, benign, hamartomatous polyps; more common in the stomach and small bowel. It is the most common polyposis syndrome to involve the small intestine but these have no malignant potential. Intussusception is a common presentation. It can also affect the large bowel where there is a risk of malignant transformation. The risk of extraintestinal malignancy is increased, for example in the ovary, thyroid, testis, pancreas and breast.

Cronkhite-Canada syndrome, a type of non-hereditary syndrome, and Cowden syndrome can also affect the entire GI tract with hamartomatous polyps. Familial adenomatous polyposis syndrome (FAPS) is a hereditary condition characterised by hundreds of adenomatous polyps of the large bowel. Juvenile polyposis syndrome also causes hundreds of juvenile hamartomatous polyps affecting the entire GI tract.

(The Final FRCR Complete Revision Notes Page 181)

22. (d) Ultrasound and DMSA if recurrent infection

NICE guidelines on paediatric urinary tract infections (UTI) are intermittently updated and the current guidelines are listed for review in December 2024. In both the previous and current guidance for a typical *Escherichia coli* infection, in a child of 11 months who is responding to treatment, the guidance suggests no imaging is required. US and DMSA only becomes necessary if the UTI is recurrent.

If the infection is atypical (non-*E. coli*) or there are other concerning features such as sepsis, abdominal mass, unresponsiveness to treatment, raised creatinine or poor urine flow, then urgent US is indicated.

Similarly, if a child is less than 3 months old and has a UTI, then paediatric referral and imaging would be indicated.

(The Final FRCR Complete Revision Notes Page 358)

National Institute for Health and Care Excellence (NICE). 2007 (updated 2018). *NICE Clinical Guideline 54. Urinary Tract Infection in Under 16s: Diagnosis and Management.*

23. (a) Endplate: Low T1, High T2, enhancement present, Disc: T2 low

Modic endplate changes are subdivided into three types, ranging from acute to chronic appearances. In the early phases, (Type I) there is inflammation causing low T1 and high T2 endplate signal. Endplate enhancement can be present. In contrast to discitis, the disc will demonstrate low T2 signal.

Modic Type II endplate changes are related to fat deposition and therefore T1 signal is high and T2 signal is intermediate to high.

Following this, the endplates become hypointense on both T1 and T2 sequences due to sclerosis (Type III). As with Modic Type I changes, the disc should stay low signal on T2 sequences.

(The Final FRCR Complete Revision Notes Pages 83, 444)

24. (b) Alcoholic gastritis

The stomach can be challenging to assess on imaging, particularly if not well-distended. Abnormally thickened gastric folds are described as above 3–5 mm at the prepyloric region and >5–10 mm at the fundus. The most common cause of thickened gastric folds is alcoholic gastritis.

In contrast to this, atrophic gastritis causes inflammation and atrophy of the gastric glands causing loss of rugae and a smooth, featureless stomach.

Another cause of thickened folds is lymphoma, which is the most common malignant cause. Other findings would include diffuse stomach wall thickening and ulceration causing wall irregularity.

Crohn's disease and Zollinger-Ellison syndrome can also cause thickened folds, along with multiple ulcers and a cobblestone appearance in the former. Zollinger-Ellison causes hypersecretion of gastric acid so there can be high volumes of fluid in the stomach which dilute the contrast.

(The Final FRCR Complete Revision Notes Page 153)

25. (b) Endotracheal tube tip position

Always remember lines and tubes on a plain film and always remember ABC (airway, breathing, circulation). Although a left apical cap is suspicious for aortic transection and is a very urgent finding, the airway is potentially compromised due to the incorrect placement of the endotracheal tube, especially with a concomitant large right pneumothorax.

Bilateral pleural effusions in the context of trauma should be considered to represent haemothoraces, and right lung consolidation is presumed to represent lung contusion.

Radiographic findings associated with aortic transection include left apical pleural cap, mediastinal widening (over 8 cm above the level of the carina and more than 25% the width of the chest), indistinct aortic arch contours, filling in of the aortopulmonary window, tracheal deviation towards the right and depression of the left main bronchus.

(The Final FRCR Complete Revision Notes Page 5)

26. (d) Semimembranosus tendon and medial head of gastrocnemius

Baker's cysts are associated with osteoarthritis of the knee and extend from the joint space, often with a beaked appearance, between the medial head of gastrocnemius and the semimembranosus tendon. They can present as a mass or with pain. A ruptured Baker's cyst can cause acute presentations, and ruptured popliteal aneurysms and deep vein thrombosis would be the main differentials.

Radiographic appearances can include increased soft tissue density at the posterior aspect of the knee on the lateral view.

On ultrasound these lesions can be discriminated from a popliteal artery aneurysm by their anatomical location but also due to lack of vascularity. Baker's cysts will be anechoic with posterior acoustic enhancement. They can contain loose bodies.

MRI reveals a fluid signal lesion at the posterior aspect of the knee extending from the joint between the **m**edial head of gastrocnemius and the semi**m**embranosus tendon – remember the '**m**'s of medial head and semimembranosus go together.

(The Final FRCR Complete Revision Notes Page 67)

27. (a) Salmonella

The underlying organism in infectious colitis may be predicted by the segment of the bowel affected.

The typical inpatient and antibiotic history associated with *Clostridioides difficile* (previously known as *Clostridium difficile*) colitis does not fit with the history in this case. Furthermore, it tends to cause a diffuse colitis with gross mural thickening.

(The Final FRCR Complete Revision Notes Page 182)

Table 1.7: Causative organisms and segment of colon most likely to be affected in infectious colitis

Organism	Segment of large bowel affected
Salmonella	Ascending colon
Shigella	Sigmoid colon
Cytomegalovirus	Ileocolic
Herpes simplex virus	Proctitis

Source: Reprinted with permission from V Helyar and A Shaw, *The Final FRCR: Complete Revision Notes*, CRC Press, Taylor & Francis Group, 2018, p. 182.

28. (b) CT abdomen as next available outpatient appointment

The ultrasound features are of an angiomyolipoma – an echogenic, often cortically based exophytic lesion containing fat, as well as vessels and muscle. The figure 4 cm is important to remember; below this size these lesions should be followed up to assess for interval growth. Once greater than 4 cm in size, the risk of haemorrhage increases and embolisation or partial nephrectomy should be considered. Although ultrasound imaging demonstrates typical features, these lesions need prompt CT to characterise fully and confirm the diagnosis. It can sometimes be difficult to exclude renal cell carcinoma (RCC), particularly those containing microscopic fat or if the angiomyolipoma is lipid poor. MRI may be helpful in these cases. Features such as calcification and necrosis would tend to favour RCC. In this instance, further staging imaging could then be completed.

(The Final FRCR Complete Revision Notes Page 246)

29. (a) Epididymitis

Testicular torsion is always a concern with scrotal pain and swelling. Although an urgent ultrasound is frequently requested, this may not reveal a significant abnormality, especially in cases of intermittent torsion. Therefore appropriate clinical assessment is vital. In this case, the left epididymis is swollen and heterogenous with increased vascularity, and this is consistent with epididymitis.

Torsion of the appendix testis has similar symptoms to testicular torsion. Specific findings may not be evident on ultrasound and it is sometimes a diagnosis of exclusion; however occasionally the appendix may be visible as a small structure at the upper pole of the testicle with internal echoes which is hypoechoic compared to the adjacent testicle. A hydrocele and scrotal wall oedema may also be present.

The small, thin-walled lesion at the epididymal head has features of a cyst with anechoic echotexture and posterior acoustic enhancement. In this position, this is likely to be an epididymal cyst.

Findings that would be suggestive of orchitis would be hypoechoic echotexture and hypervascularity within the testicle itself. There may also be swelling and scrotal wall oedema. Orchitis is most commonly associated with epididymitis but can occur in isolation; for example in mumps. Although the left testicle is marginally bigger, there is frequently physiological asymmetry and without the other findings, orchitis cannot be confidently diagnosed.

(The Final FRCR Complete Revision Notes Pages 278, 357)

30. (a) Inform neurosurgical team

The epidural collection has the signal characteristics of hyperacute blood; T1 isointense to cord and T2 bright. In the context of recent trauma this is consistent with epidural haemorrhage. This is a surgical emergency and therefore the neurosurgeons should be informed urgently. Haemorrhage causes blooming on T2* MRI sequences and although this may be helpful to confirm the diagnosis, it could also delay treatment. If the neurosurgeons want any further clarification then this could always be performed following discussion with them.

With a history of fever and other infective symptoms then an epidural abscess could be considered and microbiology input may be required. Epidural abscess usually have low T1 signal, high T2 signal and peripheral enhancement.

Contrast enhanced imaging would not be indicated in this case as the history and radiological findings are consistent and additional sequences may delay appropriate management.

(The Final FRCR Complete Revision Notes Page 450)

31. (e) Treated lymphoma

The differential diagnosis of tiny lung nodules and calcified mediastinal lymph nodes could include sarcoidosis and silicosis (these are the most common causes) as well as histoplasmosis and amyloidosis (these are comparatively rare).

Treated lymphoma may demonstrate calcification of the mediastinal and hilar nodes; pulmonary nodules are not a typical feature and there is no history provided in the main stem.

Silicosis typically demonstrates 'eggshell' calcification of the nodes and lung. Parenchymal findings are varied from nodules to larger opacities and fibrosis.

Previous histoplasmosis infection can cause multiple calcified pulmonary nodules (2–5 mm in size) and eggshell calcification of the lymph nodes; in some cases the calcified lymph node may erode into an airway.

Sarcoidosis can demonstrate calcification of the lymph nodes, usually at advanced stage of the pulmonary disease; fibrosis is the more typical parenchymal finding in the late stage of disease.

(The Final FRCR Complete Revision Notes Pages 33, 45–46, 53)

32. (c) Increased tracer uptake on all three phases

Bone scans are sensitive but not specific for osteomyelitis. The bone scan will often be abnormal before any radiographic changes are evident. The three phases are angiographic, tissue and osseous phases. Osteomyelitis will demonstrate increased tracer uptake on all three phases due to increased blood flow to the region, increased tracer uptake within the adjacent inflamed soft tissues and then increased uptake within the bone itself. This is in contrast to cellulitis where uptake would only be increased on the angiographic and tissue phases.

The most sensitive test for osteomyelitis is MRI which can reveal bone marrow oedema as the earliest change. After several days a low T1 signal area, representing intraosseous or subperiosteal abscess, may be evident with surrounding intermediate T1 signal which enhances (penumbra sign).

Radiographic features are often delayed and include soft tissue swelling, periosteal reaction and soft tissue gas.

(The Final FRCR Complete Revision Notes Page 68)

33. (a) Carmen meniscus

It is important to know the different imaging characteristics of benign and malignant gastric ulcers. Carmen meniscus is a sign caused by malignant ulcers; there are heaped-up margins causing an inner ulcer margin, which is convex towards the lumen and causes subsequent lenticular pooling of barium in the ulcer, whereas a benign ulcer has a smooth concave shape without heaped-up margins. The gastric folds therefore do not reach the edge of a malignant ulcer as they do in a benign ulcer.

Hampton's line, associated with benign ulcers, is a radiolucent line seen at the edge of the ulcer. A way to remember these two signs is Carmen = Carcinoma and Hampton = Harmless.

Lesser curve ulcers are more typically associated with benign ulcers, whereas malignant ulcers tend to be found on the greater curve. Benign ulcers tend to be exoluminal, extending beyond the gastric contour, whereas malignant ulcers are endoluminal and do not. Similarly smooth gastric folds are benign features, whereas irregular folds are more concerning.

(The Final FRCR Complete Revision Notes Page 155)

34. (b) Eagle-Barrett syndrome

Eagle-Barrett syndrome, also known as prune-belly syndrome due to hypoplasia of the abdominal wall muscles, causes a constellation of findings including urinary tract anomalies and cryptorchidism. The urinary tract can be affected by renal dysplasia, posterior urethral valve, urachal diverticulum, an enlarged trabeculated bladder and vesicoureteral reflux.

Posterior urethral valves are indicated by the presence of a thickened bladder and sometimes bilateral hydronephrosis and hydroureter due to vesicoureteral reflux. A micturating cystourethrogram will find a dilated posterior urethra and a valve may be visualised. The other findings in this case of small kidneys and cryptorchidism make Eagle-Barrett syndrome more likely than just a solitary posterior urethral valve.

Edwards and Patau syndrome can be associated with Eagle-Barrett syndrome; however there are no other features to suggest that these are more likely. Patau syndrome is also associated with cryptorchidism, and Edwards syndrome is associated with ureteral duplication and horseshoe kidney.

Bladder exstrophy leads to herniation of the bladder through the anterior abdominal wall and it is also associated with cryptorchidism in males.

(The Final FRCR Complete Revision Notes Page 356)

35. (e) GCS < 15 at 2 hours post injury

Indications for an immediate CT scan within 1 hour, according to updated 2019 NICE guidelines, include GCS < 13 at initial assessment or GCS < 15 at 2 hours post injury. Other risk factors include possible basal skull fracture, post-traumatic seizure, focal neurology and more than one episode of vomiting post head injury.

Indications for scanning within 8 hours include loss of consciousness, more than 30 minutes retrograde amnesia, age ≥65, anticoagulation or history of coagulopathy and dangerous mechanism of injury.

The radiology report should be available within 1 hour of the scan being performed.

National Institute for Health and Care Excellence (NICE). 2014 (updated 2019). NICE Clinical Guideline 176. Head injury: assessment and early management

36. (c) MRI abdomen

The characteristics of the case in this question are suggestive of neuroblastoma; the patient is <2 years old and the mass is large, displacing the bowel and kidney and encasing the vasculature. On ultrasound it has areas which likely represent calcification. The mass extends adjacent to the vertebral column, and neural foraminal involvement is important to establish as it may impact management if neurosurgical input is required. Neuroblastoma frequently metastasises, commonly to the liver and bone. CT is frequently employed in the diagnosis and staging of neuroblastoma. To assess distant extent, MIBG has traditionally been the investigation of choice; however PET/CT has been used in some centres. Technetium-99m bone scans can also be helpful.

In this case, MRI abdomen would be the best modality to assess local disease extent and particularly neuroforaminal involvement.
(The Final FRCR Complete Revision Notes Page 354)

37. (c) Myxoma
This is a typical description of a cardiac myxoma, which is the most frequent primary cardiac tumour in adults. It is typically attached to the interatrial septum within the atria, on the left (75–80%) more than right. Rarely it can be sited in the ventricles. Myxomas can be part of Carney's complex which is a multiple endocrine neoplasia syndrome comprising multiple, often cardiac, myxomas and skin pigmentation.
Both fibroma and rhabdomyoma are more typically in the ventricles with rhabdomyoma the most common cardiac tumour in childhood, and can be associated with tuberous sclerosis.
Metastases are 20–40 times more common than primary cardiac tumours but with the typical description of the atrial myxoma, this is less likely. The most common primary tumours to metastasise to the heart include melanoma, lung and breast.
Thrombus is a possibility, especially on a CT pulmonary angiogram study; however the description, particularly the enhancement on the MRI, makes this unlikely.
(The Final FRCR Complete Revision Notes Page 8)

38. (a) Abrupt change in median nerve diameter
Carpal tunnel syndrome can be associated with conditions such as acromegaly, hypothyroidism, pregnancy, rheumatoid arthritis and diabetes. It presents with pain and paraesthesia in the hand in the distribution of the median nerve. Tinel test (tapping the median nerve) and Phalen test (paraesthesia exacerbated by wrist flexion) are used to aid diagnosis.
The most specific sign on MRI is enlargement of the nerve. Other findings include bowing of the flexor retinaculum, flattening and/or enhancement of the nerve and oedema within the nerve or carpal tunnel and loss of fat within the carpal tunnel.
Ultrasound can be used and can also show bowing of the flexor retinaculum and nerve compression causing flattening distally and enlargement of the nerve just proximal to the flexor retinaculum.
(The Final FRCR Complete Revision Notes Page 69)

39. (b) Small bowel tuberculosis
Differentiating tuberculosis (TB) from Crohn's disease can sometimes be challenging on imaging; however, Table 1.8 summarises the main differentiating features. Hypoattenuating lymph nodes can be seen in TB and small bowel lymphoma. Lymphoma of the small bowel most classically affects the ileum. In this case, the presence of dense ascites and predominant caecal involvement points towards a diagnosis of TB. Yersiniosis and actinomycosis classically affect the appendix, mimicking appendicitis.
(The Final FRCR Complete Revision Notes Pages 183, 162)

Table 1.8: Differentiating Tuberculosis from Crohn's Disease

Features of Tuberculosis
TB involves the caecum > terminal ileum
Causes caecal retraction
Is associated with low-attenuation mesenteric lymph node enlargement
Causes hyperattenuating ascites

Source: Reprinted with permission from V Helyar and A Shaw, *The Final FRCR: Complete Revision Notes.* CRC Press, Taylor & Francis Group, 2018, p. 184.

40. (a) Cystoscopy
The patient has haematuria and although the upper tracts have normal CT appearances, the lower tract requires direct visualisation to complete the assessment. The urinary bladder cannot be accurately assessed on CT and although sometimes focal bladder wall thickening is visible, this is not always the case and cystoscopy is still indicated.

Similarly, if a bladder lesion is identified on cystoscopy, screening of the upper tracts is always indicated with CT urogram for synchronous proximal lesions.

The right renal lesion is in keeping with a hyperdense cyst which falls into the Bosniak 2 category and does not require further action. Therefore staging CT, biopsy or follow-up would not be appropriate.

(The Final FRCR Complete Revision Notes Pages 248, 266)

41. (d) Nephroblastomatosis

Nephroblastomatosis is the presence of embryonic renal tissue beyond 36 weeks' gestation. It is known to be a risk factor for nephroblastoma (Wilms tumour). The appearances are either of a lesion which can have plaque-like or nodular appearance, low on T1 and T2 weighted sequences with minimal enhancement compared to the adjacent renal parenchyma.

In comparison, a Wilms tumour is usually T2 hyperintense and heterogenous in appearance with areas of necrosis and haemorrhage. Enhancement would be greater than nephroblastomatosis and inhomogeneous. Wilms tumours are also frequently large at diagnosis.

Mesoblastic nephromas typically involve the renal sinus and are also usually more heterogenous in appearance; it is therefore difficult to confidently differentiate them from a Wilms tumour on conventional imaging.

Multilocular cystic nephromas are multicystic renal lesions which classically herniate into the renal hilum.

A prominent column of Bertin can be mistaken for a renal mass. They are continuous with the renal cortex and on MRI demonstrate the same signal characteristics and enhance comparably.

(The Final FRCR Complete Revision Notes Page 353)

42. (a) Diffuse axonal injury

This is a severe intracranial injury secondary to axonal shearing caused by deceleration and rotational forces. Typical distribution is at the grey–white matter junction due to the relative difference of mass of these two structures (grade I injury). Grade II injury involves the corpus callosum and grade III the brainstem. Initial CT can be normal in up to 85% of cases and MRI is most sensitive. Gradient echo or susceptibility weighted imaging is most sensitive however there will also be FLAIR hyperintensity in the affected areas.

(The Final FRCR Complete Revision Notes Page 361)

43. (d) Pleural effusion

The patient in the main stem has developed acute respiratory distress syndrome (ARDS). Lung injury, which may be direct or indirect, causes alveolar damage and filling of the alveolar spaces with protein-rich fluid. In the initial exudative phase there is airspace filling with fluid which is seen on radiographs as patchy, and peripheral airspace opacification which can develop into confluent dense consolidation. On CT, the consolidation is mostly in the dependent aspect of the lung (consolidation in the non-dependent aspect of the lung is in keeping with non-ARDS causes of consolidation). A fibrotic phase can then occur as early as 1 week later. On radiograph, reticular opacities may be seen, and on CT the fibrosis has an anterior distribution (due to the effects of barotrauma). Tractional dilatation of the airways therefore tends to occur in an anterior distribution. Pleural effusions are not usually seen in ARDS.

(The Final FRCR Complete Revision Notes Page 16)

44. (e) Syringomyelia

The question describes a case of Charcot arthropathy or neuropathic joint. The patient presents with a swollen joint but importantly it is painless. The five D's are:

normal bone **D**ensity
Debris
Dislocation
joint **D**istension
articular cartilage **D**estruction

The site of a Charcot joint can help point towards an underlying diagnosis, and involvement of shoulder or other upper limb joint is most likely to be caused by syringomyelia. The ankle and foot is most commonly affected in diabetic-related Charcot arthropathy, and traumatic spinal cord injury can cause similar appearances of the spine. Neurosyphilis is a less common

cause now, but most commonly affects the knee joint. Chronic alcohol excess tends to be associated with changes in the foot.
(The Final FRCR Complete Revision Notes Page 70)

45. (a) Adenomyomatosis
The patient has symptoms and sonographic signs of cholecystitis with gallbladder wall thickening (>3 mm) and pericholecystic fluid. Adenomyomatosis is associated with gallstones and causes both diffuse or focal thickening of the gallbladder wall. On ultrasound, bright echoes may be seen in the wall with 'comet tail' ring down artefact from Rokitanky-Aschoff sinuses. The main differential for wall thickening, particularly when focal, is gallbladder carcinoma. MRI can be helpful in differentiating the two diagnoses, with the finding of multiple curvilinear foci of T2 hyperintensities (string of beads sign) in the wall being highly specific and the hallmark for adenomyomatosis.
Gangrenous cholecystitis can develop secondary to ischaemia and necrosis of the gallbladder wall and is more likely in diabetic patients; however these MRI appearances are typical for adenomyomatosis. Mural gas on T2 weighted imaging would appear hypointense rather than the hyperintensities described in this patient.
Gallbladder polyps are frequently incidental findings and are polypoid ingrowths into the lumen rather than an area of thickening.
The finding of a Phrygian cap is an incidental anatomic variant where there is folding at the fundus which can produce a thickened or septated appearance on ultrasound. Cross-sectional imaging usually helps to confirm the diagnosis in challenging cases.
(The Final FRCR Complete Revision Notes Page 195)

46. (a) Disc material extending >90° circumference and >3 mm beyond the vertebral body margin impinging the left L2 nerve
A broad based protrusion is when the disc material extends >3 mm beyond the vertebral body margin over an area extending >90° but <180° over the circumference of the vertebral body.
This is in contrast to a focal protrusion which is <90° and a broad based bulge which is >180°.
In the lumbar spine the nerve roots exit below the matching pedicle, so at L2/3, the L2 nerve exits. In the cervical spine there is a mismatch so at C2/3 the C3 nerve root exits below the C2 pedicle.
(The Final FRCR Complete Revision Notes Page 443)

47. (d) Multicystic dysplastic kidney
Multicystic dysplastic kidney is an obstructed non-functioning kidney which manifests as an enlarged multicystic kidney lacking normal renal parenchyma. The cysts may have rim calcification. If it is bilateral it is incompatible with survival. When unilateral, the contralateral side is commonly associated with vesicoureteral reflux.
The appearance may be difficult to differentiate from a hydronephrotic kidney; however, the absence of tracer uptake on the MAG3 study indicates there is no functioning renal tissue and therefore helps to differentiate the two.
Congenital mesoblastic nephroma are most commonly predominantly solid lesions.
Autosomal recessive polycystic kidney disease is associated with bilateral enlarged kidneys and multiple tiny cysts. Hepatic fibrosis is also a feature.
Multilocular cystic nephromas typically have a thick fibrous capsule and multiple septations which may demonstrate vascularity. The lesion may compress surrounding normal renal parenchyma. A typical characteristic is herniation into the renal pelvis, although with large lesions this may be difficult to appreciate.
(The Final FRCR Complete Revision Notes Page 353)

48. (c) Extradural haematoma
Extradural haematomas are usually lentiform in shape, secondary to skull fractures and characteristically do not cross sutures. The blood is located between the skull and the dura. They can be arterial; for example secondary to middle meningeal artery injury, or venous, and the history is commonly of a head injury followed by a lucid interval prior to reduced consciousness.
In contrast, subdural haematomas are sited between the dura and the arachnoid mater. They are usually venous bleeds, crescenteric in shape and due to their subdural location can cross sutures but not dural attachments. The superior sagittal sinus is bounded by a dural lining and the observation in this case that the haematoma crosses the midline and displaces the superior sagittal

sinus indicates that it is extradural rather than subdural.

Subarachnoid haemorrhage is located between the arachnoid membranes and pia mater. Common sites to see subarachnoid haemorrhage are around the circle of Willis, Sylvian fissures, interhemispheric fissure or foramen magnum.

Intraparenchymal haematoma would be intra-axial and therefore is not a suitable answer for this case.

(The Final FRCR Complete Revision Notes Page 362)

49. (a) Arrhythmogenic right ventricular dysplasia

This is a rare cause of arrhythmia and sudden death in young adults. MRI features include right ventricular thinning and dilatation with wall motion abnormality and high T1 fat signal in the right free wall.

Dilated cardiomyopathy is the most common cardiomyopathy causing dilatation of all cardiac chambers and widespread reduced contractility. It tends to be a diagnosis of exclusion.

An established myocardial infarct could demonstrate low T1 and T2 signal in the wall due to scarring with associated wall thinning and motional abnormality; however, in this age group it is less likely.

MRI findings of hypertrophic cardiomyopathy would include left ventricular hypertrophy with systolic anterior motion of the mitral valve. It is another cause of arrhythmia and sudden death in young adults.

Restrictive cardiomyopathy is caused by diastolic filling impairment and the ventricles are typically small due to causes such amyloidosis, sarcoidosis and haemochromatosis.

(The Final FRCR Complete Revision Notes Page 9)

50. (b) CT chest

The patient has signs of dermatomyositis with a rash and inflammation of striated muscle. It tends to affect patients around the age of 50 years. Inflammatory changes of the muscles can lead to soft tissue calcification which typically is sheet-like in appearance, although can manifest as non-specific subcutaneous calcification.

On MRI the muscles can have high T2 and STIR signal, indicating oedema with low signal related to any calcification. With long-standing disease the muscles may undergo fatty infiltration.

Dermatomyositis is associated with underlying malignancy, most commonly oesophageal, melanoma, genitourinary and lung. However, the majority have interstitial lung disease with a cryptogenic organising pneumonia type pattern causing peripheral subpleural consolidation and nodularity. Patients also have high risk of myocardial ischaemia and thromboembolic events.

Therefore, all the answers could potentially be correct; however the most suitable answer is a CT chest to look for underlying interstitial lung disease, as this is the most common association.

(The Final FRCR Complete Revision Notes Page 71)

51. (d) Superior mesenteric artery syndrome

Superior mesenteric artery (SMA) syndrome, also known as Wilkie syndrome, is a rare condition where the D3 segment of the duodenum is compressed between the SMA and aorta. It is associated with severe weight loss, lumbar lordosis and pregnancy. Sagittal reconstructions of a CT angiogram are suggestive of the diagnosis if there is a tight angle between the SMA and aorta (6–22° whereas normal would be 28–65°), the distance between the aorta and SMA is reduced to 2–8 mm (normal 10–34 mm) and there is proximal dilatation of the duodenum.

Nutcracker syndrome is due to compression of the left renal vein as it passes between the SMA and aorta. Mesenteric ischaemia would be unlikely in a patient of this age. The history is not typical for a duodenal ulcer and this would not explain the duodenal narrowing or proximal dilatation. Irritable bowel syndrome would be a diagnosis of exclusion.

(The Final FRCR Complete Revision Notes Page 186)

52. (a) CT cystogram

The patient has pelvic fractures, haematuria and free fluid in the pelvis. The density of the fluid is not consistent with acute haemorrhage and would be more in keeping with urine, and therefore urinary bladder injury needs to be excluded. There is a urinary catheter in situ and therefore a CT cystogram can be performed to evaluate further. If the fluid was high density and there was a concern regarding acute haemorrhage clinically then triple phase CT could be considered; however, in this case there has already been contrast administered which will confuse the findings, as a true non-contrast scan could not be obtained.

Confirmation and characterisation of any urinary bladder injury is important as it will impact further management. Extraperitoneal rupture, characterised by contrast extravasation into the extraperitoneal space, which can extend into the thighs, anterior abdominal wall and scrotum, is treated conservatively. However, intraperitoneal rupture, when contrast extravasates around bowel loops, would require surgical intervention. Subserosal bladder rupture is less common but suggested when there is elliptical contrast extravasation adjacent to the bladder.

Sometimes a delayed phase CT can be helpful to obtain an excretory phase of contrast and helps exclude urine leak, for example from the ureters; however, the urinary bladder will be more uniformly opacified and better distended on a CT cystoscopy.

(The Final FRCR Complete Revision Notes Page 249)

53. (e) Tuberculosis

Chronic end-stage renal tuberculosis tends to manifest as amorphous foci of calcification forming throughout the kidney sometimes associated with the process of autonephrectomy. The kidney often appears shrunken with a thinned cortex. The other available answers – hyperparathyroidism, hypothyroidism, sarcoidosis and multiple myeloma – are all associated with medullary calcification, which is the most common form of nephrocalcinosis. The most common causes of medullary nephrocalcinosis are hyperparathyroidism, renal tubular acidosis and medullary sponge kidney.

(The Final FRCR Complete Revision Notes Page 352)

54. (c) Pterygoid plates

Le Fort fractures are midface fractures involving the pterygoid plates. The fractures are categorised as Type I–III.

Type I is known as a floating palate, Type II a floating maxilla and Type III is the most severe and is separation of the base of skull and midface, otherwise known as 'floating face' or 'craniofacial disjunction'. When facial fractures are bilateral there may be asymmetry in the Le Fort fracture types.

(The Final FRCR Complete Revision Notes Page 364)

55. (b) Pleural effusion

The underlying diagnosis is *Pneumocystis jiroveci*, a fungal infection seen in immunocompromised patients. In the context of HIV, patients have CD4 count <200 cells/mm^3. The most common imaging abnormality is perihilar ground glass opacification and foci of consolidation, features which may or may not be accompanied by fine reticulation. Pneumatocoeles and subpleural blebs are also a common feature, usually in the upper zones. Occasionally the rupture of these cysts or blebs cause pneumothorax, which would be considered pathognomonic of *P. jiroveci* in the case described. Pleural effusions are rarely seen in this infection, and lymph node enlargement is also uncommon and so should prompt alternative differential diagnosis.

(The Final FRCR Complete Revision Notes Page 34)

56. (c) Facet joint ankylosis

Diffuse idiopathic skeletal hyperostosis (DISH) is often an incidental finding on radiographs but reports suggest it can be associated with stiffness and decreased mobility. The classic appearance is flowing osteophytes affecting ≥4 contiguous vertebrae, commonly in the thoracic spine tending to occur on the right side of the vertebral bodies as aortic pulsation inhibits ossification on the left.

In contrast to degenerative change of the spine, intervertebral disc spaces are preserved. If DISH affects the cervical spine it can cause dysphagia. There can be calcification of the anterior and posterior longitudinal ligaments but the facet joints are spared, as are the sacroiliac joints (unlike ankylosing spondylitis). Calcification can occur elsewhere, for example along tendons and ligaments such as the calcaneus, patella, iliac crest and around the elbow. Patients with spinal fusion are at increased risk of fracture following trauma.

(The Final FRCR Complete Revision Notes Page 72)

57. (d) ^{111}In Octreotide study

The top differential for a distal small bowel tumour containing calcification with low density lymph node involvement is a carcinoid. These are most common in the gastrointestinal tract, particularly the terminal ileum, followed by the rectum and colon. They can be plaquelike or polypoidal and tend to hyper enhance. Similarly, any liver metastases hyper enhance on an arterial phase study compared to the portal venous phase, when they may become difficult to appreciate. Up to 70% of the primary tumours contain calcification. Carcinoids can affect the mesentery causing the typical 'spoke wheel' appearance of desmoplastic reaction. The symptoms are often non-specific.

The most appropriate answer is ^{111}In-Octreotide study which aids diagnosis, detects occult tumours and helps to assess disease extent enabling appropriate treatment planning. An arterial phase CT chest and abdomen may aid diagnosis of distant metastases, including arterially enhancing liver lesions, but a ^{111}In-Octreotide study is recommended at baseline for all patients with these tumours. 5-HIAA serum levels can be raised in functioning tumours but this serum marker will not aid treatment planning in terms of disease extent. 18F-FDG PET/CT is not routinely used in carcinoid tumours as uptake can be low, particularly in low grade lesions, due to relatively low metabolic rate. MIBG scans are used in the investigation of phaeochromocytomas and not for carcinoid tumours.

(The Final FRCR Complete Revision Notes Page 158)

58. (a) Early enhancement following gadolinium

Patients who have previously had back surgery, for example discectomy or laminectomy, and develop back pain often require repeat MRI to distinguish between recurrent disc prolapse and postoperative epidural fibrosis. This is an important distinction to make as recurrent prolapse would be treated surgically whereas surgeons would be reluctant to intervene for postoperative fibrosis. It can be difficult to distinguish between the two entities on non-contrast imaging as both have low T1 signal, although fibrosis tends to have irregular borders and evidence of thecal retraction towards the area of interest. In contrast to this, a disc would typically have a smoother border. Following gadolinium administration, scarring enhances early whereas a disc will either not enhance or enhance late. Enhancement of the fibrosis diminishes after a few years. DWI and ADC imaging are not routinely performed for spinal imaging. High T2 signal in a disc is associated with discitis.

(The Final FRCR Complete Revision Notes Page 72)

59. (d) The ureter draining into the vagina is associated with the upper pole moiety

The anatomy in this case represents a double collecting system. A bifid ureter is two ureters that unite before the urinary bladder. A duplicated system is associated with a normally inserting ureter which arises from a lower pole moiety and an ectopic ureter which arises from an upper pole moiety. The ectopic ureter can insert elsewhere in the urinary bladder, usually more inferiorly and medially, or as in this case into nearby structures such as the vagina, which can lead to incontinence. The upper pole moiety can be obstructed due to the presence of a ureterocoele. This can inferiorly displace the lower pole moiety, leading to the 'drooping lily' appearance. The lower pole ureter is frequently affected by vesicoureteral reflux.

(The Final FRCR Complete Revision Notes Page 351)

60. (b) Sensorineural hearing loss

Temporal bone fractures are split into longitudinal, transverse and mixed fractures. Transverse fractures are less common but more likely to lead to vertigo and sensorineural hearing loss secondary to CN VIII injury. CN VII can also be affected causing facial paralysis.

Longitudinal fractures are more likely to lead to conductive hearing loss with involvement of the ossicles and tympanic membrane.

(The Final FRCR Complete Revision Notes Page 365)

61. (c) Hydatid cysts

The description is that of hydatid cysts. The described serpiginous structure is known as the 'water lily sign', which represents a floating membrane within the cyst fluid. Whilst the liver is the most common site for cyst formation, the lungs are the second most common. The lower lobes are more commonly affected. Unlike in the liver, pulmonary hydatid cysts rarely calcify. There may occasionally be an air-fluid level due to communication with the bronchial tree.

Bronchogenic cysts are solitary and found within the mediastinum adjacent to the main airways. Pericardial cysts are also usually solitary and found adjacent to the pericardium, within the cardiophrenic angle. Surrounding inflammatory change would be expected in the case of pulmonary abscess with a thicker wall and less smoothly marginated than a cyst.

Secondary infection of a hydatid cyst can lead to abscess formation.
(The Final FRCR Complete Revision Notes Page 36)

62. (e) *Streptococcus viridans*
The MRI features are typical for pyogenic discitis and associated vertebral osteomyelitis. *S. viridans* discitis is associated with the immunocompromised and intravenous drug users and can have accompanying endocarditis.
The most common causative organism for discitis in the general population is *Staphylococcus aureus*, and blood cultures are positive in around 50–70% of cases. In patients with sickle cell disease, Salmonella should be considered. Candida is less common. *Burkholderia pseudomallei* is more commonly encountered in locations such as southeast Asia and Australasia.
Spondylodiscitis caused by *Mycobacterium tuberculosis* (TB) (also known as Pott disease) would also be within the differential for this patient, although this is a relatively acute presentation and usually TB discitis tends to have a longer history without much systemic upset. It is not unusual for the chest radiograph to be normal in TB discitis. There can be reduction in vertebral body height causing a 'gibbus' deformity. Subligamentous spread is also a feature with the potential for skip lesions. The lower thoracic/upper lumbar spine is more commonly involved, whereas the lumbar spine is most frequently affected in pyogenic discitis. Intervertebral disc height is usually quite well preserved in TB discitis compared to pyogenic discitis. Paravertebral collections are possible in both pyogenic and TB discitis but they are more likely to calcify in the latter.
(The Final FRCR Complete Revision Notes Page 72)

63. (b) Colon
The patient has metastatic liver lesions and spread from a cholangiocarcinoma, colonic, pancreatic or oesophageal carcinoma are all possible. Liver metastases in prostate cancer would be more unusual. The presence of endocarditis and blood cultures which have grown *Streptococcus bovis* are highly suspicious for an underlying colonic malignancy. Patients with colorectal cancer may present with metastatic disease, particularly if the colonic primary is right sided. Left sided tumours tend to present earlier with altered bowel habit.
(The Final FRCR Complete Revision Notes Page 160)

64. (c) Lymphoma
The most common metastatic lesion to the breast is associated with lymphoma, followed by melanoma, choriocarcinoma and renal cell carcinoma. In men, prostate cancer is commonly a cause of breast metastases. It is also possible with other malignancies such as colon, ovarian and gastric cancers.
Metastases are usually multiple and bilateral. They are frequently well-defined, solid lesions on imaging and may demonstrate posterior acoustic enhancement. In contrast to this, primary breast malignancy is typically ill defined and hypoechoic with posterior acoustic shadowing, although appearances can be variable and hence biopsy is vital to determine the cause of most solid breast lesions.
(The Final FRCR Complete Revision Notes Page 285)

65. (b) Expiratory chest radiograph
A unilateral lucent lung with evidence of hyperinflation (indicated by the increased rib spacing), suggests a possible ball-valve obstruction causing air trapping. This, along with the short history of cough, is suspicious for an aspirated foreign body. Foreign bodies are frequently radiolucent but an expiratory film will help to confirm air trapping. Bronchoscopy is the treatment of choice.
Differentials for a unilateral lucent lung include MacLeod syndrome, Poland syndrome, congenital lobar emphysema and pulmonary sling. MacLeod syndrome is often an incidental finding but the lung appears small rather than hyperinflated and there are typically reduced vascular markings. There is typically a matched ventilation-perfusion defect.
Asthma and viral infections can cause hyperinflation; however this would cause bilateral changes rather than the unilateral appearance on this radiograph.
Pulmonary sling, also known as an aberrant left pulmonary artery, is a congenital vascular malformation where the left pulmonary artery arises from the right pulmonary artery. In its path to the contralateral side, it can compress the right main bronchus causing air trapping. Arterial phase CT can help to delineate the anatomy.
(The Final FRCR Complete Revision Notes Page 323)

66. (d) Amyloid angiopathy

This condition is due to beta-amyloid protein deposition in small vessel walls of the cortical, subcortical and leptomeningeal regions leading to spontaneous multifocal peripheral cortical and subcortical haemorrhage. Patient are typically elderly and normotensive. On MRI there are usually multiple cerebral microhaemorrhages evident on susceptibility weighted imaging at the grey–white matter junction and in the cerebellum. Acute haemorrhage can lead to lobar haemorrhage, subarachnoid blood and more chronically, superficial siderosis.

Hypertensive haemorrhage tends to occur in the basal ganglia whereas amyloid angiopathy spares this region.

First presentation of an arteriovenous malformation would be unusual in this age group and they are more commonly solitary. There may be prominent feeding or draining vessels.

Haemorrhagic metastases would be within the differential particularly in more mature patients. The presence of acute haemorrhage along with features of more chronic microhaemorrhages is more indicative of amyloid angiopathy than metastatic disease.

Herpes encephalitis can lead to cortical microhaemorrhage but the distribution is typically the bilateral temporal lobes and this diagnosis would not account for the frontal haemorrhage. Other signal changes such as cortical T2 hyperintensity and restricted diffusion would be likely.

(The Final FRCR Complete Revision Notes Page 365)

67. (a) Carotid Doppler ultrasound

The patient has features of Takayasu arteritis which is a large vessel inflammatory arteritis involving the aorta and its major branches although rarely the infrarenal aorta and hence the inferior mesenteric artery or iliac vessels. Patients can present with non-specific symptoms. It is more common in women than men and tends to affect young adults. Typically imaging demonstrates arterial wall thickening and enhancement causing stenosis, associated aneurysmal dilatation and potentially occlusion.

Takayasu often involves the pulmonary arteries causing peripheral pruning and can also affect the carotid arteries, hence a carotid Doppler ultrasound is the most appropriate investigation out of the available options.

A circle of Willis CT is not currently indicated. A CT pelvis and lower limb Doppler ultrasound would also not be indicated normally in Takayasu's due to the distribution of the disease. An MRA renal arteries may show high STIR signal in the vessel wall indicating oedema, but the CT findings are already highly suggestive of a large vessel arteritis such as Takayasu.

(The Final FRCR Complete Revision Notes Page 16)

68. (b) Bone marrow biopsy

The patient has an abnormal radiograph with a normal bone scan. The differentials for this include metabolically inactive bone lesions such as bone cysts and islands, osteoporosis, new fractures (<48 hours old), multiple myeloma or metastases with no osteoblastic activity. Therefore, the most likely cause is multiple myeloma and the most appropriate answer is a bone marrow biopsy.

Most bony breast cancer deposits do demonstrate tracer uptake on nuclear medicine bone scans; however some breast cancers and other osteolytic metastases, such as from renal, thyroid or lung cancer, can be non-avid. However, these cancers tend to create photopenic foci.

Osteomyelitis can cause lytic lesions on radiographs but the multiplicity is not typical and therefore blood culture would not be appropriate. Similarly Paget's disease and hyperparathyroidism can cause abnormal radiographic appearances with lytic lesions but the bone scan would usually be abnormal in these conditions, demonstrating focal and generalised increased uptake, respectively.

(The Final FRCR Complete Revision Notes Page 68)

69. (d) Kaposi sarcoma

Kaposi sarcoma is a low grade tumour which can affect the skin, lungs or gastrointestinal tract. It is an AIDS-defining illness and the most common neoplasm in these patients. It usually requires the CD4 count to drop <200 cells/mm^3. The characteristic skin tumours are purple lesions and these help to differentiate it from other AIDS-defining illnesses. Any part of the gastrointestinal tract can be affected but the stomach, duodenum and proximal small bowel are most commonly involved.

Mycobacterial disease and lymphoma typically have hypoattenuating nodes.
(The Final FRCR Complete Revision Notes Page 242)

70. (b) Autosomal recessive
The case describes a typical case of autosomal recessive polycystic kidney disease (ARPKD). The renal cysts are often very small and may not be distinguished on ultrasound. Instead the kidneys may appear enlarged and hyperechoic. Hepatic fibrosis is an associated finding which may manifest as a coarse hepatic echotexture or periportal increased echogenicity. The finding of hepatosplenomegaly and reversal of hepatic vein flow is consistent with portal hypertension. The pancreas and liver may or may not contain cysts. ARPKD is associated with Caroli syndrome and hence the intrahepatic biliary duct dilatation in this case.
(The Final FRCR Complete Revision Notes Page 350)

71. (b) Jejunoileal fold pattern reversal
The most specific radiological sign in coeliac disease is jejunoileal fold pattern reversal. So called due to jejunisation of the ileum, this means that there are an increased number of ileal folds to compensate for reduced jejunal folds. Fluoroscopic imaging in coeliac disease can also demonstrate changes secondary to increased fluid secretion, such as flocculation and dilatation; however, these are not as specific. There can also be an absence of valvulae conniventes, otherwise known as the 'moulage sign' and regions of small bowel intussusception.
Crowding of the valvulae conniventes, reduced peristalsis and small bowel sacculation is more commonly associated with scleroderma. Crowding of the valvulae conniventes in scleroderma is often referred to as a 'hidebound' appearance – the bowel folds are not thickened. This is in contrast to a 'stack of coin' appearance where the folds are smoothly thickened and can be seen in conditions associated with haemorrhage into the bowel wall, such as coagulopathies, ischaemia and vasculitides.
Sacculation can also be associated with ischaemic bowel insults and Crohn's disease.
(The Final FRCR Complete Revision Notes Page 160)

72. (e) Subacute sclerosing panencephalitis
The patient has a history consistent with measles infection. The buccal spots are Koplik spots and are highly characteristic for measles. The associated asymmetrical subcortical and deep white matter changes and volume loss are consistent with subacute sclerosing panencephalitis. This typically affects the temporoparietal region but can become diffuse, affecting the basal ganglia and corpus callosum.
Acute demyelinating encephalomyelitis (ADEM) is within the differential, especially with a history of infective illness; however this rarely involves the basal ganglia and is not associated with atrophy. Acute haemorrhagic leukoencephalopathy is a severe variant of ADEM characterised by significant oedema and small white matter haemorrhages.
Herpes simplex encephalitis affects the temporal lobes, often bilaterally, as well as commonly involving the frontal lobes and insular cortex with gyral and leptomeningeal enhancement rather than the patchy white matter enhancement described in this case.
Japanese encephalitis typically demonstrates bilateral thalamic involvement, which can lead to haemorrhage, as well as involvement of other both supra and infra tentorial structures.
(The Final FRCR Complete Revision Notes Page 416)

73. (c) Paratracheal
The presence of Reed-Sternberg cells is in keeping with a diagnosis of Hodgkin lymphoma. Over 80% of patients with Hodgkin lymphoma have involvement of the thorax at the first presentation. Most commonly, the anterior mediastinum and paratracheal nodes are involved. Less frequently the subcarinal, perioesophageal and internal mammary nodes may also be involved. Hilar lymph node enlargement usually occurs in the context of mediastinal lymphadenopathy.
Lymphoma is staged using the Cotswolds Modification of the Ann Arbor Staging System and treatment response is assessed using the Lugano classification and Deauville scale.

- **Stage I** is when there is a single affected nodal group.
- **Stage II** is when there are multiple involved nodal groups, all on the same side of the diaphragm.
- **Stage III** is when these groups span both sides of the diaphragm.

- **Stage IV** is when extra-nodal disease sites become affected, such as the liver, bone marrow or cerebrospinal fluid.
- Other letters may be used including '**A**' when a patient is asymptomatic and '**B**' when they have symptoms such as fevers, weight loss and night sweats.
- **E** is used when there is extra-nodal extension adjacent to a known nodal site.
- **S** indicates splenic involvement.
- **X** is used when there is a nodal mass >10 cm.

(The Final FRCR Complete Revision Notes Page 35)

74. (d) Lateral osseous bump, 65°, Labral tear

There are two subtypes of femoroacetabular impingement (FAI); cam FAI is more common in young men versus pincer FAI which is associated more with middle-aged females. Cam FAI is caused by a non-spherical femoral head impacting against the acetabulum; typically there is a flattening at the junction between the femoral head and neck with an osseous bump just lateral to the physeal scar. This is associated with subsequent degenerative change and labral tears. Cartilage and labral injuries tend to be positioned anterior-superiorly. The alpha angle is frequently cited and an angle >55–60° (depending on the article) is considered abnormal.

Pincer FAI is due to a deep acetabulum; therefore the coverage of the femoral head is increased and leads to abnormal contact between the femoral head/neck junction and the overhanging acetabulum. Chondral injury is more typically circumferential versus the anterior-superior position in cam FAI. It is also possible to have a combined type of FAI.

(The Final FRCR Complete Revision Notes Page 74)

75. (b) Middle rectal vein

The most frequent location for colorectal cancer is the rectosigmoid colon followed by descending, transverse and then ascending colon and caecum. Left sided tumours may present with fresh red rectal blood; however, bleeding from right sided tumours is often occult and therefore patients may present with anaemia.

In this question the low attenuation liver lesions are longstanding and of unlikely clinical significance. In contrast, the multiple bilateral lung nodules are concerning. The presence of lung metastases in the absence of convincing liver lesions makes a rectal primary site most likely as the drainage of the rectum is via the pelvic veins directly into the inferior vena cava. Consequently, metastatic spread can bypass the portal venous system and the liver, causing lung metastases. The superior rectal vein drains into the portal venous system but the middle and inferior rectal veins drain directly into the inferior vena cava.

(The Final FRCR Complete Revision Notes Page 160)

76. (e) Unenhanced CT abdomen

The patient has bilateral renal lesions. The lesion on the right kidney is consistent with a Bosniak 2F cyst with thin septae and nodular calcification; this will require CT follow-up. Once septae or walls become thickened and nodular with measurable enhancement then the cyst falls into the Bosniak 3 category and many patients will undergo invasive management, either surgery or radiofrequency ablation.

The lesion associated with the left kidney is hyperdense. This CT is enhanced, likely portal venous phase imaging for this clinical indication, so we need to establish whether this hyperdensity is enhancement or due to the inherent density of the lesion. A hyperdense renal cyst should not significantly change density between the unenhanced and the enhanced sequences. A soft tissue mass would demonstrate a significant difference being lower density on the unenhanced and then increasing following contrast administration.

The patient should be fully worked up prior to being discussed at the multidisciplinary team meeting and therefore although the patient will require follow-up for the right Bosniak 2F lesion, the unenhanced CT should be performed in the first instance to complete the imaging and complete characterisation of the lesion.

(The Final FRCR Complete Revision Notes Page 250)

77. (c) Langerhans cell histiocytosis

The constellation of clinical signs and symptoms are consistent with Hand-Schüller-Christian disease which is the chronic systemic form of Langerhans cell histiocytosis. It can manifest with bone lesions, hepatosplenomegaly, diabetes insipidus, proptosis and dermatitis. The majority of bone lesions in Langerhans cell histiocytosis have variable appearances, with both lucency and sclerosis depending on the stage of the disease. However, skull lesions typically have a bevelled 'hole within a hole' appearance and vertebral involvement leads to vertebra plana, which is the most common cause of vertebra plana in children.

Sarcoidosis and tuberculosis can cause diabetes insipidus with other systemic signs and symptoms, including musculoskeletal manifestations. Sarcoidosis can affect the eyes too but usually affects the lacrimal glands rather than causing proptosis.

Graves disease can cause exophthalmos and skeletal changes, such as thyroid acropachy, but it is not associated with the other clinical signs in this case.

Diabetes mellitus is a cause of increased thirst in children but does not account for the other changes.

(The Final FRCR Complete Revision Notes Page 324)

78. (d) T1 sagittal and coronal, T1 post contrast sagittal and coronal, T1 coronal with dynamic contrast

The coronal and sagittal planes give the most information. Coronal dynamic post-contrast T1 sequences are also crucial for imaging potential microadenomas. Post-contrast imaging is always acquired on T1 sequences rather than with T2. Using a small field of view can also be helpful.

The normal pituitary gland has anterior and posterior components. The anterior pituitary is T1 and T2 isointense. The posterior pituitary is T1 hyperintense and T2 hypointense. Post-contrast imaging helps to detect microadenomas which are usually hypo enhancing compared to the rest of the gland.

(The Final FRCR Complete Revision Notes Page 404)

79. (a) Recommendations for the categorisation of carotid artery stenosis is as follows:

(The Final FRCR Complete Revision Notes Page 10)

Table 1.9: Grey-Scale and Doppler Ultrasound Criteria for Diagnosis of Carotid Artery Stenosis (The Society of Radiologists in Ultrasound 2003)

ICA Stenosis	ICA PSV (cm/sec)	ICA/CCA PSV Ratio	ICA EDV (cm/sec)	Plaque estimate (%)
Normal	<125	<2.0	<40	None
<50%	<125 cm/sec	<2.0	<40	<50
50–69%	125–230	2.0–4.0	40–100	≥50
≥70%	>230	>4.0	>100	≥50
Near occlusion	High, low or undetectable	Variable	Variable	Visible
Total occlusion	Undetectable	Not applicable	Not applicable	Visible, no detectable lumen

Source: Data from Grant EG, Benson CB, Moneta GL et al. Carotid artery stenosis: Grayscale and Doppler Ultrasound Diagnosis-Society of Radiologists in Ultrasound Consensus Conference. *Ultrasound Quarterly.* 2003;19(4):190–198.

80. (c) Multiple lytic skull lesions

The case describes vertebra plana. The most common cause in children is Langerhans cell histiocytosis (LCH) which among other findings can cause lytic skull lesions. LCH can cause aggressive looking osseous lesions with a laminated or 'onion skin' periosteal reaction, as described in Answer D. However, the skull is more commonly affected in LCH than the long bones. The femoral appearances in the available answer are concerning for Ewing's sarcoma which is another, less common cause of vertebra plana.

The other available answers describe other potential causes of vertebra plana in children including neuroblastoma which could cause the finding of an abdominal mass adjacent to the aorta on abdomen ultrasound. Raised inflammatory markers are non-specific but would be associated with infection, including osteomyelitis and tuberculosis.

Multiple abnormal lymph nodes would be suspicious for lymphoma; however in lymphoma there may be multi-level spine involvement.

(The Final FRCR Complete Revision Notes Pages 101, 324)

81 (d) Spleen

Splenic injury is most common following a blunt force trauma causing abdominal injury. Hepatic injury is more common following penetrating trauma. The history in this case also indicates the potential for significant haemorrhage which would fit with splenic injury. Regardless, careful scrutiny of all the abdominal viscera is required. If splenic injury is identified then consideration of injuries in other adjacent structures is important, for example the left kidney, pancreatic tail and left hemidiaphragm. Splenic (and other abdominal visceral) injury is graded with the American Association for the Surgery of Trauma (AAST) grading system.

(The Final FRCR Complete Revision Notes Page 240)

82 (b) MacLeod syndrome

MacLeod syndrome, also known as Sywer-James syndrome, is thought to occur secondary to childhood infectious bronchiolitis. Previous infections with mycoplasma pneumoniae and viral infections are thought to play a role. It causes a unilateral, often small, lucent lung with reduced vascularity and expiratory air trapping. It can be an incidental finding in adulthood.

The history in this case is not typical for congenital lobar over inflation (CLO), which was previously known as congenital lobar emphysema. CLO usually presents in neonates with respiratory distress. It most commonly affects the left upper lobe, followed by the right middle and upper lobes. It tends to cause marked mediastinal shift.

Pulmonary agenesis causes an absent lung on one side with no vasculature. Therefore, this usually causes a dense hemithorax with mediastinal shift towards the affected side due to cross-herniation from the contralateral side.

Poland syndrome is a congenital unilateral absence of the pectoralis muscles. It would not cause a small unilateral hemithorax and would also not impact the vasculature.

Scimitar syndrome does not typically cause a lucent lung; however, the lung is commonly small, with associated ipsilateral mediastinal shift and anomalous venous drainage. This is most commonly into the inferior vena cava which causes a 'scimitar' appearance in the right lower zone.

(The Final FRCR Complete Revision Notes Page 325)

83 (c) They sometimes contain an intracystic nodule

Rathke cleft cysts are benign, incidental, midline lesions associated with the pituitary gland. Intracystic nodules are pathognomic for these lesions and are typically non-enhancing and small. Rathke cleft cysts neither calcify nor demonstrate restricted diffusion. There may be minimal peripheral rim enhancement. They rarely extend beyond the sella.

(The Final FRCR Complete Revision Notes Page 405)

84 (d) Repeat ultrasound in 3 weeks

The radiological findings are suggestive of adrenal haemorrhage. This often presents as an asymptomatic abdominal mass, and depending on the age of the haemorrhage it can have variable sonographic appearances. Acutely they may appear more solid with internal echoes but over time blood products liquify and they become more heterogenous with cystic components. Chronically they may calcify. The main differential is neuroblastoma which can have similar appearances of a solid appearing mass. One distinguishing feature is the history, and in this case there is a history of a traumatic birth. Secondly, the lack of vascularity is indicative of adrenal haemorrhage rather than neuroblastoma. On follow-up ultrasound, adrenal haemorrhage will decrease in size over time, whereas neuroblastoma will increase in size. Therefore prompt follow-up ultrasound is important. Ultrasound guided biopsy would not be indicated and MRI is usually reserved for challenging cases. MIBG is often used in the staging of neuroblastoma.

(The Final FRCR Complete Revision Notes Page 349)

85 (d) Non-specific interstitial pneumonia (NSIP)

Rheumatoid arthritis can be associated with both usual interstitial pneumonia (UIP) pattern of disease as well as NSIP. The features described on the CT are more typical for NSIP. Radiological overlap between the two diseases can occur; however the UIP pattern is associated with honeycomb destruction of the parenchyma compared to the predominantly ground glass opacification seen in NSIP. The immediate subpleural sparing is considered specific for NSIP and traction dilatation occurs due to the fibrotic process pulling the small airways open. Although UIP is associated with an apicobasal gradient, the parenchymal changes are typically peripheral rather than diffuse, as can be the case in NSIP.

Subacute hypersensitivity pneumonitis can manifest as ground glass subpleural nodularity with subpleural sparing, representing infiltrate into the small airways. There may also be mosaicism secondary to air trapping. In the chronic stage, features of lung fibrosis can occur, although this is more typically in the upper zones.

The predominant imaging finding in cryptogenic organising pneumonia is ground glass change and dense consolidation.

Lymphocytic interstitial pneumonia is very rare and more typically associated with Sjogren syndrome or HIV. The main imaging finding is ground glass opacification and perivascular cysts.

(The Final FRCR Complete Revision Notes Pages 37–39)

86 (a) Gaucher disease

The patient is around the typical age for presentation and has classical radiological features of Gaucher disease: hepatosplenomegaly, paranasal sinus obliteration due to medullary expansion and Erlenmeyer flask deformity of the proximal humerus. Erlenmeyer flask deformity has a limited number of differentials which can be remembered with the mnemonic 'Lead GNOME':

Lead poisoning
Gaucher disease
Niemann-Pick disease
Osteopetrosis
Metaphyseal dysplasia
Ematological conditions such as thalassaemia

Osteopetrosis can cause medullary hyperexpansion and hepatosplenomegaly but the bones are typically sclerotic and fracture easily. Similarly, Niemann-Pick disease can cause hepatosplenomegaly; however, Gaucher disease is more common than Niemann-Pick. Granulomatosis with polyangiitis (previously known as Wegener granulomatosis) is a cause of paranasal sinus obliteration and sarcoidosis is a cause of hepatosplenomegaly but neither cause Erlenmeyer flask deformities.

(The Final FRCR Complete Revision Notes Page 76)

87 (b) Duodenal involvement

The appearances of gastric lymphoma can be varied; however, wall thickening tends to be more diffuse and thicker than with gastric carcinoma. Extensive wall thickening and submucosal infiltration can extend into the duodenum. There is less likely to be perigastric fat invasion and gastric outlet obstruction than with gastric carcinoma.

Atrophic gastritis is a risk factor for gastric carcinoma, along with pernicious anaemia. *Helicobacter pylori* infection is associated with both gastric carcinoma and lymphoma.

Both gastric carcinoma and lymphoma tend to metastasise to the liver first. Regional adenopathy is common in both malignancies but the lymph nodes in gastric lymphoma are usually larger and more extensive than with gastric carcinoma, potentially extending below the level of the renal vein.

(The Final FRCR Complete Revision Notes Pages 168–169)

88 (a) Adenomyosis

Adenomyosis tends to affect perimenopausal women and is a cause of heavy periods. It is caused by ectopic endometrial tissue within the myometrium. The whole uterus can be affected, appearing bulky and thickened, or it can be more focal, as in this case. There is thickening of the junctional zone >12 mm (the region between the endometrium and myometrium) and there are frequently cystic T2 hyperintensities in this region. There may also be areas of T1 hyperintensity with recent haemorrhage.

Endometrial cancer can be a cause of abnormal uterine bleeding. The endometrium in this case is 7 mm. Normal endometrial thickness pre-menopause is up to 16 mm, depending on the stage of the menstrual cycle, and post menopause it can measure up to 3–4 mm.

Imaging features are not typical for a leiomyoma (fibroid), which are usually T2 hypointense and on T1 sequences are intermediate to low signal. Leiomyosarcoma is suspected in fibroids with atypical imaging features and irregular borders.

Endometriosis can have a variety of appearances but features such as ovarian endometriomas, kissing ovaries, adhesions and areas of high T1 haemorrhage within the pelvis are common.

(The Final FRCR Complete Revision Notes Page 270)

89 (c) Fracture of the acromion of the scapula

The most specific injuries for non-accidental injury (NAI) include fractures of the distal third of the clavicle, posterior rib fractures, sternum, scapula and metaphyseal 'corner' fractures.

Moderately specific fractures include bilateral fractures, injuries of differing ages, spiral fractures, complex skull fractures and vertebral fractures or subluxations. Fractures of digits in non-mobile children (such as in this case) would also fit within this category.

Fractures such as those at the mid-clavicle, linear skull fractures and greenstick fractures have low specificity for NAI.

(The Final FRCR Complete Revision Notes Page 330)

90 (c) CADASIL

Cerebral autosomal dominant arteriopathy with subcortical infarctions and leukoencephalopathy (CADASIL) is an autosomal dominant vasculopathy. Patients between 30 and 50 years present with recurrent transient ischaemic attacks and stroke. On MRI there are often multiple areas of subcortical white matter T2 hyperintensity with similar appearances to small vessel disease. However, patients with CADASIL are younger and lack vascular risk factors. Anterior temporal lobe and external capsule involvement is common. Occipital lobe involvement is unusual. CADASIL is eventually associated with cerebral atrophy and dementia.

The history does not fit with Susac syndrome; this condition affects women, causing a triad of encephalopathy, retinal artery occlusions and sensorineural hearing loss.

MELAS (mitochondrial encephalomalacia with lactic acidosis and stroke-like episodes) presentation can be similar to CADASIL with recurrent stroke; however there are other symptoms and signs such as lactic acidosis, encephalopathy and seizures. The distribution differs too, with parietal and occipital lobe involvement more common.

Although acute demyelinating encephalomyelitis (ADEM) can cause subcortical T2 white matter hyperintensity, it usually presents differently with fever, seizure, reduced GCS and headache.

Amyloid angiopathy affects an older age group and acute presentations with stroke-like symptoms is due to haemorrhage rather than ischaemic infarcts. Additionally, there is blooming on susceptibility weighted images from chronic microhaemorrhages.

(The Final FRCR Complete Revision Notes Page 367)

91 (e) Post-transplant lymphoproliferative disease

Post-transplant lymphoproliferative disease affects around 10% of solid organ recipients, peaking around 1 year or 5 years post-transplant. It is thought to be secondary to B or T cell proliferation related to Epstein-Barr virus infection. Presentation can be non-specific and may include fever. Pulmonary manifestations include pulmonary nodules which can cavitate. It can also affect the brain, liver and bowel. Appearances may look similar to lymphoma with lymph node enlargement.

Infection is the most common post cardiac transplant complication and aspergillus infection can present as pulmonary nodules; however, this tends to occur within the first couple of months following transplant. Nocardia is another possible causative agent.

Drug reactions causing pulmonary manifestations are possible but they tend to cause more non-specific changes, and any small nodules would tend to be associated with ground glass opacification and consolidation.

Lymphocytic interstitial pneumonitis is associated with autoimmune disorders and can resemble lymphoma with lymphadenopathy. Pulmonary nodules are possible as well as cysts, ground glass opacification and interlobular septal thickening.

Metastatic malignancy is possible, especially in an immunosuppressed patient; however patients should be thoroughly screened for this prior to any solid organ transplant.

(The Final FRCR Complete Revision Notes Page 8)

92 (e) Radiographs of the cervical spine

The NICE indications for CT head in a paediatric patient of this age include suspicion of non-accidental injury, post traumatic seizure, initial GCS < 14 or GCS < 15 at 2 hours following the injury, suspected open or depressed skull injury, suspected basal skull fracture or focal neurological deficit. Based on the provided information the patient does not fulfil these criteria.

The NICE indications for CT cervical spine in paediatric patients include initial GCS < 13, other areas being scanned, for example for head injury, focal neurological signs and/or paraesthesia and if there was an urgent definitive diagnosis of cervical spine injury required, for example prior to surgery. In this case, the answer is no to all of these and therefore due to the neck pain and mechanism of injury the patient would be suitable for three-view cervical spine radiographs in the first instance. If there is still a strong suspicion of injury or if the films are suboptimal, then CT should be considered.

The ALARA principal is important when considering imaging in paediatric trauma patients and the Royal College of Radiologists have published useful guidance based on the NICE algorithms.

The Royal College of Radiologists. 2014. Paediatric trauma protocols.
https://www.rcr.ac.uk/publication/paediatric-trauma-protocols

National Institute for Health and Care Excellence (NICE). 2014 (updated 2019). NICE Clinical Guideline 176. Head injury: assessment and early management.
https://www.nice.org.uk/guidance/cg176

93 (b) Typhlitis

Typhlitis (or neutropenic enterocolitis) is a serious, potentially life threatening, acute inflammation of the bowel that typically involves the caecum, appendix and terminal ileum. It is usually seen in children who are neutropenic secondary to immunosuppression following treatment of lymphoma or leukaemia. Classically there is concentric bowel wall thickening with surrounding mesenteric inflammatory fat stranding. Pneumatosis can also be present.

The history in this case is particularly suggestive of typhlitis. Although the appendix is affected, the more extensive involvement of the caecum and terminal ileum makes acute appendicitis less likely. Similarly, although Crohn's disease favours the terminal ileum it is frequently multifocal with skip lesions, stricturing and extraintestinal manifestations. Bowel lymphoma is usually non-Hodgkin and small bowel involvement is more likely than large bowel involvement; it also usually affects an older age group. Necrotising enterocolitis is a condition affecting preterm neonates.

(The Final FRCR Complete Revision Notes Page 187)

94 (b) Dentigerous cyst

The mandibular cyst in this case is unilocular and related to the dentition. This narrows the differentials to a radicular cyst or a dentigerous cyst. A radicular cyst, also known as a periapical cyst, is related to the root of the tooth whereas a dentigerous cyst is related to an unerupted or impacted tooth and is in a pericoronal position.

Unilocular cysts which are not related to the teeth have differentials depending on the age of a patient. Generally if the patient is >40 years old, consider diagnoses such ameloblastoma, myeloma or metastases. Ameloblastoma typically has a 'bubbly' appearance and can cause root resorption. If the patient is younger (<30 years), consider odontogenic keratocysts and simple bone cysts. The appearance of a multilocular cyst raises the possibility of an aneurysmal bone cyst or odontogenic keratocyst. In the case of multiple odontogenic keratocysts consider Gorlin-Goltz syndrome.

(The Final FRCR Complete Revision Notes Page 442)

95 (a) Catheter passes inferiorly from umbilicus into pelvis, turning cephalad with the tip at the level of T9

Umbilical arterial catheters should pass from the umbilicus inferiorly into the pelvis before turning cephalad and going into the aorta. The aim is for the tip to be sited within the aorta in either a high or low position, but not between the levels of T10-L3 which is where the main aortic branches arise.

In contrast to this, umbilical venous catheters should pass superiorly from the umbilicus into the umbilical vein, portal vein, ductus venosus and then into the hepatic vein and inferior vena cava. The tip should ideally lie at the junction of the inferior vena cava and right atrium, which is usually around the level of the diaphragm at T8/9.

(The Final FRCR Complete Revision Notes Page 332)

96 (c) Bone erosion

Haemangiopericytomas are rare, aggressive tumours of the meninges. They are often solitary. Their appearances can be very similar to meningioma with T1 and T2 isointensity and a dural tail but should be suspected if there are atypical features such as bone erosion or if a lesion lacks common characteristics of a meningioma such as calcification or adjacent hyperostosis. Meningiomas are usually homogenous in appearance. In contrast to this, the vascular nature of haemangiopericytomas means that there are often visible flow voids. Meningiomas are associated with increased alanine levels on MRI spectroscopy but this is absent in a haemangiopericytoma.

(The Final FRCR Complete Revision Notes Page 401)

97 (a) Actinomycosis

Actinomycosis is a bacterial infection which is relatively uncommon, usually affecting those who have chronic debilitating illnesses, poor oral hygiene (the organism is usually spread to the thorax following aspiration from the oropharynx) or alcoholism. Most cases of actinomycosis are seen in the cervicofacial region (50–65%). The thorax is the second most common site, accounting for 15–30%. In the thorax it usually presents as chronic consolidation with low attenuation foci centrally, representing abscess formation. Actinomycosis is able to spread beyond connective tissue planes, hence the described chest wall invasion and periostitis of the adjacent ribs. Patients with previous history of lung destruction secondary to previous infection, such as tuberculosis, are more susceptible to the infection. Furthermore, the presence of sulphur granules within the specimen is also highly suggestive for diagnosis of the infection (although this may also be seen in infection with other fungal-like organisms).

Heo SH, Shin SS, Kim JW et al. Imaging of actinomycosis in various organs: a comprehensive review. RadioGraphics. 2014;34(1):19–33.

Han JY, Lee KN, Lee JK et al. An overview of thoracic actinomycosis: CT features. Insights Imaging. 2013;4(2):245–252.

98 (c) Joint aspiration

The patient has an underlying diagnosis of gout which is associated with hyperuricaemia. Although 24-hour urine collection can demonstrate high urine uric acid levels, the gold standard test is joint aspiration to confirm the presence of monosodium urate crystals.

The MRI findings are consistent with gouty tophi which are usually low on T1 sequences, heterogeneously low on T2 weighted imaging and enhance following gadolinium administration. Tophi can erode into adjacent bone causing marrow oedema, and there can be oedema adjacent to the typical punched out marginal erosions. Gout has a predilection for certain tendons around the knee including the patellar and popliteus tendons.

Serum parathyroid hormone levels would confirm hyperparathyroidism which can cause calcific soft tissue lesions particularly in secondary hyperparathyroidism. 18F-FDG PET/CT could help to confirm FDG avidity in potentially malignant conditions such as a synovial sarcoma however appearances and history are not typical for this. A CT chest, abdomen and pelvis would not be indicated.

(The Final FRCR Complete Revision Notes Page 77)

99 (c) FDG-PET/CT study

Serum CEA is used to monitor patients following treatment for colorectal cancer but it can also be raised in other cancers and in conditions such as inflammatory bowel disease and liver disease. This patient is young and although asymptomatic it would be important to ascertain if there is evidence of disease recurrence so prompt management can be administered if appropriate.

A CT cologram is used for asymptomatic screening and following a failed colonoscopy but its use is not appropriate in this setting. Furthermore, rectal cancer is better visualised and locally staged using MRI rather than CT. An MRI pelvis could be helpful in the identification of recurrence more than 6 months following surgery, with the latter demonstrating higher T2 signal intensity compared to post-surgical fibrosis. FDG-PET/CT is also helpful in recurrence as there will be increased tracer uptake compared to post-surgical changes.

An MRI liver may be helpful in assessing for metastatic spread; however with T3N1bM0 disease it is important to exclude local recurrence, and an FDG-PET/CT should also identify any distant disease, for example in the liver.

(The Final FRCR Complete Revision Notes Page 160)

100 (d) Grade IV

The laceration is >1 cm which means it is at least Grade III. The low density fluid around the kidney is consistent with a urine leak which immediately elevates it to a Grade IV. Similarly a segmental vascular injury, including infarcts, and active bleeding beyond Gerota fascia would also fit within the Grade IV category.

Grade V injuries include a shattered kidney, main renal artery laceration, thrombosis and complete avulsion of the renal pelvis which devascularises the kidney.

Grade I includes contusion and haematoma. Grade II extends to include a parenchymal laceration up to 1 cm without a urine leak or a non-expanding perirenal haematoma confined to Gerota fascia. Grade III is a laceration >1 cm, again without a urine leak or a vascular injury contained within Gerota fascia.

Current guidance (2018) suggests to advance one grade for bilateral injuries up to Grade III. Surgical management is considered for Grades III and above.

(The Final FRCR Complete Revision Notes Page 251)

The American Association for the Surgery of Trauma. 2018 revision. AAST Kidney Injury Scale. Table 8. https://www.aast.org/library/traumatools/injuryscoringscales.aspx#kidney

101 (e) Proximal oesophageal atresia with distal fistula

Tracheo-oesophageal fistula and oesophageal atresia are associated with other VACTERL anomalies. The typical finding which indicates this problem is a coiled nasogastric tube on a chest radiograph. The most frequent type (85% of cases) is Type C which is proximal oesophageal atresia with a distal tracheo-oesophageal fistula. The second most common type is Type A which is isolated oesophageal atresia. The three other types are rare. The finding of gas in the stomach suggests the presence of a distal fistula or an 'H-type' fistula where there is no oesophageal atresia.

(The Final FRCR Complete Revision Notes Page 346)

102 (c) *Mycobacterium tuberculosis*

The distribution of findings is typical for tuberculous meningitis. It typically affects the basal cisterns with leptomeningeal enhancement and purulent material in the basal cisterns which can lead to hydrocephalus, the early signs of which are evident in this case. There is also the potential for cranial nerve palsies, particularly the third, fourth, and sixth nerves. The patient in this case has a right third nerve palsy.

A differential with a similar distribution of changes is neurosarcoidosis. Neurosarcoidosis most commonly causes parenchymal changes but it can cause leptomeningeal enhancement and cranial nerve palsies, particularly the facial and optic nerves. Fever also makes an infective cause more likely in this case. Serum angiotensin converting enzyme is frequently raised in sarcoidosis.

Streptococcus pneumoniae is one of the most common causes of bacterial meningitis in adults. CT imaging is often normal and lumbar puncture should be considered if clinical suspicion is high. Imaging can be helpful in complicated cases when there is development of hydrocephalus, abscess or subdural effusion. Thin, generalised leptomeningeal enhancement may be seen rather than the thickened basal enhancement in this case.

Group B streptococcus is the most common cause of meningitis in neonates and therefore does not fit with the patient in this case.

Viral meningitis is often self limiting and not associated with reduced conscious level or cranial nerve palsies. It most commonly affects children or immunocompromised adults.

(The Final FRCR Complete Revision Notes Page 410)

103 (d) Polyarteritis nodosa

Polyarteritis nodosa is a vasculitic process affecting small and medium sized arteries causing stenoses and aneurysmal dilatation. This most commonly affects the kidneys but can also affect other solid abdominal organs as well as the gastrointestinal tract, CNS and heart. Males are affected more commonly. It can present with non-specific symptoms such as fever, weight loss and malaise but also more acutely with bleeding and infarct.

Behçet's disease affects both arteries and veins. The classical presentation includes a triad of ocular inflammation along with oral and genital ulceration. The central nervous system and cardiorespiratory and gastrointestinal systems can also be involved.

Fibromuscular dysplasia also typically affects the kidneys but affects medium and small vessels causing arterial stenoses, along with intervening dilated segments creating the typical 'string of beads' appearance. It can be asymptomatic or present with refractory hypertension.

Goodpasture syndrome is characterised by pulmonary haemorrhage and glomerulonephritis. Patients usually present due to the pulmonary manifestations.

Takayasu disease is a large vessel arteritis causing stenosis, aneurysmal dilatation and potentially occlusion.

(The Final FRCR Complete Revision Notes Page 13)

104 (b) Incompletely ossified sternum

Cleidocranial dysostosis is associated with completely absent clavicles or absence of the lateral portion of them. There is delayed ossification of midline structures causing delayed skull suture closure, enlarged fontanelle and an incompletely ossified sternum. The pubic symphysis may appear widened due to delayed or absent ossification of the pubic bone. Small, high scapulae, supernumerary ribs and a narrowed thorax are also features. There may be hemivertebrae and hypoplasia of the iliac bones. Other bones may be short or absent, such as the radius, fibula and terminal phalanges. Wormian bones and dental abnormalities are also features.

Decreasing interpedicular distance is associated with achondroplasia and thanatophoric dysplasia. Pectus excavatum is associated with various conditions including Marfan syndrome, Ehlers-Danlos, neurofibromatosis 1 and osteogenesis imperfecta. Platyspondyly is a feature of Morquio syndrome, osteogenesis imperfecta and thanatophoric dysplasia. Shortened horizontally orientated ribs are associated with asphyxiating thoracic dysplasia.

(The Final FRCR Complete Revision Notes Page 107)

105 (b) Increased rupture risk is associated with cirrhosis

Splenic artery aneurysms are often incidental findings and associated with atherosclerosis, cirrhosis, portal hypertension, infection, pregnancy, trauma and pancreatitis. In the latter two cases, the aneurysms are pseudoaneurysms rather than true aneurysms. Treatment should be considered above 1.5 cm in diameter and imaging follow-up is required for smaller aneurysms. Factors which increase the risk of bleeding and warrant intervention include rapidly increasing size, pregnancy and symptomatic aneurysms.

(The Final FRCR Complete Revision Notes Page 240)

Khosa F, Krinsky G, Macari M et al. Managing incidental findings on abdominal and pelvic CT and MRI, Part 2: White paper of the ACR Incidental Findings Committee II on vascular findings. Journal of the American College of Radiology. 2013;10(10):789–794.

106 (b) Axial proton density fat saturation

Chondromalacia patellae is caused by patella cartilage degeneration leading to knee pain, often in young women, which is exacerbated by certain movements such as squatting, kneeling or climbing stairs.

Knee radiograph may demonstrate degenerative changes or effusion, but is often normal.

MRI is the best modality to assess for the condition; for assessing cartilage either T2 or proton density fat saturation sequences are most helpful. Focal increased signal in the cartilage along with cartilage irregularity is abnormal. T1 weighted sequences may show low signal in the adjacent patella if there is marrow oedema.

STIR imaging is best for assessing inflammatory changes such as occult fracture, marrow oedema and soft tissue inflammation.

Post gadolinium sequences can be helpful when assessing the synovium.

(The Final FRCR Complete Revision Notes Pages 70, 84)

107 (e) Ventricular septal defect

The child has a number of VACTERL associations which include Vertebral anomalies, Anorectal malformations, Cardiac defects, Tracheo-oesphageal fistula, Renal and Limb anomalies. Usually three are required to fulfil the diagnostic criteria. Vertebral anomalies may be picked up incidentally on radiographs and therefore careful assessment is necessary. The most common cardiac anomaly is a ventricular septal defect followed by an atrial septal defect.

(The Final FRCR Complete Revision Notes Page 332)

108 (a) T2*

Cavernomas are venous malformations with a low risk of haemorrhage and therefore many are incidental lesions. However, when symptomatic they can present with headaches and seizures. T2* or gradient echo are the best sequences to help diagnose cavernomas as they demonstrate blooming or susceptibility artefact. On T1 post contrast they can have a 'popcorn'

appearance with central enhancement. On T2 weighted imaging they show peripheral low signal intensity due to haemosiderin deposition.
(The Final FRCR Complete Revision Notes Page 367)

109 (d) Primary ciliary dyskinesia
Kartagener syndrome is a type of primary ciliary dyskinesia, typically consisting of a triad of dextrocardia, bronchiectasis and sinusitis. It has an autosomal recessive mode of inheritance. It is also associated with infertility in males, reduced fertility in females, transposition of the great vessels, pyloric stenosis, post-cricoid web and epispadias. The patient has presented with pneumonia which is caused by ciliary dysfunction and can be a recurrent problem in patients with this condition.
Post infective bronchiectasis is the most common acquired cause of bronchiectasis, including allergic bronchopulmonary aspergillosis (ABPA).
Recurrent aspiration and immunodeficiency such as hypogammaglobulinaemia also cause bronchiectasis, but are not associated with dextrocardia.
Cystic fibrosis is the most common congenital cause of bronchiectasis.
(The Final FRCR Complete Revision Notes Page 39)

110 (a) Adductor magnus
The ischial tuberosity is the origin of the hamstring muscles. These include biceps femoris, semimembranosus and semitendinosus. The 'hamstring portion' of the adductor magnus muscle also arises from this site.
Avulsion fractures are more common in children due to their immature skeleton, and appearances may be subtle with just small bone flakes visible on close inspection.
Avulsion fracture sites of the other tendons around the pelvis and proximal femora are listed below.

Gracilis – inferior pubic ramus
Iliopsoas – lesser trochanter of the femur
Rectus femoris – anterior inferior iliac spine
Tensor fascia lata – anterior superior iliac spine
Sartorius – anterior superior iliac spine
(The Final FRCR Complete Revision Notes Page 104)

111 (e) Organo-axial gastric volvulus
The vomiting, abdominal pain, retrocardiac air-fluid level, inability to pass a nasogastric tube and raised lactate is consistent with gastric volvulus. The elevated lactate is concerning for ischaemia. Organo-axial gastric volvulus is more common in adults and often associated with a diaphragmatic defect, sometimes following trauma or with a para-oesophageal (rolling) hiatus hernia. The previous chest radiograph demonstrating an air-fluid level is suggestive of this. This type of volvulus can be chronic and asymptomatic; however, the appearance of the air-fluid level increasing and its position, along with the other clinical symptoms and signs, suggests that the stomach has volved and become trapped above the diaphragm.
Mesentero-axial gastric volvulus is more common in children and also more frequently associated with vascular compromise due to twisting of the mesentery.
Epiphrenic diverticulum can occur secondary to conditions with oesophageal dysmotility and raised oesophageal pressure, such as achalasia. The presentation in this case is not typical as they often present with dysphagia and regurgitation.
This patient does likely have a hiatus hernia and subsequent aspiration pneumonia could cause raised inflammatory markers and a raised lactate; however, this would not account for the abdominal pain, vomiting and inability to pass a nasogastric tube.
A lung abscess is a differential for an air-fluid level in the thorax; however the other features in this case are not typical.
(The Final FRCR Complete Revision Notes Page 171)

112 (d) Papillary carcinoma
The mass has imaging features of papillary carcinoma of the kidney which is the second most common malignant renal tumour following the clear cell subtype. Papillary tumours are often hypovascular and poorly enhancing, hence the minimal change in density following contrast administration during the CT. The MRI findings of homogenous hypointensity on T1

and T2 weighted images are also consistent with this diagnosis.

Clear cell carcinomas are usually T2 hyperintense; they enhance more and can be more heterogenous in appearance. Similarly, oncocytomas are usually heterogenous and can also demonstrate a central scar and pseudocapsule.

Renal lymphoma frequently causes multiple masses and diffuse renal infiltration rather than a discrete mass. Like papillary carcinoma it can be poorly enhancing; however it is usually T1 hypointense and T2 iso- or hyperintense.

A haemorrhagic renal cyst would typically be T1 hyperintense and T2 hypointense. An uncomplicated cyst would not enhance and, in contrast to the lesion in this case, it would not demonstrate restricted diffusion. Layering of debris may be seen within a haemorrhagic cyst.

(The Final FRCR Complete Revision Notes Page 258)

113 (b) MRI whole spine

The imaging appearances are characteristic of a medulloblastoma with a posterior fossa mass which is hyperdense on CT and demonstrates restricted diffusion on MRI. The demographics are also typical (age <5 and male). Fifty percent of patients with medulloblastoma will have leptomeningeal metastases at presentation. Therefore, whole spine imaging is recommended as part of the workup.

(The Final FRCR Complete Revision Notes Page 393)

114 (c) Pseudotumour

Pseudotumours most commonly involve the lacrimal glands but can involve the extraocular muscles, commonly the lateral rectus muscle. They involve the whole muscle including the tendon, whereas thyroid ophthalmopathy spares the tendon.

Pseudotumours are iso- to hypointense on T1 imaging and hypointense on T2 imaging whereas true tumours, such as lymphoma, are usually T2 hyperintense. Lymphoma also tends to be painless, in contrast to the presentation in this case.

Metastases are often extraconal but can infiltrate into the intraconal region. They are not usually centred on the extraocular muscles and would also usually be T2 hyperintense.

Rhabdomyosarcoma originates from the extraocular muscles but is usually a paediatric tumour, is usually T2 hyperintense and due to its aggressive nature may be associated with adjacent bone destruction.

(The Final FRCR Complete Revision Notes Page 439)

115 (a) Artery of Adamkiewicz

The distribution of neurological symptoms suggests an anterior spinal cord infarct. The artery of Adamkiewicz can have a variable origin usually arising between T9 and L2. It is the dominant arterial supply to the lumbosacral cord segments. Occlusion of this artery should be considered in patients with sudden onset chest pain caused by aortic dissection and evolving neurological symptoms. It can also be damaged during spinal surgery or abdominal aortic aneurysm repair.

The artery of Percheron is variant anatomy of the posterior cerebral circulation which is characterised by a single artery arising from the posterior cerebral artery supplying the bilateral thalami and midbrain.

The posterior spinal arteries are paired arteries arising from the vertebral or posterior inferior cerebellar arteries and they supply the posterior columns of the spinal cord. Occlusion of these arteries can lead to contralateral loss of vibration, proprioception and two-point discrimination.

The recurrent artery of Heubner is also known as the medial striate artery and can be seen on angiography as the largest perforating branch of the anterior cerebral artery, arising from the A1 or A2 segments.

(The Final FRCR Complete Revision Notes Page 3)

116 (a) Faecal calprotectin levels

The question describes bilateral symmetrical sacroiliitis with syndesmophytes which are also symmetrical and marginal. The differentials for bilateral symmetrical sacroiliitis include ankylosing spondylitis, inflammatory bowel disease and rheumatoid arthritis. Hyperparathyroidism can also mimic these appearances.

With regard to syndesmophyte formation, they tend to either be non-marginal and asymmetric;

for example in psoriatic and reactive arthritis, or marginal and symmetrical; for example in ankylosing spondylitis and inflammatory bowel disease.

Therefore, the likely answers for this question would either be ankylosing spondylitis or inflammatory bowel disease. Ankylosing spondylitis is more common in males and you would expect other associated changes on radiographs of the spine. Therefore, inflammatory bowel disease is most likely to be the underlying diagnosis. Faecal calprotectin levels are commonly used in the diagnosis of inflammatory bowel disease.

Anti-CCP levels are more sensitive and specific than rheumatoid factor (RF) in the diagnosis of rheumatoid arthritis. HLA B27 is associated with the RF seronegative arthropathies including ankylosing spondylitis and psoriatic arthritis. Parathyroid hormone levels could be investigated in suspected hyperparathyroidism, and punch skin biopsy is sometimes used to help diagnose psoriasis.

(The Final FRCR Complete Revision Notes Pages 63 and 91–93)

117 (d) Long axis of the distended loops arises from the right lower quadrant

Differentiating sigmoid from caecal volvulus on plain abdominal radiograph can be challenging. However, it is important to distinguish between the two as the management can differ greatly. Typically caecal volvulus occurs in younger patients (30–60 years) than sigmoid volvulus. Radiographs shows marked caecal distension, preservation of haustral markings and the distended loop arises from the right lower quadrant and usually extends towards the left upper quadrant. Sometimes the caecum can twist axially and remain in the right lower quadrant.

In contrast to this, the bowel wall in sigmoid volvulus is ahaustral and the bowel loop has a different position; it arises from the pelvis extending cranially towards the left hemidiaphragm. The apex of the loop can sometimes reach the level of the thoracic spine and overlaps the hepatic border. It has been described as a 'coffee bean' appearance.

(The Final FRCR Complete Revision Notes Page 188)

118 (b) Maximum pressure generated of 120 mmHg within the colon

Pneumatic reduction of intussusception is attempted to try and avoid the need for surgery; however, recurrence and procedural failure is possible. Most cases of recurrence reoccur within 72 hours. Contraindications include peritonitis, pneumoperitoneum and hypovolaemic shock. Children should be fluid resuscitated prior to attempting the procedure and a member of the surgical team should be present. The risks, as mentioned previously, are failure and recurrence as well as perforation. Pneumatic reduction is more likely to be successful if there is a shorter duration of symptoms (<24 hours) but longer than this is not a contraindication.

Three attempts can be made, with three minutes between each attempt. The maximum pressure within the colon should not exceed 120 mmHg.

(The Final FRCR Complete Revision Notes Pages 341, 342)

119 (e) Posterior midline diverticulum proximal to cricopharyngeus

A pharyngeal pouch, otherwise known as a Zenker's diverticulum, originates from the midline posteriorly above the level of cricopharyngeus. This is more common and more likely to be symptomatic than a Killian-Jamieson diverticulum which arises more laterally, often on the left side, and below cricopharyngeus. These are both examples of 'false' diverticula because the outpouching does not contain all layers of the oesophageal wall but is mucosa protruding through a muscular defect.

A pulsion diverticulum is most commonly seen in the distal oesophagus and is associated with high pressures, for example in diffuse oesophageal spasm. The diverticulum may be present along with a 'corkscrew oesophagus' appearance.

(The Final FRCR Complete Revision Notes Page 164)

120 (d) Contrast enhancement extending into the sulci

Both lepto and pachymeningeal metastases are possible in breast cancer. Pachymeningeal disease is durally based and may be secondary to adjacent skull lesions or via lymphatic or haematogenous spread. The dura appears thickened around the brain in a curvilinear distribution and enhances following contrast.

Leptomeningeal disease is characterised by fine nodular post contrast enhancement of the

surface of the brain which, unlike pachymeningeal disease, extends into the sulci. Signal abnormality may also be evident on FLAIR and DWI/ADC sequences. It is sometimes described as having a 'sugar coated' 'sugar-coated' appearance. It can be secondary to primary intracranial malignancies or secondary to haematogenous spread from primary cancers such as breast or lung. Parenchymal brain lesions are not a feature of either pachymeningeal or leptomeningeal diseasedisease; however, there may be associated adjacent cerebral oedema.
(The Final FRCR Complete Revision Notes Page 394)

PAPER 2

1. An athletic 28 year old man presents with intermittent claudication affecting the right leg particularly when running or playing sports. Examination is normal with present lower limb pulses. The vascular team query popliteal artery entrapment syndrome and request further imaging to evaluate further and help plan surgical management.

   What would be the most appropriate test?

   a. Angiography
   b. AP and lateral right knee radiographs
   c. Arterial phase CT
   d. MRI
   e. Ultrasound

2. A 49 year old dialysis patient is referred to the rheumatology clinic with back and joint pain involving bilateral shoulders and hips. Radiographs of the hips and shoulders demonstrate erosions and subchondral cyst formation. Joint space is well preserved. An MRI spine reveals normal alignment. There is a low T1 and T2 signal lesion at the inferior endplate of the L3 vertebral body adjacent to the L3/4 disc. This lesion enhances following contrast. The L3/4 disc returns normal MRI signal. Similar low signal intra-articular nodules are seen on MRI of the right shoulder.

   Which finding would indicate the most appropriate diagnosis?

   a. Congo red staining of synovial fluid
   b. Cartilage pigmentation on arthroscopy
   c. Growth of *Staphylococcus aureus* on blood culture
   d. Serum parathyroid hormone levels
   e. Weakly positive birefringent crystals on polarised light microscopy of synovial fluid

3. A 60 year old female with a recent diagnosis of scleroderma presents with dysphagia to both solids and liquids. A barium swallow is performed.

   What is the most likely radiological finding?

   a. Improvement of the flow of barium following the ingestion of warm fluid
   b. Narrowing of the distal oesophagus
   c. Aperistalsis of the lower oesophagus
   d. Oesophageal diverticulum
   e. Mucosal ulceration

4. A 23 year old cyclist is on the Intensive Care Unit following a road traffic collision. Thirty-six hours previously he was knocked off his bike by a car at approximately 20 mph. Initial admission CT demonstrated a right subcapsular renal haematoma.

   The team call you for an ultrasound urinary tract, including Doppler assessment, due to uncontrollable hypertension and increasing right flank pain which has developed over the past 4 hours. Ultrasound shows an unobstructed right kidney with a substantial right subcapsular collection. There is vascularity within the kidney and the arterial trace shows forward flow in diastole with a resistive index of 0.9. Appearances of the left kidney and bladder are within normal limits.

   What is the most likely diagnosis?

   a. Page kidney
   b. Pseudoaneurysm
   c. Renal artery stenosis
   d. Renal vein thrombosis
   e. Ureteric obstruction

5. A 3 year old child is seen with a painless right upper quadrant mass which can be balloted. An ultrasound confirms a heterogenous right upper quadrant lesion with cystic and solid components measuring up to 10 cm centred on the right kidney.

   What is the most likely diagnosis?

   a. Mesoblastic nephroma
   b. Multilocular cystic nephroma

c. Nephroblastoma
d. Neuroblastoma
e. Rhabdoid tumour

6. A 35 year old man was assaulted several months previously, experiencing head trauma. He now presents with reduced visual acuity in his left eye and also describes pulsatile exophthalmos. An MRI of the orbits is performed.

   What is the most likely finding?

   a. Orbital mass
   b. Dilated superior ophthalmic vein
   c. Thrombosis of the cavernous sinus
   d. Optic nerve enlargement
   e. Aneurysm of the ophthalmic artery

7. A 55 year old man reviewed in the Infection and Immunity clinic has marked cachexia and is generally unwell. He is known to have HIV and has poor compliance with antiretrovirals; his CD4 count is 154 cells/mm^3 (500–1400 cells/mm^3). A chest radiograph is abnormal, and the patient is referred for a CT chest abdomen pelvis to investigate further. CT reveals multiple perihilar and peribronchovascular ill-defined nodular opacities with surrounding ground glass opacification and marked bilateral enhancing hilar lymph node enlargement. The abdomen and pelvis are normal. He is considered too unwell for a bronchoscopy and so you suggest a gallium scan to aid diagnosis. The thoracic abnormalities are not tracer avid.

   Which diagnosis is most consistent with the above clinical information?

   a. Cytomegalovirus
   b. Kaposi sarcoma
   c. Lymphoma
   d. *Mycobacterium avium*
   e. *Pneumocystis* pneumonia

8. A 55 year old female rheumatology clinic patient is sent for hand radiographs. These show distal phalangeal cortical irregularity and widening of the joint spaces with marginal erosions at the middle and distal interphalangeal joints. Adjacent soft tissue swelling is also demonstrated and there is periosteal reaction along the diaphyses of some of the middle phalanges. The metacarpal phalangeal joints have normal appearances. Bone density is well preserved. You also note the patient is awaiting radiographs of the right shoulder and left knee due to pain and swelling.

   What is the most likely diagnosis?

   a. Erosive osteoarthritis
   b. Gout
   c. Psoriatic arthritis
   d. Reactive arthritis
   e. Rheumatoid arthritis

9. A 28 year old female patient with frequent abdominal discomfort, diarrhoea and weight loss has a positive faecal calprotectin test. Following a recent exacerbation of symptoms, an MRI abdomen is performed which demonstrates multiple radiological features of Crohn's disease.

   Which MRI sequence is most helpful in identifying fistulae?

   a. T1 weighted sequence
   b. T2 weighted sequence
   c. Fat supressed T1 weighted sequence
   d. Fat supressed T2 weighted sequence
   e. Diffusion weighted imaging

10. A 44 year old female patient with hereditary spastic paraplegia is unable to tolerate a transvaginal ultrasound and has an MRI pelvis for intermenstrual bleeding. On the most inferior slices a lesion is seen adjacent to the proximal right femur. The patient denies any pain in this area. The duty radiologist suggests extending the MRI imaging to include the entire

area of abnormality. The mass is approximately 50 mm, with very low peripheral T1 and T2 signal. Centrally the T1 signal is isointense to muscle and T2 signal is heterogenous. On STIR sequences there is marked peripheral hyperintensity in the surrounding muscle.

Which test is most likely to confirm benignity?

a. CT angiogram of the lower limb
b. Nuclear medicine bone scan
c. Radiograph of the proximal femur
d. Ultrasound guided biopsy
e. Post contrast MRI sequence

11. A neonate with dyspnoea has a chest radiograph which demonstrates a large lower zone opacity. An MRI scan helps confirm a congenital diaphragmatic hernia containing abdominal fat and viscera.

Where is the diaphragmatic defect most likely to be?

a. Left posterolateral
b. Left posteromedial
c. Right anterolateral
d. Right anteromedial
e. Right posterolateral

12. A day 2 postpartum woman in Intensive Care has a CT brain followed by an MRI brain after she was neurologically inappropriate during a sedation hold. The patient experienced a period of hypertension secondary to pre-eclampsia which has now resolved. Clinically the differential lies between posterior reversible encephalopathy syndrome (PRES) and a posterior circulation infarct.

Which of the following would be most consistent with the finding of an acute posterior cerebral artery territory infarct rather than PRES?

a. Low density on CT
b. Microhaemorrhage
c. Occipital lobe distribution
d. Restricted diffusion
e. T2 hyperintensity

13. A 55 year old male patient of average weight with a 15 year pack year smoking history has an incidental finding of a nodule on a chest radiograph. CT confirms a 17-mm right middle lobe lung nodule and MDT discussion suggests CT guided lung biopsy. On the day the patient is positioned, the skin is cleaned and 10 mL 1% lidocaine is injected into the skin and soft tissues; however the patient continues to experience discomfort and requests more local anaesthetic.

What is the maximum additional volume of 1% lidocaine you can safely administer to this patient?

a. 0 mL
b. 5 mL
c. 10 mL
d. 15 mL
e. 25 mL

14. A 10 year old boy's spinal radiograph demonstrates posterior vertebral body scalloping, beaking of the vertebral bodies at the anteroinferior corners and shortened pedicles with a decreased interpedicular distance.

Which of the following underlying congenital skeletal anomalies is consistent with these findings?

a. Achondroplasia
b. Asphyxiating thoracic dysplasia
c. Hurler syndrome
d. Morquio syndrome
e. Thanatophoric dysplasia

15. A 33 year old woman has an abdominal ultrasound for investigation of non-specific abdominal pain. The spleen is normal in size but there is a hyperechoic 3-cm nodule within it. The patient goes on to have a MRI abdomen. The nodule shows low T1 and high T2 signal. Following contrast administration there is peripheral enhancement on arterial phase imaging. Delayed images show progressive central enhancement of the nodule.

    What is the most likely diagnosis?

    a. Metastasis
    b. Lymphoma
    c. Abscess
    d. Sarcoidosis
    e. Haemangioma

16. A CT aorta in an emergency department patient with hypertension and abdominal pain describes an indeterminate adrenal lesion. An MRI adrenals is requested and the lesion demonstrates characteristic features of a phaechromocytoma.

    Which of the following radiological features fits with this diagnosis?

Table 2.1:

	T1 Signal	T2 Signal	Enhancement	Out-of-Phase Sequence
a	Hypointense	Hyperintense	Avid	Signal loss
b	Hypointense	Hyperintense	Minimal	Signal loss
c	Hyperintense	Hypointense	Avid	No signal loss
d	Hyperintense	Hyperintense	Minimal	No signal loss
e	Hypointense	Hyperintense	Avid	No signal loss

17. A neonate is diagnosed with pyloric stenosis following presentation with vomiting. This is confirmed following an upper gastrointestinal (GI) fluoroscopic study and ultrasound scan.

    Which of the following radiological findings correlates with this diagnosis?

    a. Corkscrew appearance on upper GI contrast study
    b. Muscle wall thickness of 2 mm on ultrasound
    c. Pyloric canal length of 15 mm on ultrasound
    d. Pyloric transverse diameter of 10 mm on ultrasound
    e. Pyloric volume of 1.6 cm^3 on ultrasound

18. A 36 year old woman presents with sudden onset headache and visual disturbance. On examination she is found to have bilateral homonymous hemianopia and left third cranial nerve palsy. A diagnosis of pituitary apoplexy is suspected.

    Regarding imaging in suspected pituitary apoplexy, which of the following statements is most accurate?

    a. CT is sensitive for the diagnosis
    b. High T1 signal helps differentiate it from other pituitary masses
    c. Macroscopic haemorrhage is uncommon
    d. The pituitary gland rarely demonstrates restricted diffusion on MRI
    e. The pituitary gland usually shows peripheral enhancement

19. A 45 year old male is under investigation for haematuria and proteinuria. He also has episodes of chest pain, shortness of breath and new haemoptysis. The renal team perform a renal biopsy which shows focal glomerulonephritis and a serologic cytoplasmic ANCA test is positive. A CT chest has features supportive of the diagnosis.

    Which of the following findings is most commonly seen on CT chest in this condition?

    a. Airway wall thickening
    b. Increased mediastinal or hilar lymph node enlargement

c. Nodules with cavitation
d. Nodules without consolidation
e. Pleural effusion

20. A 73 year old man trips on ice and both hands go through a glass door pane. He attends the emergency department with bruising, swelling and lacerations of both hands. Radiographs confirm soft tissue swelling, no radiopaque foreign body and no acute fracture. There is periosteal reaction noted at the metadiaphyseal regions of the metacarpals and phalanges bilaterally.

    What would be the most appropriate next step?

    a. Chest radiograph
    b. Echocardiogram
    c. Liver ultrasound
    d. Nuclear medicine bone scan
    e. Radiograph of both wrists

21. A 55 year old female patient presents with a short history of abdominal pain, vomiting and a distended abdomen. A contrast enhanced CT abdomen pelvis confirms small bowel obstruction secondary to intussusception. The patient undergoes laparotomy which identifies a polypoid lesion as the lead point. Note is made of multiple other polypoid lesions in the small bowel and areas of darker skin on her fingers and toes. The patient reports a positive family history for an underlying genetic condition with her sister, brother and father also affected. Her sister is currently undergoing treatment for cervical adenoma malignum.

    What is the most likely underlying diagnosis?

    a. Carney complex
    b. Cowden syndrome
    c. Cronkhite-Canada syndrome
    d. Neurofibromatosis 1
    e. Peutz-Jeghers syndrome

22. The clinical team come to discuss the case of a neonate with you who had abnormal antenatal scans showing an anterior abdominal wall defect. The patient has been diagnosed with Turner syndrome.

    Which of the following group of features is most likely associated with the anterior abdominal wall defect?

Table 2.2:

	Position of Defect	Peritoneal Covering	Herniated Liver	Associated Bowel Complications
a	Midline	Absent	Yes	Yes
b	Midline	Present	Yes	No
c	Midline	Present	No	Yes
d	Right paramedian	Absent	No	No
e	Right paramedian	Present	Yes	No

23. A 62 year old woman, with known gallstones, presents to the emergency department with abdominal pain and vomiting. An abdominal radiograph is performed which shows bowel obstruction, pneumobilia and a densely calcified abdominal mass. The doctors suspect the patient has gallstone ileus.

    What is the most likely site of bowel obstruction?

    a. D2
    b. Proximal ileum
    c. Caecum

d. Terminal ileum
e. Sigmoid colon

24. An MRI is performed for an Ear, Nose and Throat clinic patient with right haemotypanum and conductive hearing loss. There is a well-defined mass in the right middle ear without evidence of adjacent bone involvement. This is predominantly high signal on T1 and T2 weighted sequences with a rim of peripheral low signal. Hyperintensity is maintained on a fat supressed sequence. There is mild peripheral enhancement but no restricted diffusion.

What is the most likely underlying cause?

a. Cholesterol granuloma
b. Cholesteatoma
c. Chondrosarcoma
d. Glomus tympanicum
e. Mucocoele

25. A 28 year old female non-smoker presents to the emergency department with acute onset shortness of breath and left sided chest pain. She had a chest radiograph which demonstrates a left sided pneumothorax. The acute medical team site a chest drain and she undergoes a high resolution CT chest. The CT shows the drain sited appropriately with almost complete resolution of the pneumothorax. Within the lungs there are multiple, bilateral thin-walled cysts. These are uniform in size, distributed in all zones and have normal intervening lung parenchyma.

What is the most likely underlying diagnosis?

a. Birt-Hogg-Dubé syndrome
b. Lymphocytic interstitial pneumonia
c. *Pneumocystis jiroveci*infection
d. Pulmonary Langerhans cell histiocytosis
e. Tuberous sclerosis

26. A 42 year old female patient without significant past medical history presents to her GP with a 3 week history of feeling increasingly tired and feverish with generalised aches and pains. On examination, the chest is clear and the abdomen is soft and non-tender. The GP notes characteristic tender swollen red patches on both her lower limbs. A chest radiograph is requested and reports bilateral prominent hila but the lungs are clear.

Which diagnosis is most appropriate?

a. Chronic lymphocytic leukaemia
b. Löffler syndrome
c. Löfgren syndrome
d. Sapho syndrome
e. Sever disease

27. A contrast enhanced CT abdomen and pelvis is performed for a 49 year old female patient with abdominal pain. Previous medical history includes smoking, hypertension, type 2 diabetes and a community acquired pneumonia which was treated by the GP 2 weeks previously. The CT identifies bowel wall thickening and hyperenhancement along with pericolic fat stranding and a small amount of free fluid. These changes affect the entire colon and rectum.

Which radiological feature is more suggestive of inflammatory bowel disease rather than pseudomembranous colitis?

a. Bowel wall thickening
b. Free fluid
c. Mucosal hyperenhancement
d. Pericolic fat stranding
e. Rectal involvement

28. A 53 year old female patient has a contrast enhanced CT abdomen pelvis for non-specific abdominal pain. This identifies multiple small, ill-defined, bilateral renal lesions which are hyperdense to the adjacent renal parenchyma. The kidneys are unobstructed. You also report an ill-defined 16 mm splenic lesion and 12 mm short axis retrocrural and retroperitoneal

lymph node enlargement. The other solid abdominal viscera are within normal limits. The imaged lung bases demonstrate multiple pulmonary nodules.

What is the most likely primary malignancy?

a. Breast
b. Lung
c. Lymphoma
d. Melanoma
e. Gastrointestinal tract

29. The neonatal intensive care unit request a written report for a radiograph of a baby who has just undergone endotracheal intubation.

When reviewing the position of the endotracheal tube, which of the following statements is correct?

a. The tube tip should be projected approximately 1.5 cm distal to the carina
b. The tube tip should be projected approximately 1.5 cm proximal to the carina
c. The tube tip should be projected approximately 3 cm proximal to the carina
d. The tube tip should be projected around the level of T4
e. The tube tip should be projected at the level of the superior clavicular line

30. A 10 year old boy presents with a sudden reduction in GCS following a week-long history of headaches, nausea and vomiting. A CT head shows hydrocephalus and a large cystic mass in the posterior fossa. An MRI brain is performed. This demonstrates a well-defined cystic mass arising from the cerebellum. There is also a small solid component which is isointense on T1 weighted imaging and hyperintense to the adjacent cerebellum on T2 weighted imaging. It shows avid contrast enhancement on T1 post contrast.

Which diagnosis is most consistent with this description?

a. Cerebellar abscess
b. Ependymoma
c. Medulloblastoma
d. Pilocytic astrocytoma
e. Pleomorphic xanthoastrocytoma

31. A 52 year old male patient presents with symptoms of shortness of breath and pedal oedema. Echocardiogram shows reduced contractility and ejection fraction. The only previous imaging is a radiograph of the left hand 2 years previously. This was performed for trauma and did not show a fracture but did report osteopenia and chondrocalcinosis, as well as osteophytes. The cardiac MRI demonstrates reduced myocardial signal intensity. You notice on the MRI scout images that the liver has an irregular contour.

What is the most likely diagnosis?

a. Amyloidosis
b. Alcohol related dilated cardiomyopathy
c. Haemochromatosis
d. Haemosiderosis
e. Sarcoidosis

32. A 56 year old male patient has 6 months of increasing thoracic back pain. A lumbar spine radiograph performed at first presentation was normal. A more recent MRI lumbar spine shows vertebral body collapse at T12. Marrow signal at T12 is hypointense to the intervertebral disc on T1 and T2 weighted images with no hyperintensity on the STIR sequence.

Which other feature would most appropriately correlate with these findings?

a. Convex margin of the posterior vertebral body
b. Post-contrast enhancement in the vertebral body
c. Multiple further fractures
d. Retropulsion of bone fragments
e. Vacuum phenomenon of the intervertebral disc

33. A 56 year old man with a background of hepatitis C undergoes a routine surveillance liver ultrasound. There is a 3-cm hyperechoic lesion in segment VI of the liver. A CT liver is performed. The lesion is arterially enhancing with rapid contrast washout. The case is discussed at the regional hepatocellular carcinoma MDT meeting.

    Which of the following statements are true regarding the management of hepatocellular carcinoma?

    a. Transarterial chemoembolisation (TACE) is a curative treatment option
    b. TACE and thermal ablation cannot be used together
    c. TACE is indicated in Child-Pugh score C and D patients
    d. TACE may be used for large, unresectable tumours
    e. Thermal ablation is a curative treatment option

34. Antenatal scans for a 3 day old baby demonstrated polyhydramnios. A chest radiograph following a difficult insertion of a nasogastric tube depicts a coiled tube projected over the mediastinum. The patient has surgical management for oesophageal atresia. A subsequent upper gastrointestinal water soluble contrast study demonstrates a good result but reveals a short narrowing of the duodenum at D2. There are normal calibre gas-filled distal small and large bowel loops. A couple of hemivertebrae are noted.

    What is the most likely cause?

    a. Annular pancreas
    b. Duodenal atresia
    c. Duodenal diverticulum
    d. Duodenal web
    e. Pancreas divisum

35. An MRI brain has been performed for a 32 year old neurology outpatient with worsening parkinsonism and ataxia. A recent CT brain found no focal abnormality. The MRI demonstrates T2 hyperintensity in the caudate nuclei, lateral thalami, putamina and tegmentum with sparing of the red nuclei and substantia nigra.

    What is the most likely diagnosis?

    a. Haemochromatosis
    b. Menke's disease
    c. Pantothenate kinase-associated neurodegeneration
    d. Creutzfeldt-Jakob disease
    e. Wilson disease

36. A chest radiograph for a febrile 6 year old child with a cough demonstrates left lower lobe air space opacification with air bronchograms. There is no evidence of cavitation or significant volume loss and no pleural effusion. The right lung is clear. Heart size is normal.

    What is the most likely causative organism?

    a. Group B streptococcus
    b. *Haemophilus influenzae*
    c. *Klebsiella*
    d. *Listeria*
    e. *Pneumococcus*

37. A 42 year old male patient presents to the urgent care centre with a 2 month history of increasing shortness of breath on exertion. His past medical history includes scoliosis and an episode of spontaneous pneumothorax 20 years previously. Chest radiograph is in keeping with pectus excavatum but is otherwise normal with no pneumothorax. An echocardiogram reports reduced ejection fraction and an aortic root diameter of 57 mm.

    What is the most likely unifying diagnosis?

    a. Beals syndrome
    b. Homocystinuria
    c. Loeys-Dietz syndrome

d. Marfan syndrome
e. Multiple endocrine neoplasia

38. A 72 year old male patient presents to the emergency department with facial bruising and swelling. Radiographs of his facial bones reveal a fracture of the nasal bone and soft tissue swelling. You also notice a couple of lucent areas in the partially imaged skull which are well-defined without surrounding sclerosis. In his right proximal ulna there is bony expansion and a lytic lesion extending along the cortex. Subsequent nuclear medicine bone scan reveals tracer uptake in all these regions, particularly peripherally in the skull lesions. There is also diffuse uptake throughout the L3 vertebral body.

What is the most likely underlying diagnosis?

a. Fibrous dysplasia
b. Langerhans cell histiocytosis
c. Myeloma
d. Metastatic disease
e. Paget's disease

39. A 32 year old woman complains of right upper quadrant pain. Ultrasound demonstrates a well-defined solitary lesion in the right lobe of the liver.

What further imaging features would favour a diagnosis of focal nodular hyperplasia rather than hepatic adenoma?

a. No uptake of hepatobiliary contrast agent on MRI
b. T1 hyperintensity on MRI
c. Lesion size greater than 10 cm
d. Central T2 hyperintense scar on MRI
e. Reduced tracer uptake on Tc99m sulphur colloid scan

40. A 35 year old male patient with no fixed abode is admitted with bilateral flank pain and haematuria. The flank pain is worse on the right side. An abdominal radiograph reveals no urinary tract calcification; however, there is coarse calcification in the left upper quadrant. The left femoral head is noted to be flattened and sclerotic.

Renal ultrasound identifies mild right hydronephrosis but no calcified calculi. There are similar findings following an unenhanced CT urinary tract. A contrast enhanced CT urogram is then performed which identifies a few small filling defects in the right renal pelvis.

Which of the following conditions accounts for the findings in this case?

a. Acute tubular necrosis
b. Indinavir calculi
c. Papillary necrosis
d. Pyeloureteritis cystica
e. Pyonephrosis

41. A trauma CT scan is completed for a child following a road traffic collision. There are multiple pelvic fractures and evidence of haemorrhage within the pelvis. The CT has features of hypoperfusion complex.

Which of the following is NOT consistent with hypoperfusion?

a. Hyper enhancing kidneys
b. Increased adrenal gland enhancement
c. Increased splenic enhancement
d. Small calibre aorta
e. Thickened jejunal wall with hyperdense mucosa

42. A 53 year old presents with a 2 day history of seizures, reduced conscious level and fever. There is no history of trauma or significant medical history. An admission CT head 2 days previously was normal. An MRI reveals signal abnormality in the cingulate gyrus and asymmetrical signal in the insula cortices and posterior temporal lobe white matter and cortex with predominantly T2 and FLAIR hyperintensity. There is restricted diffusion in the areas of FLAIR hyperintensity and subtle gyral enhancement. There are small punctate foci

of T2 hypointensity which are high signal on T1 sequences. The basal ganglia have normal appearances.

What is the most likely underlying cause?

a. Autoimmune encephalitis
b. Epstein-Barr virus encephalitis
c. Gliomatosis cerebri
d. Herpes simplex encephalitis
e. Middle cerebral artery territory infarct

43. A patient is referred to the respiratory team for follow-up of an incidental lung nodule seen in the visualised lung bases on an unenhanced CT urinary tract performed for renal colic. They have a past medical history of rheumatoid arthritis.

What is the most common finding in the thorax in rheumatoid arthritis?

a. Bronchiectasis
b. Lung nodule
c. Pleural effusion
d. Pulmonary artery hypertension
e. Pulmonary fibrosis

44. A 40 year old female patient has lumbar spine and pelvic radiographs following a trampolining accident. The emergency department junior doctor asks you to review it as he is unsure if there is abnormality of the sacrum. There are no acute fractures. There is dense subchondral sclerosis at the inferior aspects of the bilateral medial iliac bones. Sacroiliac and hip joint spaces are well preserved. There is no cortical irregularity.

What recommendation is the most appropriate?

a. MRI sacrum with T1, T2 and STIR sequences
b. No further action required
c. Nuclear medicine bone study
d. Review other previous plains films to assess for other skeletal manifestations
e. Suggest clinical correlation and consideration of rheumatology referral

45. The ultrasound of a 71 year old female patient with weight loss and abdominal bloating demonstrates large volume ascites. Past medical history includes hyperlipidaemia. A CT chest abdomen pelvis reveals bibasal atelectasis in the lungs with a couple of 3 mm lung nodules unchanged from a CT pulmonary angiogram 3 years previously.

In the abdomen and pelvis there is large volume of septated fluid with a density ranging from 0 to 12HU. Scalloping of the hepatic and splenic contours is evident; however no parenchymal splenic or hepatic lesions are identified. There are several calcified peritoneal foci and multiple small lymph nodes.

What is the most likely diagnosis?

a. Peritoneal lymphomatosis
b. Peritoneal mesothelioma
c. Sclerosing peritonitis
d. Pseudomyxoma peritonei
e. Tuberculosis

46. A 54 year old male undergoes a follow-up MRI brain with spectroscopy. He has a left frontal lobe glioblastoma diagnosed 6 months previously that was treated with chemoradiotherapy. The scan shows a substantial increase in size of the peripherally enhancing component of the tumour. There is surrounding vasogenic oedema causing mass effect.

Which of the following features indicate tumour progression as opposed to pseudo progression?

a. Elevated ADC values
b. Elevated Cho/NAA ratio
c. Increased lactate peak

d. Increased lipid peak
e. Reduced cerebral blood volume

47. A neonate is born at 38 weeks' gestation following elective caesarean section and develops respiratory distress at 5 hours following delivery. A chest radiograph demonstrates normal lung volumes and heart size with perihilar airspace opacification, a small right pleural effusion and a trace of fluid in the fissures. The baby starts improving clinically after 48 hours.

What is the most likely cause of this child's illness?

a. Beta-haemolytic streptococcal pneumonia
b. Meconium aspiration
c. Patent ductus arteriosus
d. Surfactant deficiency disease
e. Transient tachypnoea of the newborn

48. An MRI head is performed for a trauma patient on neurosurgical intensive care who is 5 days post-surgical decompression of a large right subdural haematoma following multiple skull fractures.
The MRI shows a small right subdural collection, much smaller than the collection prior to decompression. It has intermediate T1 and high T2 signal. The collection demonstrates restricted diffusion and peripheral enhancement.
Anterior to the left frontal lobe there is a thin, crescentic, T1 hyperintense collection which was not evident on the admission CT. There is no significant mass effect.
On susceptibility weighted imaging (SWI) there are a couple of small areas of hypointensity at the grey–white matter interface in both hemispheres and in the corpus callosum.
In the posterior fossa at the left cerebellopontine angle there is a 25-mm extra-axial lesion which demonstrates high T2 and low T1 and FLAIR signal without diffusion restriction or enhancement. It was also evident on the admission CT. After reviewing sagittal sequences you note that the cerebellar tonsils descend 4 mm below the foramen magnum.

In terms of clinical relevance, which finding is most important to prioritise in your report?

a. Bilateral regions of parenchymal SWI signal hypointensity
b. Cerebellar tonsil position
c. Left cerebellopontine angle lesion
d. New collection adjacent to left frontal lobe
e. Right subdural collection

49. A 46 year old male non-smoker presents with increased shortness of breath on exertion. Chest radiograph demonstrates hyperexpansion with bilateral predominantly lower zone lucency. The pleural spaces are clear and mediastinal appearances are within normal limits. Pulmonary function tests are abnormal and reveal an obstructive pattern. A blood test confirms the diagnosis.

What other imaging would be important in this patient?

a. Cardiac MRI
b. Carotid Doppler ultrasound
c. Echocardiogram
d. Abdominal ultrasound
e. Renal Doppler ultrasound

50. A 42 year old male patient with ongoing right foot pain following a tennis injury 1 year ago has an MRI requested by the orthopaedic consultant. The request form queries whether this may represent sinus tarsi syndrome.

What MRI finding would confirm this diagnosis?

a. Böhler's angle $<20^\circ$
b. Destruction of the sinus tarsi
c. Blooming artefact in the sinus tarsi on gradient echo sequences
d. High STIR signal in the calcaneus
e. Low T1 and low T2 signal in the sinus tarsi

51. A 45 year old male presents with acute, severe abdominal pain. This is localised to the right lower abdomen. A CT abdomen pelvis demonstrates a well-defined 3.5-cm area of homogenous, high attenuation fat with stranding within the mesentery adjacent to the ascending colon. The adjacent colon and small bowel are normal.

    What is the most likely diagnosis?

    a. Desmoid tumour
    b. Diverticulitis
    c. Epiploic appendagitis
    d. Omental infarction
    e. Mesenteric vein thrombosis

52. A 24 year old patient has an MRI pelvis following an abnormal cervical smear and subsequent examination under anaesthetic and biopsy reveals squamous cell carcinoma. The patient tests positive for human papilloma virus. The patient is going to be discussed at the gynaecology MDT meeting.

    Which initial staging imaging is most appropriate?

    a. CT chest/abdomen and MRI pelvis
    b. CT chest and MRI abdomen/pelvis
    c. CT chest/abdomen/pelvis and US pelvis
    d. 18F-FDG PET/CT and CT chest/abdomen/pelvis
    e. 18F-FDG PET/CT and MRI pelvis

53. A 15 month old with abdominal distension has an abdominal ultrasound. This identifies a large right upper quadrant mass, inseparable from the liver. The lesion contains multiple anechoic, septated cysts. The septae demonstrate vascularity. The kidneys, pancreas and spleen have normal appearances. There is no free fluid. The aorta is normal calibre. Serum alpha-fetoprotein is normal.

    What is the most likely diagnosis?

    a. Hepatic adenoma
    b. Hepatoblastoma
    c. Infantile haemangioendothelioma
    d. Mesenchymal hamartoma
    e. Metastatic Wilms tumour

54. A 30 year old male is referred by the neurologists with a several month history of headache. He was found to have papilloedema. An MRI brain shows a well-defined intraventricular mass. This appears to arise from the septum pellucidum. It is T1 isointense and T2 hyperintense with multiple cystic regions. There is blooming artefact on susceptibility weighted imaging. It shows mild, heterogenous T1 enhancement.

    What is the most likely diagnosis?

    a. Central neurocytoma
    b. Choroid plexus papilloma
    c. Ependymoma
    d. Intraventricular meningioma
    e. Subependymal giant cell astrocytoma

55. A 21 year old male student has a chest radiograph prior to going travelling which reveals an incidental smooth, rounded mediastinal mass at the level of the hila. Subsequent CT chest shows that this is a well-defined, thin walled lesion in the middle mediastinum just caudal to the carina and anterior to the oesophagus with a density of 11HU. It does not enhance following contrast administration.

    What is the most likely diagnosis?

    a. Bronchogenic cyst
    b. Enlarged subcarinal lymph node
    c. Enteric cyst

d. Neurenteric cyst
e. Pericardial cyst

56. A 27 year old male presents to the emergency department with right wrist pain. There is no history of trauma, there is point tenderness on examination. A plain film of the wrist is performed which demonstrates increased sclerosis of the lunate bone. The ulnar is also noted to be approximately 5 mm shorter than the radius.

    What is the most likely diagnosis?

    a. Blount disease
    b. Freiberg disease
    c. Kienböck disease
    d. Köhler disease
    e. Preiser disease

57. A CT abdomen pelvis is performed for a 76 year old GP patient who is feeling well in himself but has deranged liver function tests. It has been reported as having a liver with an increased attenuation of around 100HU. A recent ultrasound abdomen showed no gross abnormality. There is no previous CT imaging for comparison.

    Which of the following conditions would NOT be associated with this radiological finding?

    a. Amiodarone hepatotoxicity
    b. Thalassaemia
    c. Hepatic amyloidosis
    d. Previous Thorotrast use
    e. Wilson disease

58. A 45 year old female has a staging CT scan of the chest, abdomen and pelvis following a recent diagnosis of breast cancer. Within the visualised proximal left femur there is a low density lesion seen in the subtrochanteric region. It has a thin sclerotic margin and there is the impression of a central calcified nidus, although the lesion is not completely imaged. Further assessment with MRI is performed; the lesion demonstrates high T1 signal, and there is a low signal intensity rim.

    What is the most likely diagnosis?

    a. Chondromyxoid fibroma
    b. Fibrous dysplasia
    c. Intraosseous ganglion cyst
    d. Intraosseous lipoma
    e. Metastasis

59. An 8 year old girl has had a couple of small volume episodes of rectal bleeding following an upper respiratory tract infection 1 week prior to this. An abdominal ultrasound identifies a pseudo kidney appearance in the right upper quadrant. During the scan both kidneys are also noted to be enlarged and mildly hyperechoic with reduced corticomedullary differentiation. The liver and spleen have normal appearances. The child reports arthralgia and has a rash on the back of her legs.

    Which of the following is the most likely diagnosis?

    a. Eosinophilic granulomatosis with polyangiitis (Churg-Strauss)
    b. Granulomatosis with polyangiitis (Wegener granulomatosis)
    c. IgA vasculitis (Henoch-Schönlein purpura)
    d. Intussusception
    e. Systemic lupus erythematosus

60. An MRI brain is performed for a stroke patient confirming a right middle cerebral artery territory infarct. Whilst reviewing the acquired images you note a well-defined midline nasopharyngeal mass, just deep to and elevating the mucosa of the posterior nasopharynx between the heads of the longus colli muscles. The mass is homogenous, T1 isointense and T2 hypointense. There is no restricted diffusion. Looking at a previous MRI from 1 year earlier, this was present at that time and has not changed.

    What is the most likely underlying cause?

a. Branchial cleft cyst
b. Ranula
c. Rathke cleft cyst
d. Thyroglossal duct cyst
e. Tornwaldt cyst

61. A 23 year old female has a CT abdomen pelvis to investigate right iliac fossa pain, which shows features of acute appendicitis. Additionally there is an abnormality reported in the visualised anterior mediastinum and so there is further investigation with a CT chest. The finding is of a well-defined lesion which is predominantly cystic and contains foci of density including fat and calcification. There is no other significant finding seen in the chest and there is no previous imaging for comparison.

What is the most likely diagnosis?

a. Lymphoma
b. Teratoma
c. Thymoma
d. Thymolipoma
e. Thymus hyperplasia

62. A 7 year old male is under investigation for vitamin C deficiency. Wrist radiographs demonstrate sclerotic epiphyseal margins, loss of epiphyseal density, dense metaphyseal lines and an exuberant periosteal reaction.

What additional feature might be present on cross sectional imaging?

a. Cloaca
b. Coarsened trabeculae
c. Haemarthrosis
d. Involucrum
e. Sequestrum

63. A 76 year old man presents with painless, obstructive jaundice. A liver ultrasound examination shows an echogenic soft tissue mass centred on the biliary hilum. There is focal thickening and dilatation of the right hepatic lobe bile ducts and the walls appear hyperechoic. There is dilatation up to the second order ducts in the right lobe. A subsequent MRCP demonstrates high T2 signal within the dilated right lobe bile duct walls. The hilar lesion shows delayed contrast enhancement. Cholangiocarcinoma is suspected.

According to the Bismuth classification what would be the grade of the cholangiocarcinoma?

a. I
b. IIB
c. IIIA
d. IIIB
e. IV

64. A 25 year old female patient with breast implants has a 4 week history of a painless left breast lump. Following a GP appointment she is referred to the 2 week wait breast services at her local hospital for triple assessment.

What does triple assessment involve?

a. Examination, imaging, biopsy
b. Examination, ultrasound, biopsy
c. Examination, ultrasound guided biopsy, MDT discussion
d. Mammogram, breast ultrasound, axilla ultrasound
e. Mammogram, ultrasound, biopsy

65. A 6 month old boy is sent for an MRI as an investigation for an enlarged head circumference. This demonstrates hydrocephalus.

Which statement regarding congenital aqueduct stenosis is most accurate?

a. The posterior fossa has normal appearances
b. The third, lateral and fourth ventricles are dilated
c. Presence of a T2 flow void at the aqueductal level is highly suspicious
d. Ultrasound is not useful in the diagnosis of the condition
e. Post contrast MRI sequences are most helpful

66. A 25 year old female with known polycystic kidney disease presents with sudden onset severe occipital headache. An unenhanced CT head shows acute subarachnoid blood in the interhemispheric fissure. A ruptured intracranial aneurysm is suspected.

What is the most likely site of intracranial aneurysm?

a. Pericallosal artery
b. Right middle cerebral artery
c. Basilar tip
d. Anterior communicating artery
e. Posterior communicating artery

67. A 56 year old female smoker has ongoing shortness of breath and reduced exercise tolerance. She is known to have a diagnosis of Sjögren syndrome. The GP requests a high resolution CT to assess for interstitial lung disease. The CT shows diffuse ground glass opacification.

Which interstitial lung disease is most commonly associated with Sjögren syndrome?

a. Acute interstitial pneumonia
b. Desquamative interstitial pneumonia
c. Lymphocytic interstitial pneumonitis
d. Non-specific interstitial pneumonia
e. Usual interstitial pneumonitis

68. A 3 year old girl is under investigation for abnormality of the facial bones. She has a plain film which demonstrates well-defined multilocular, expansile, cystic osseous lesions. The working diagnosis is cherubism.

Which of the following is most accurate?

a. It always affects the mandible
b. The changes are histologically indistinguishable from ameloblastoma
c. It is usually unilateral
d. The condition is idiopathic
e. Tooth development is usually unaffected

69. You are asked to review the pelvic MRI of a 38 year old woman with chronic pelvic pain and suspected endometriosis. There is a well-defined, thin walled lesion located between the sacrum and rectum. It is multiloculated and demonstrates high T2 and intermediate T1 weighted signal. There is no evidence of high T1 signal in the pelvis on fat suppressed sequences. There is minimal wall enhancement following contrast administration. There is no distal ureteric dilatation. Appearances of the vagina, cervix, uterus and ovaries are within normal limits with a corpus luteum on the right. A few bilateral common and external iliac lymph nodes measure up to 5 mm in short axis. There is a trace of pelvic free fluid. The imaged bones have normal appearances.

Based on the imaging findings, what is the most likely diagnosis?

a. Anterior sacral meningocele
b. Dermoid cyst
c. Duplication cyst
d. Endometrioma
e. Tailgut cyst

70. You are the duty radiologist covering inpatient CT when you get a call to come to the CT scanner immediately. A 53 year old man was having a contrast enhanced CT abdomen and pelvis for fever and left sided abdominal pain. Following the scan, the patient has become acutely short of breath and wheezy and has swollen lips and eyes. The CT radiographer has already called switchboard to request the emergency medical team to attend. You assess the

patient with an ABCDE approach and diagnose anaphylaxis. You follow the anaphylaxis treatment algorithm.

What is the most appropriate next step?

a. High flow oxygen via a non rebreathe mask
b. 500 µg of 1:1000 intramuscular adrenaline
c. 1 mg of 1:10,0000 adrenaline via intravenous injection
d. 10 mg slow intravenous injection of chlorphenamine
e. 200 mg hydrocortisone via intravenous injection

71. A 55 year old man has an MRCP as an investigation for recurrent pancreatitis. A previous CT demonstrates generalised pancreatic atrophy. At MRCP the main pancreatic duct measures 7 mm and there is a enhancing solid nodule with low signal on T2 weighted imaging in the pancreatic head. No calcification is associated with this when reviewed alongside the previous CT.

What is the most likely diagnosis?

a. Branch duct intraductal papillary mucinous papillary neoplasm
b. Main duct intraductal papillary mucinous neoplasm
c. Insulinoma
d. Serous cystadenoma
e. Mucinous cystadenoma

72. A 36 year old woman with neurofibromatosis type 1 has an MRI brain and whole spine as part of her annual follow-up.

Which of the following findings would NOT be expected in her condition?

a. Diffusely thickened, enhancing optic nerve
b. Enhancing bilateral cerebellopontine angle masses
c. Expanded spinal dura causing posterior vertebral scalloping
d. Kyphoscoliosis
e. Multiple, bilateral cerebral white matter high T2/FLAIR signal lesions

73. A 25 year old asymptomatic male doctor requires a chest radiograph to apply for a visa to work in Australia. The chest radiograph is performed which is of good quality, although slightly rotated to the left side. It demonstrates increased transradiancy of the whole right hemithorax. Lung markings are present; however there is paucity of the vascular markings on the right when compared to the left side. The hilum of the right side is thought to be marginally smaller than on the left; however this is difficult to determine accurately due to the rotation.

What is the most likely aetiology?

a. Large pulmonary embolus
b. MacLeod syndrome
c. Poland syndrome
d. Pneumothorax
e. Rotated chest radiograph

74. A 50 year old male is under investigation by the endocrinology team for a hormonal disorder. A chest radiograph is performed. There is a well-defined lucent and expansile lesion in the lateral aspect of a left sided rib. CT chest demonstrates the lesion well. There is no associated periosteal reaction. Further scrutiny of the distal clavicle demonstrates subperiosteal bone resorption. Following a period of treatment, the lucent lesion resolves.

What is the most likely diagnosis?

a. Brown tumour
b. Fibrous dysplasia
c. Haemangioma
d. Metastasis
e. Myeloma

75. A 31 year old male is referred for an abdominal ultrasound by the gastroenterologists. He presented with pruritis and was noted to have elevated alkaline phosphatase (ALP) and gamma glutamyl transferase (GGT). Ultrasound shows multiple dilated intra- and extrahepatic ducts. There is increased echogenicity of the portal triads. An MRCP shows irregular stricturing of both the intra- and extra hepatic ducts with dilatation between strictures.

    What is the most likely diagnosis?

    a. Primary biliary cirrhosis
    b. Choledochal cyst
    c. Primary sclerosing cholangitis
    d. Ischaemic cholangiopathy
    e. Cholangiocarcinoma

76. A 50 year old male is involved in a road traffic collision. He was driving a car at approximately 50 mph and collided with an oncoming vehicle. A trauma CT shows multiple rib fractures, a right lower lobe lung contusion, a grade III liver laceration and free fluid in the pelvis. In addition, there is a nodular focus of hyperdensity seen in the body of the right adrenal gland which has density of 70HU, and there is peri-adrenal fat stranding. The left adrenal gland is normal.

    Which of the following has caused these appearances in the right adrenal gland?

    a. Adrenal calcification
    b. Adrenal haemorrhage
    c. Adrenal hyperplasia
    d. Adrenal laceration
    e. Myelolipoma

77. A 4 year old girl is referred to the paediatric neurologists for investigation of recurrent seizures and global developmental delay. An MRI brain shows a thick band of abnormal T1 hyperintense, T2 hypointense signal intensity deep to the cerebral cortex. It parallels the cortex in contour and signal intensity. There is diminished overlying gyral sulcation and many of the cortical sulci are shallow.

    Which of the following conditions correlates best with these features?

    a. Band heterotopia
    b. Polymicrogyria
    c. Schizencephaly
    d. Subependymal heterotopia
    e. Subcortical heterotopia

78. An 82 year old, unkempt woman who lives alone is admitted with acute confusion. On clinical examination she is noted to be ataxic. A CT head is unremarkable. MRI brain demonstrates bilateral high T2 and FLAIR signal within the mammillary bodies and medial thalami. Further high signal is seen within the pons. Following gadolinium administration there is enhancement of the mammillary bodies bilaterally.

    What is the most likely diagnosis?

    a. Cerebral lymphoma
    b. Leigh syndrome
    c. Osmotic demyelination syndrome
    d. Pontine glioma
    e. Wernicke encephalopathy

79. A 45 year old male smoker has a high resolution CT to investigate chronic cough. The only finding is a mixed ground glass nodule in the right upper lobe measuring 9 mm in diameter.

    Which of the following parameters is the most powerful in predicting invasive adenocarcinoma over adenocarcinoma in situ or minimally invasive adenocarcinoma?

    a. Nodule diameter
    b. Nodule location
    c. Nodule mass

d. Nodule multiplicity
e. Nodule volume

80. A 27 year old male presents with a firm lump arising around the left elbow. Elbow radiographs demonstrate a pedunculated bony outgrowth from the humerus consisting of the cortex and medulla. MRI confirms the presence of a cartilage cap. The most likely diagnosis is considered to be a benign osteochondroma.

Which of the following is most likely to be true?

a. The bony protrusion is directed away from the joint
b. The humerus is most commonly affected
c. The cartilage cap is 2.2 cm in thickness
d. There are likely to be multiple osteochondromas
e. The stem is prone to fracture

81. A 55 year old male with a background of type 2 diabetes has an abdominal ultrasound due to deranged serum liver function tests. This shows a diffusely echogenic liver. There is attenuation of the ultrasound beam with poor visualisation of the portal venous architecture.

Which of the following features is most likely given the likely underlying condition?

a. Liver density of 10HU more than the spleen on unenhanced CT
b. Increased tracer uptake on Tc99m sulphur colloid scan
c. Liver reflectivity less than that of the renal cortex on ultrasound
d. Hypoenhancement of the liver relative to the spleen on contrast CT
e. Signal dropout of the liver on out-of-phase MRI sequence

82. A 6 month old girl is referred for investigation for suspected congenital cytomegalovirus (CMV) infection due to delayed neurological development.

Which of the following features is more typically associated with congenital rubella infection than with congenital CMV infection?

a. Hepatomegaly
b. Hydrocephalus
c. Cardiac anomaly
d. Microcephaly
e. Ultrasound showing hyperechoic foci in a periventricular distribution

83. The MRI brain of a 47 year old female neurology inpatient is reviewed. The patient is cardiovascularly stable and immunocompetent. The MRI has features of multiple sclerosis.

However, there is also a left temporal lobe lesion. It is T2 hyperintense but the central signal is T1 hypointense. There is surrounding white matter oedema, mass effect and a complete rim of peripheral enhancement. Restricted diffusion is present peripherally, but not centrally. MRI perfusion finds that relative cerebral blood flow is markedly increased both in and surrounding the lesion.

What is the most likely diagnosis of the left temporal lobe lesion?

a. Abscess
b. Glioblastoma
c. Lymphoma
d. Metastases
e. Tumefactive multiple sclerosis

84. An 18 month old girl, born by elective caesarean section at term, is referred to the ophthalmologists due to leukocoria. A CT orbits shows a large, calcified retrolental mass in the left globe. An MRI of the orbits is performed, and the mass is T1 isointense and T2 hypointense. Following gadolinium administration there is heterogenous enhancement.

What is the most likely diagnosis?

a. Capillary haemangioma
b. Cavernous haemangioma

c. Retinoblastoma
d. Retrolental fibroplasia
e. Rhabdomyosarcoma

85. An emergency department doctor asks you to review the chest radiograph of a 22 year old woman presenting with shortness of breath and green sputum. There is patchy consolidation with relatively symmetrical perihilar and upper lobe tubular opacities. There is elevation of the oblique fissures and hila bilaterally. The film demonstrates a right sided tunnelled central venous catheter.

What is the most likely diagnosis?

a. Allergic bronchopulmonary aspergillosis
b. Drug induced lung disease
c. Invasive aspergillosis
d. Tracheobronchopathia osteochrondroplastica
e. Granulomatosis with polyangiitis (Wegener granulomatosis)

86. A 56 year old with left wrist pain has radiographs taken. The report suggests the presence of a periosteal reaction at the distal radius and recommends further assessment with an MRI scan.

Which of the following features is most likely to be associated with a benign periosteal reaction?

a. Codman's triangle (elevated periosteum)
b. Lamellated
c. Onion skin
d. Soap bubble
e. Sunray

87. An 18 month old boy presents to the emergency department with his parents following two episodes of bright red blood in his nappy. He is cardiovascularly stable. There is no significant medical history and he was born at term by an uncomplicated vaginal delivery. The paediatric team suspect Meckel's diverticulum and ask for your advice regarding imaging.

Which is the most appropriate test to confirm the diagnosis?

a. Angiography
b. CT angiography
c. Small bowel fluoroscopy
d. 99mTc-Na-pertechnetate scintigraphy
e. Ultrasound

88. A 31 year old female patient has an MRI pelvis following a completed miscarriage. The sonographer in the early pregnancy assessment unit was concerned about a uterine anomaly and so an MRI was arranged. The uterine cavity is bisected by soft tissue extending to the internal cervical os. The external fundal uterine contour is convex. There is one cervix, one vagina and two ovaries and fallopian tubes.

Which Müllerian duct anomaly does this patient have?

a. Arcuate uterus
b. Bicornuate uterus
c. Septate uterus
d. Unicornuate uterus
e. Uterus didelphys

89. A 4 year old girl presents with fever, rash, conjunctivitis and bilateral cervical lymph node enlargement. Chest radiograph demonstrates bilateral atelectasis and a small right pleural effusion. A diagnosis of Kawasaki disease is made.

Which of the following radiological findings would be consistent with this diagnosis?

a. Abdominal aortic wall thickening
b. Calcified splenic artery aneurysm
c. Enlarged kidneys with loss of corticomedullary differentiation
d. Renal artery microaneurysms
e. Thin-walled dilated gallbladder

90. A 25 year old man with a background of Cowden syndrome presents to the neurologist with left sided dysarthria and ataxia. An MRI brain is arranged. This shows a mass-like appearance of the left cerebellum with widened left cerebellar folia and a striated appearance. The affected area is T1 hypointense and T2 hyperintense and demonstrates high signal on both DWI and ADC. The lesion does not enhance. Supratentorial appearances are within normal limits.

    What is the most likely diagnosis?

    a. Cerebellitis
    b. Cerebellar infarction
    c. Cerebral lymphoma
    d. Demyelination
    e. Lhermitte-Duclos disease

91. A 56 year old female is under investigation for increasing shortness of breath. She has a CT chest which shows symmetrical honeycomb destruction of the parenchyma in the lower lobes with scattered ground glass opacification and basal volume loss. The oesophagus is markedly patulous.

    What is the most likely diagnosis?

    a. Achalasia
    b. Non-specific interstitial pneumonitis
    c. Recurrent aspiration
    d. Scleroderma
    e. Usual interstitial pneumonitis

92. A 67 year old male presents with a 1 year history of pain and new bladder dysfunction. On plain film there is a large lytic, expansile lesion within the sacrum with internal calcification. A CT neck chest abdomen pelvis is performed – the lesion is confirmed to be solitary and there is no evidence of visceral disease. The lesion demonstrates a narrow zone of transition, a mixed density, with areas of low attenuation and calcification, and it enhances. MRI pelvis shows a lobulated sacral mass, which is high signal on T2 with multiple foci of T1 high signal.

    What is the most likely primary bone tumour?

    a. Chondrosarcoma
    b. Chordoma
    c. Metastasis
    d. Osteosarcoma
    e. Sacrococcygeal teratoma

93. A 70 year old female has a CT abdomen and pelvis due to right upper quadrant pain and leucocytosis. This demonstrates gallbladder wall thickening.

    Which of the following features favours a diagnosis of xanthogranulomatous cholecystitis over gallbladder carcinoma?

    a. Pericholecystic infiltration into the liver
    b. Biliary obstruction
    c. Regional lymphadenopathy
    d. Multiple, hypodense intramural nodules
    e. Cholelithiasis

94. A 45 year old woman attends the neurology clinic with right-sided hearing loss and facial paraesthesia. She also complains of intermittent dizziness. An MRI brain shows a large mass at the right cerebellopontine angle which is high signal on T2 weighted imaging. Differentials include vestibular schwannoma, epidermoid cyst and meningioma.

    Which of the following sequences would be most helpful in deciding if the mass is an epidermoid cyst?

    a. DWI
    b. FLAIR

c. STIR
d. SWI
e. T2

95. A neonate who was diagnosed with truncus arteriosus in the antenatal period has a chest radiograph.

Which of the following radiographic features is most likely to be observed in this child?

Table 2.3:

	Heart Size	Lungs	Aortic Arch
a	Enlarged	Plethoric	Right sided
b	Enlarged	Plethoric	Left sided
c	Enlarged	Normal	Left sided
d	Enlarged	Normal	Left sided
e	Normal	Plethoric	Right sided

96. A 7 year old boy is referred to a paediatric neurologist with lower than normal IQ and recurrent seizures. He is noted to have a facial rash. A diagnosis of tuberous sclerosis is suspected and an MRI brain is performed which confirms the diagnosis.

Which of the following imaging findings is most likely to be present in this child?

a. Focal areas of signal intensity in the deep white matter
b. Subcortical calcification
c. Optic nerve gliomas
d. Subependymal giant cell astrocytoma
e. Prominent leptomeningeal enhancement

97. A 23 year old motorcyclist is brought into hospital following a road traffic collision at 50 mph with a car. The patient requires stabilising before being brought to the CT scanner for a trauma scan. The paramedics report an open fracture to the left femur and suspect thoracoabdominal injuries. The emergency department team ask you to review a portable chest radiograph; this demonstrates an appropriately sited endotracheal tube and a nasogastric tube with the tip projected over the left lower hemithorax. There are several left sided rib fractures and increased density in the left lower zone obscuring the contour of the left hemidiaphragm. The mediastinal width is 6 cm.

Which of the following injuries would you suspect from the radiographic appearances?

a. Aortic rupture
b. Diaphragmatic rupture
c. Fat embolism
d. Tracheobronchial rupture
e. Oesophageal rupture

98. A 4 year old patient is currently under the paediatric team for investigation of severe iron deficiency anaemia, thought to be secondary to poor nutritional state. In view of safeguarding concerns, a skeletal survey and CT head are performed.

Which of the following findings is LEAST likely to be seen?

a. Hair-on-end appearance of the skull
b. Osteoporosis of the long bones
c. Rodent facies
d. Sparing of the occiput
e. Widening of the diploe and thinning of the inner and outer tables

99. A 34 year old woman presents to the emergency department with right upper quadrant pain. Blood tests show she has elevated inflammatory markers and deranged liver function tests.

An abdominal ultrasound finds that the gallbladder is distended, thick walled and oedematous. The common bile duct measures 12 mm in diameter, extending down to the level of the cystic duct. A 3-mm echogenic mass is seen in the cystic duct. It demonstrates posterior acoustic shadowing. MRCP is performed which confirms the ultrasound findings and the absence of any common bile duct stones.

What is the most accurate diagnosis?

a. Acute cholecystitis
b. Mirizzi syndrome
c. Gallbladder polyp
d. Adenomyomatosis
e. Choledochocele

100. You are asked to review the first screening mammogram for an asymptomatic patient. They have had no previous breast imaging previously. There is calcification in the breasts.

Which of the following types of calcification is most concerning for malignancy?

a. Bilateral scattered coarse calcification
b. Branching linear calcification extending from the right upper outer quadrant towards the nipple areolar complex
c. Calcification with a layered appearance, dependent on the MLO view in the right upper outer quadrant
d. Coarse dystrophic calcification in right upper inner quadrant
e. Tram-like serpiginous calcification in the left upper outer quadrant extending towards the nipple areolar complex

101. A neonate is born at term with respiratory distress. The initial radiograph shows a hazy, mass-like opacity in the left upper zone. Follow-up radiographs show a hyperlucent left upper zone with mass effect and contralateral mediastinal shift.

What is the most likely diagnosis?

a. Bronchial atresia
b. Bronchogenic cyst
c. Congenital lobar over inflation
d. Congenital pulmonary airway malformation
e. Mucous impaction

102. A middle-aged male patient with a low CD4 count, secondary to poorly controlled HIV infection, is admitted as an inpatient due to deteriorating neurological function. An MRI brain reveals normal cerebral volume and no evidence of hydrocephalus. There are multifocal white matter abnormalities with high T2 signal and low T1 signal. This is primarily affecting the right parieto-occipital region, and to a lesser degree the left parietal lobe and subcortical right frontal lobe. There is no associated mass effect, no enhancement and minor peripheral restricted diffusion.

What is the most likely diagnosis?

a. Cerebral toxoplasmosis
b. Cytomegalovirus encephalitis
c. HIV encephalopathy
d. Posterior reversible encephalopathy syndrome
e. Progressive multifocal leukoencephalopathy

103. A 56 year old male who retired from the mining industry 10 years ago has investigations for worsening shortness of breath. The CT chest shows tiny calcified nodules predominantly in the upper lobes. In the right mid-zone the nodules coalesce and there is upper lobe fibrosis with volume loss and elevation of the hila bilaterally. The hila lymph nodes demonstrate eggshell calcification.

What is the most likely diagnosis?

a. Caplan syndrome
b. Coal workers' pneumoconiosis

c. Hypersensitivity pneumonitis
d. Pulmonary alveolar proteinosis
e. Silicosis

104. A baby is stillborn with obvious skeletal abnormalities including shortening and bowing of the femora and humeri with metaphyseal flaring. The child is short in length and plain films also reveal platyspondyly, trident acetabula and squared iliac wings.

The features are considered to be in keeping with thanatophoric dysplasia. What type of dwarfism are these imaging appearances consistent with?

a. Acromelic
b. Mesomelic
c. Metatrophic
d. Micromelic
e. Rhizomelic

105. A Meckel diverticulum is diagnosed incidentally on an MRI small bowel performed for a patient with Crohn's disease.

Where is the diverticulum most likely to have been visualised?

a. Antimesenteric border of the distal jejunum
b. Antimesenteric border of the distal ileum
c. Antimesenteric border of the proximal ileum
d. Mesenteric border of the distal ileum
e. Mesenteric border of the proximal jejunum

106. A 15 year old female with physical features of a short neck and low posterior hairline has restricted neck movement. She has an MRI of the spine, which demonstrates scoliosis, spinal stenosis within the cervical spine, partial fusion of C2 and C3 as well as the presence of hemivertebrae.

What is the most likely diagnosis?

a. Ankylosing spondylitis
b. Homocysteinuria
c. Juvenile idiopathic arthritis
d. Klippel-Feil syndrome
e. Turner syndrome

107. A 12 year old boy is referred to the paediatric cardiologists with shortness of breath and palpitations. On examination he is found to have an ejection systolic murmur heard loudest at the left upper sternal border. He is suspected of having an atrial septal defect.

Which of the following radiological signs would be indicative of an atrial septal defect?

a. Enlarged left atrium
b. Enlarged aortic arch
c. Enlarged right atrium
d. Enlarged left ventricle
e. Lower zone vascular prominence

108. A 62 year old presents with worsening headaches, dysarthria and confusion. A CT brain shows an ill-defined, hypoattenuating mass arising from the midline with a large amount of surrounding vasogenic oedema. The patient then has an MRI brain. Again, there is a large, solitary central mass which involves the corpus callosum and crosses the midline. The mass shows ring-like post contrast T1 enhancement. There is minimal restricted diffusion.

What is the most likely diagnosis?

a. Cerebral lymphoma
b. Cerebral metastasis
c. Demyelination
d. Glioblastoma multiforme
e. Toxoplasmosis

109. A 72 year old female patient with right lower limb intermittent claudication has a CT angiogram of her lower limbs which identifies widespread vascular calcification with a short tight stenosis of her right common iliac artery. The patient is prepared for an interventional radiology procedure to stent the stenotic segment. Endovascular access is straightforward and the stenosis is confirmed with digital subtraction angiography. Following positioning of the stent and dilatation of the stenosis, the patient's blood pressure suddenly drops and the patient becomes tachycardic.

What is the most appropriate immediate management?

a. CT angiogram of the lower limbs
b. Deploy embolisation coils at the site of the stenosis
c. Re-inflate the balloon at the site of stenosis
d. Re-inflate the balloon proximal to the stenosis
e. Remove the vascular access sheath, wire and balloon

110. A 12 year old male attends the GP with his mother. He complains of knee pain and swelling. He plays football regularly but doesn't recall any specific trauma. The GP refers him for a plain film, which shows increased radiolucency of the infrapatellar fat pad, fragmentation of the tibial tubercle, loss of the sharp margin of the patellar tendon and anterior soft tissue swelling.

Which of the following is LEAST likely to be seen on the subsequent MRI?

a. Anterior cruciate ligament tear
b. Bone marrow oedema on STIR sequence
c. Distension and fluid in the deep infrapatellar bursa
d. Oedema in the soft tissues and the Hoffa fat pad
e. Thickening of the distal patellar tendon

111. A 67 year old female presents with a palpable abdominal mass. A CT abdomen pelvis demonstrates a large retroperitoneal soft tissue mass containing fat density as well as soft tissue density.

Which of the following is most accurate?

a. Distant metastases are a rare finding in leiomyosarcoma
b. The myxoid type subtype of liposarcoma typically shows low T2 signal
c. Liposarcoma are the most common retroperitoneal sarcoma
d. Calcification is rare in malignant fibrous histiocytoma.
e. Retroperitoneal angiosarcoma has rarely metastasised at presentation

112. A 32 year old female patient had a living donor renal transplant 3 years previously in France and has now relocated to the UK. Her GP refers her for transplant follow-up and the patient has an outpatient renal ultrasound. This identifies the transplant kidney in the right iliac fossa. There is a 10-mm upper pole simple renal cyst and no hydronephrosis. There is good global perfusion of the kidney with an arterial resistive index of 0.6 and forward flow in diastole. Normal colour Doppler flow is evident in the renal vein. There is a 50-mm avascular, thin-walled, anechoic structure which appears separate from, but adjacent to, the kidney.

Based on the imaging characteristics, what is the most likely diagnosis?

a. Abscess
b. Haematoma
c. Lymphocele
d. Seroma
e. Urinoma

113. A 14 year old boy is referred to the paediatricians for recurrent chest infections. A chest radiograph shows a wedge-shaped opacity within the medial right lower zone. Bronchopulmonary sequestration is suspected, and a CT thorax is arranged.

Which of the following features favour a diagnosis of intralobar sequestration over extralobar sequestration?

a. Associated diaphragmatic hernia
b. Venous drainage to pulmonary veins

c. Enclosed in its own pleura
d. Presents in neonates
e. Systemic arterial supply from the aorta

114. A 40 year old woman is referred to the neurologists. She has a history of postural headaches which are relieved by lying down. An MRI brain shows sagging of the midbrain with reduced volume in the basal cisterns. The cerebellar tonsils are also low lying. The reporting radiologist suspects a diagnosis of intracranial hypotension and advises a T1 post gadolinium sequence.

What is the most likely pattern of meningeal enhancement?

a. Cortical gyral enhancement
b. Diffuse leptomeningeal enhancement
c. Diffuse, smooth dural enhancement
d. Focal dural enhancement
e. Focal, nodular leptomeningeal enhancement

115. A 36 year old male patient is under the care of the respiratory team. He has a high resolution CT chest which demonstrates bilateral hilar and mediastinal lymph node enlargement. There is nodular interlobular septal thickening in the right lower zone. The patient undergoes an endobronchial ultrasound and lymph node biopsy which confirms the diagnosis.

What is the most likely diagnosis?

a. Lymphoma
b. Stage 1 sarcoidosis
c. Stage 2 sarcoidosis
d. Stage 4 sarcoidosis
e. Stage 5 sarcoidosis

116. A 7 year old is taken to the emergency department with a painful left elbow. Plain films are performed and the referring junior doctor asks you for your interpretation of the imaging.

Which of the following ossification centres is LEAST likely to be seen in this patient?

a. Capitellum
b. External epicondyle
c. Internal epicondyle
d. Radial head
e. Trochlear

117. A 22 year old female presents with fever, general malaise and right upper quadrant pain. She has recently returned from southeast Asia. Bloods tests reveal an eosinophilia. An ultrasound demonstrates an anechoic, 6-cm cyst within the right lobe of the liver. The cyst has thin, perceptible walls with several smaller adjacent cysts.

What is the most likely diagnosis?

a. Pyogenic abscess
b. Amoebic abscess
c. Hydatid cyst
d. Schistosomiasis
e. Fungal abscess

118. You are asked to review the MRI head of a patient with an abnormal posterior fossa. The clinical team suspects a Chiari II malformation.

Which of these descriptions correctly describes a Chiari II malformation?

a. Absent cerebellum and herniation of the occipital lobe through the foramen magnum
b. An occipital and/or high cervical encephalocele
c. Displacement of the medulla and cerebellar vermis through the foramen magnum
d. Peg-like cerebellar tonsils displaced into the upper cervical canal through the foramen magnum

e. Severe cerebellar hypoplasia without displacement of the cerebellum through the foramen magnum

119. A 57 year old male oncology patient with T3c N1 M1 renal cell carcinoma is suspected to have acute Budd-Chiari syndrome following an admission with abdominal pain, abnormal liver function tests and rapid onset ascites. A contrast enhanced CT chest, abdomen and pelvis is performed. This confirms thrombus partially obstructing the suprahepatic inferior vena cava and there is a large volume of ascites.

What CT finding would NOT be consistent with acute Budd-Chiari syndrome?

a. Absent hepatic veins
b. Caudate lobe hypertrophy
c. Hepatosplenomegaly
d. Hyperenhancing early phase central liver enhancement
e. Increased portal vein diameter

120. A 42 year old man without significant past medical history has returned to the UK after 5 years teaching in Asia. He presents with headache and seizures. His MRI brain identifies hydrocephalus and there are multiple small bilateral parenchymal cysts. These are predominantly at the grey–white matter junction and some of them have a small amount of surrounding oedema and rim enhancement. There is also a cyst in the fourth ventricle, which appears as a small nodular focus of increased T1 signal compared to the cerebrospinal fluid. This enhances following contrast.

What is the most likely diagnosis?

a. Cryptococcus
b. Hydatid cysts
c. Neurocysticercosis
d. Toxoplasmosis
e. Tuberculosis

ANSWERS 2

1. (d) MRI

Popliteal artery entrapment syndrome is caused by symptomatic compression or occlusion of the popliteal artery by adjacent structures. It commonly presents in athletic males and is most frequently caused by the medial head of gastrocnemius or occasionally popliteus. It presents as intermittent claudication, which may be exacerbated by plantar flexion, or with thrombosis and can be bilateral in two-thirds. MRI is the favoured imaging modality because it demonstrates the underlying anatomy and aids surgical planning. Arterial phase CT and angiography would help to delineate the popliteal artery but the underlying soft tissue definition is better on MRI than CT. Similarly, ultrasound can help to demonstrate the artery and plantar flexion whilst scanning may reveal arterial compression, but MRI would still be favoured for surgical planning. A knee radiograph would not provide much benefit in this scenario.

(The Final FRCR Complete Revision Notes Page 14)

2. (a) Congo red stain following biopsy

The case describes amyloid arthropathy caused by amyloid deposition in the joints. This can be primary, or secondary to dialysis-dependent renal failure or multiple myeloma. It often presents as a large joint, bilateral, symmetrical arthropathy. Shoulder pain and carpal tunnel syndrome are common. Radiographic findings include preservation of joint space with subchondral cyst formation and well circumscribed erosions. MRI can reveal low T1 and T2 intra-articular nodules and bone lesions which enhance following contrast. Amyloid protein stains with Congo red.

Cartilage pigmentation is seen in ochronosis, otherwise known as alkaptonuria. Homogentisic acid accumulates within cartilage leading to dark pigmentation and premature degeneration.

Synovial pigmentation is a feature of pigmented villonodular synovitis due to haemosiderin staining.

Staphylococcus aureus is associated with spondylodiscitis. Amyloid lesions in the spine can resemble discitis; however, the disc would be expected to have high T2 signal rather than the low signal described in the question.

Secondary hyperparathyroidism is associated with chronic renal failure too but features include metastatic calcification and osteosclerosis with the 'rugger jersey' spine appearance.

Weakly positive birefringent crystals are associated with calcium pyrophosphate deposition disease (CPPD), also known as pseudogout. This can be commonly misdiagnosed as osteoarthritis due to overlapping features but the distribution is more unusual and chondrocalcinosis is frequently present.

(The Final FRCR Complete Revision Notes Page 62)

3. (c) Aperistalsis of the lower oesophagus

   The oesophagus is the most commonly affected part of the gastrointestinal tract in scleroderma. There is fibrosis of the smooth muscle, resulting in a dilated oesophagus with absent or reduced peristalsis in the distal two-thirds. A mediastinal air-fluid level may be apparent on frontal imaging due to poor oesophageal emptying. The upper oesophagus is composed of skeletal muscle and is therefore unaffected. Aspiration, reflux, Barrett oesophagus and distal strictures are all potential complications. Warm fluids may help the passage of contrast in achalasia but this is not a feature of scleroderma.

   (The Final FRCR Complete Revision Notes Page 180)

4. (a) Page kidney

   Arterial resistive index can be raised above normal limits (0.70 is the upper limit of normal) for several reasons in native kidneys, including renal artery stenosis, ureteric obstruction, hypotension and a perinephric fluid collection.

   In transplant kidneys problems such as transplant rejection, renal vein thrombosis, drug toxicity and acute tubular necrosis are also within the differential.

   Page kidney is a condition caused by a subcapsular collection compressing the kidney and typically presenting with flank pain and hypertension. Compression of the renal vasculature leads to activation of the renin angiotensin system.

   The history and clinical presentation in this case is key. On ultrasound there is often a distorted appearance to the kidney due to the subcapsular haematoma and an elevated resistive index. CT may show reduced enhancement of the kidney along with the perinephric collection.

   Pseudoaneurysm is possible following trauma; however, these would be more common follow a laceration. Renal artery stenosis would be unlikely to acutely develop in this clinical setting. Renal vein thrombosis is more common in transplant kidneys than native kidneys and the forward flow in diastole on the arterial trace is reassuring. The lack of hydronephrosis and the clinical history makes ureteric obstruction unlikely.

   (The Final FRCR Complete Revision Notes Page 261)

5. (c) Nephroblastoma

   Nephroblastoma (also known as a Wilms tumour) is the most common renal mass in childhood. This is usually heterogenous in appearance due to necrosis, haemorrhage and less commonly, calcification. It typically displaces adjacent structures compared to neuroblastoma which encases them. Neuroblastoma also tends to affect a slightly younger age group. Assessment of the adjacent vascular structures such as the renal vein and inferior vena cava is important. It typically metastasises to adjacent para-aortic nodes, lungs and liver.

   Mesoblastic nephroma is the commonest neonatal renal mass and usually presents before 3 months of age so does not fit with the patient in this case. It also can have a heterogenous appearance. It does not typically invade the vasculature.

   (The Final FRCR Complete Revision Notes Page 359)

6. (b) Dilated superior ophthalmic vein

   The history is suggestive of a caroticocavernous fistula; a fistula between the carotid artery and cavernous sinus. Signs include pulsatile exophthalmos, chemosis, reduced visual acuity and cranial nerve palsies (commonly III and VI). MRI findings include enlarged, oedematous extraocular muscles, a dilated superior ophthalmic vein with flow void and enlargement of the cavernous sinus. There can be enlargement of the superior orbital fissure and sella erosion when chronic.

   (The Final FRCR Complete Revision Notes Pages 369–370, 376)

7. (b) Kaposi sarcoma

   The perihilar and peribronchovascular nodular opacities describe the 'flame-shaped' nodular opacities seen in Kaposi sarcoma, accompanied by the lymph node enlargement. This condition is seen in patients with HIV and CD4 count <200 cells/mm^3.

The main differential diagnosis in this patient is lymphoma; however lymphoma associated with HIV (mostly non-Hodgkin) is usually associated with disseminated extra-nodal disease involving the CNS, GI tract and bone marrow. Lack of avidity on gallium scan is more in favour of Kaposi sarcoma. Lymphoma is gallium avid.

Pneumocystis pneumonia can occur in patients with CD4 count <200 cells/mm^3. The imaging appearances are of diffuse ground glass opacification but enhancing lymph node enlargement is not a feature.

Cytomegalovirus (CMV) can be seen in patients with CD4 >200cells/mm^3. The predominant imaging features of pulmonary CMV are multiple ground glass pulmonary nodules and consolidation. *Mycobacterium avium* is seen in patients with CD4 count <50 cells/mm^3.

(The Final FRCR Complete Revision Notes Page 33)

8. (c) Psoriatic arthritis

Psoriatic arthritis is one of the seronegative spondyloarthropathies. It most commonly affects the hands and feet and can manifest as a symmetric polyarthropathy or asymmetric oligoarthropathy at these sites. When affecting larger joints it is typically asymmetrical. The spine and sacroiliac joints are also commonly involved.

Findings in the hands and feet include a predominance for the distal joints, marginal erosions, periostitis, joint space widening and preserved bone density. As the disease progresses, changes such as terminal tuft resorption and pencil-in-cup deformity can also be seen.

Rheumatoid arthritis tends to be symmetrical with a predilection for the metacarpal phalangeal joints causing periarticular osteopenia and erosions.

Reactive arthritis (previously known as Reiter syndrome) preferentially affects young men and the feet. It can also cause periosteal reaction but has a predilection for the first metatarsal phalangeal joint and calcaneus.

Erosive osteoarthritis also typically affects the distal interphalangeal joints but causes more central erosions and marginal osteophytes leading to the 'gull-wing' appearance.

Gout is more likely to be monoarticular affecting the first metatarsal phalangeal joint. It also does not commonly cause periarticular osteopenia. The erosions are more peripherally sited than in psoriatic or rheumatoid arthritis and are well-defined with sharp overhanging edges.

(The Final FRCR Complete Revision Notes Page 91)

9. (d) Fat supressed T2 weighted sequence

MRI is helpful in Crohn's disease for monitoring disease activity and has the added benefit of no radiation, particularly for younger patients with the condition. Fistulae are possible in Crohn's disease due to transmural bowel inflammation. Bowel wall ulceration can progress to full thickness fistulae which can communicate between bowel loops as well as between bowel and bladder, perineum or sometimes the vagina.

Although all the sequences in the question may be employed for an MRI looking for manifestations of Crohn's disease, fistulae can be visualised particularly well with fat supressed T2 weighted imaging, where they appear as a high signal tract. Following contrast administration the fistulae will enhance and post contrast enhancement can also highlight other areas of disease activity within the abdomen and pelvis.

(The Final FRCR Complete Revision Notes Page 162)

10. (c) Radiograph of the proximal femur

The question describes typical MRI findings of myositis ossificans. This condition causes heterotopic bone formation, most commonly following trauma but it occurs in paraplegic patients, sometimes with no history of preceding trauma. Typical radiographic appearances include a lesion adjacent to the knee or hip with peripheral calcification. Calcification will be low signal on T1 MRI sequences and sometimes the early features can include quite marked increased STIR signal extending into the muscle.

The main imaging differential is paraosteal osteosarcoma but these tend to calcify centrally rather than peripherally and on MRI they are often low signal on both T1 and T2 sequences. Radiographs can therefore help to confirm benignity. Myositis ossificans is a 'don't touch' lesion, meaning the radiological features are characteristic and they should not be biopsied. Histology from myositis ossificans can be difficult to differentiate from a soft tissue osteosarcoma.

Nuclear medicine bone scan may show uptake in both myositis ossificans and malignant lesions and will therefore not help to differentiate. Similarly, early myositis ossificans will likely

show enhancement on both CT angiogram and MRI.
(The Final FRCR Complete Revision Notes Page 85)

11. (a) Left posterolateral
The majority of congenital diaphragmatic herniae are the Bochdalek variety. These are large, associated with other conditions such as pulmonary hypoplasia and usually in a left posterolateral position. Retroperitoneal contents such as fat, the spleen and left kidney may herniate into them. They may be diagnosed on antenatal scans.
Morgagni herniae are less common, usually smaller and in a right anteromedial position. The transverse colon and stomach may herniate. BochdaLek are Left sided and MoRgagni are Right sided. **BBBB** can be used to remember the features of Bochdalek hernia: **B**ochdalek, **b**ig, **b**ad, **b**ack and lateral.
(The Final FRCR Complete Revision Notes Page 335)

12. (d) Restricted diffusion
Posterior reversible encephalopathy syndrome (PRES) can be caused by a variety of insults, one of which is hypertension. The distribution is variable and can include more anterior structures such as the watershed zones, inferior temporal and posterior frontal lobes but it is classically described as occipitoparietal. There is T2 hyperintensity and T1 hypointensity in the affected regions due to oedema which manifests as hypodensity on CT. Given the right clinical history one differential diagnosis is a posterior circulation stroke. Microhaemorrhage can be a feature in both diagnoses; however, whereas an acute stroke would lead to restricted diffusion, this finding is not typical in PRES and can be a helpful distinguishing factor.
(The Final FRCR Complete Revision Notes Page 420)

13. (c) 10 mL
According to the British National Formulary, the maximum dose of 1% lidocaine is 3 mg/kg up to 200 mg and equates to 20 mL. For 2% lidocaine the maximum dose is therefore 10 mL. The 2018 Royal College of Radiologists guidance on sedation, analgesia and anaesthesia in radiology differs slightly and suggests 4 mg/kg (around a total of 30 mL of 1% lidocaine for an adult of typical weight) as the maximum dose. Regardless of either recommendation, the correct answer for this question is 10 mL because 20 mL is not a given option.
The maximum dose for lidocaine with adrenaline is greater at 7 mg/kg because it decreases the rate of systemic absorption. Lidocaine with adrenaline has a faster onset and is generally used for procedures where there may be a greater chance of bleeding or where bloodless fields are required, for example dental and tracheostomy procedures. Symptoms and signs of lidocaine toxicity include drowsiness, disorientation, visual and auditory disturbances, numbness and tingling of the tongue and/or mouth and a metallic taste. If untreated this can potentially lead to seizures and cardiac arrythmia. Treatment includes resuscitation with an ABCD approach, calling the appropriate medical emergency team, supportive measures and intralipid administration.
British National Formulary, Lidocaine Hydrochloride,
https://bnf.nice.org.uk/drug/lidocaine-hydrochloride.html
The Royal College of Radiologists. Sedation, analgesia and anaesthesia in the radiology department, Second edition. 2018.
https://www.rcr.ac.uk/system/files/publication/field_publication_files/bfcr182_safe_sedation.pdf

14. (a) Achondroplasia
Features associated with achondroplasia on a spinal radiograph include an anteroinferior beak causing a bullet-shaped vertebrae and posterior vertebral body scalloping. Decreasing interpedicular distance and short pedicles increases the potential risk of canal stenosis.
The mucopolysaccharidoses are associated with posterior vertebral body scalloping, and Hurler syndrome does also share a similar anteroinferior beak, but the other features make achondroplasia more likely. The vertebral body shape associated with Morquio syndrome is an anterior central beak (this could be remembered as **M**orquio – **m**iddle) and there is often platyspondyly.
Thanatophoric dysplasia is also associated with platyspondyly and the typical 'telephone handle' appearance of the long bones. It overlaps with achondroplasia as both conditions cause narrowing of the interpedicular distance.
Asphyxiating thoracic dysplasia, also known as Jeune syndrome, tends to cause more thoracic abnormalities leading to a long narrow thorax and high clavicles.
(The Final FRCR Complete Revision Notes Page 103)

15. (e) Haemangioma
    Haemangiomata are the most common benign tumours of the spleen. Imaging characteristics are identical to hepatic haemangiomas with typical centripetal enhancement.
    Sarcoidosis tends to show low signal on all MRI sequences and hypoenhancement compared to the rest of the spleen. Splenomegaly is also common.
    Similarly, splenomegaly is frequently a feature in lymphoma and the lesions are T1 and T2 low signal or isointense on MRI with hypoenhancement compared to the rest of the spleen.
    The history does not correlate with abscess, and furthermore, splenic abscesses have appearances comparable with abscesses elsewhere: high T2, low T1 and peripheral enhancement.
    Metastases can have variable appearances depending on the primary site but they are commonly low on T1 and high on T2 sequences with variable enhancement. The characteristic centripetal enhancement in this case and the solitary nature of the lesion makes a haemangioma most likely.
    (The Final FRCR Complete Revision Notes Page 238)

16. (e) T1 hypointense, T2 hyperintense, Avid enhancement, No out-of-phase signal loss
    Phaechromocytomas are paragangliomas in the adrenal glands. They can be heterogenous in appearance but are usually T1 hypointense, although areas of haemorrhage may be bright on T1 sequences. They are usually very T2 hyperintense and can have a 'salt-and-pepper' appearance due to flow voids. They have prolonged avid enhancement which is frequently heterogeneous. There is no signal loss following in- and out-of-phase imaging.
    Phaechromocytomas usually demonstrate MIBG uptake on scintigraphy and this can be helpful to detect metastatic or locally recurrent disease.
    (The Final FRCR Complete Revision Notes Page 269)

17. (e) Pyloric volume of 1.6 cm^3
    Pyloric stenosis most commonly presents in neonates with non-bilious vomiting. An olive-sized mass may be palpable in the right upper quadrant. Ultrasound will demonstrate a thickened pylorus. The diagnostic sonographic measurements can be slightly variable. The diameter of a single wall is usually >3 mm and the hypertrophied muscle will appear as a thickened hypoechoic layer surrounding internal hyperechoic mucosa. The overall pyloric transverse diameter will exceed 11 mm (13 mm in some publications) and the pyloric length will be >15–17 mm. The pyloric volume exceeds 1.5 cm^3.
    On fluoroscopy, peristaltic waves may be seen with delayed gastric emptying. The 'string' sign represents a long pylorus with a thin lumen. The 'tit' or 'shoulder' sign is caused by the thickened pylorus indenting the antrum and the pyloric entrance may be beak shaped. A 'corkscrew' appearance is associated with midgut volvulus, not with pyloric stenosis.
    (The Final FRCR Complete Revision Notes Page 347)

18. (e) The pituitary gland usually shows peripheral enhancement
    Pituitary apoplexy is caused by pituitary necrosis, which may be haemorrhagic. This is frequently secondary to an underlying pituitary lesion, such as a macroadenoma. CT is insensitive for the diagnosis, and the pituitary fossa is better imaged with MRI. The pituitary may show high T1 signal if the cause is haemorrhagic; however, this will also depend on the age of blood, and other haemorrhagic/proteinaceous/necrotic masses can also have high T1 signal. Enhancement is typically peripheral and the infarcted centre commonly demonstrates restricted diffusion.
    (The Final FRCR Complete Revision Notes Page 403)

19. (c) Nodules with cavitation
    The condition described in the main stem is ANCA associated granulomatous vasculitis or granulomatosis with polyangiitis (previously known as Wegener granulomatosis). Cytoplasmic ANCA test is specific for the diagnosis of the condition if there are typical clinical features. Clinical features include upper airway symptoms (rhinitis, sinusitis, otitis media, subglottic or bronchial stenosis), lower respiratory tract infections (cough, chest pain, dyspnoea) and glomerulonephritis (haematuria/proteinuria). The most common imaging abnormality is cavitation of nodules or consolidation. The other imaging features provided in the question are also seen in this condition but are less frequent. Nodules, masses and focal areas of opacification are associated with active inflammation. Ground glass opacification may also be seen which can represent pulmonary haemorrhage.

(The Final FRCR Complete Revision Notes Page 59)
Chung MP, Chin AY, Lee HY et al. Imaging of pulmonary vasculitis. Radiology. 2010; 255(2):322–341.

20. (a) Chest radiograph
The case describes hypertrophic osteoarthropathy (HPOA) with typical radiographic appearances of smooth periosteal reaction which can affect the metacarpals, metatarsals and phalanges. Other more frequently occurring sites include the tibia, fibula, radius, ulna, humerus and femur. HPOA may also be detected on nuclear medicine bone scan and would present as increased cortical tracer uptake in the affected bones, which can have a 'tram track' appearance.
Secondary causes are most common, with non-small cell lung cancer being the most frequent cause. Pleural fibromas, mesothelioma, bronchiectasis, cyanotic heart disease and inflammatory bowel disease can also lead to HPOA. Thyroid acropachy and venous stasis can have similar appearances to HPOA but in the latter, other signs such as vascular calcification and phleboliths may be present.
Chest radiograph is the most appropriate next step out of the available options, although echocardiogram, liver ultrasound and nuclear medicine bone scan are not unreasonable in the appropriate setting.
(The Final FRCR Complete Revision Notes Page 79)

21. (e) Peutz-Jeghers syndrome
The patient has a condition with an autosomal dominant inheritance pattern. There are several polyposis syndromes; however, the one associated with cervical adenoma malignum is Peutz-Jeghers syndrome. Multiple gastrointestinal polyps can lead to presentations for haemorrhage and bowel obstruction secondary to intussusception. Patients also frequently have oral mucocutaneous pigmentation which can also affect the fingers and toes.
Carney complex is a combination of cardiac myxomas and blue skin pigmentation tending to affect the trunk and face, including the eyes and lips. Gastrointestinal polyps are not a feature. Myxomas can occur elsewhere in the body and patients are also predisposed to testicular tumours and pituitary adenomas.
Cowden syndrome causes multiple gastrointestinal hamartomatous polyps as well as mucocutaneous lesions and increases a patient's risk of cancers such as breast and thyroid primaries.
Cronkhite-Canada syndrome is more common in males and does not have a recognised familial inheritance pattern. As well as gastrointestinal polyps, patients may have brown skin pigmentation, nail atrophy and alopecia.
Neurofibromatosis 1 can cause cutaneous café-au-lait spots, amongst other clinical signs; however, it is not associated with gastrointestinal polyps.
(The Final FRCR Complete Revision Notes Page 181)

22. (b) Midline defect, peritoneal covering present, herniated liver, no associated bowel complications
The headings in this question help to differentiate an omphalocele from gastroschisis. Turner syndrome, along with other chromosomal abnormalities, is associated with an omphalocele whereas gastroschisis is usually sporadic. An omphalocele is a midline defect with a peritoneal covering and therefore ascites may be present. In contrast to this, gastroschisis is usually to the right of the midline, has no peritoneal covering and therefore no ascites. The liver herniates infrequently in gastroschisis and is more common with an omphalocele. Unlike in gastroschisis, where the bowel is in contact with amniotic fluid, bowel complications are not a feature of an omphalocele.
(The Final FRCR Complete Revision Notes Page 338)

23. (d) Terminal ileum
Gallstone ileus has the classic radiographic triad of bowel obstruction, pneumobilia and a radiopaque intraluminal gallstone; however, the so-called Rigler's triad is only seen in 10% of cases. It occurs due to fistulation of the stone through the gallbladder wall into the bowel, most commonly the duodenum and rarely, into the colon. The gallstone most commonly obstructs at the terminal ileum.
(The Final FRCR Complete Revision Notes Page 201)

24. (a) Cholesterol granuloma
Cholesterol granulomas are a complication of chronic infection and can occur in the middle

ear, mastoid or petrous apex. Due to their cholesterol content they are T1 and T2 hyperintense but their predisposition to haemorrhage means they may have a low signal haemosiderin rim. There may be thinning of the adjacent bone. They may enhance peripherally but do not demonstrate restricted diffusion.

Cholesteatoma are an important differential for a middle ear mass but they have different signal characteristics with low T1, high T2 signal and restricted diffusion. Depending on location they may displace and erode the ossicles.

A mucocoele may exhibit similar T1 and T2 hyperintensity as a cholesterol granuloma but they would not have the low signal rim and enhancement described in this case.

Glomus tympanicum are highly vascular and demonstrate intense enhancement. Similar to paragangliomas elsewhere in the body, they can have a 'salt-and-pepper' appearance due to the presence of flow voids.

A chondrosarcoma affecting the skull base would be centred on the bone rather than on the middle ear, although these masses may erode into the middle ear. Signal would classically be T1 hypointense and T2 hyperintense with heterogenous enhancement.

(The Final FRCR Complete Revision Notes Page 431)

25. (e) Tuberous sclerosis

The imaging features are that of lymphangioleiomyomatosis (LAM), which is a rare interstitial lung disease, more common in women of childbearing age. It manifests as thin-walled cysts of uniform size with normal intervening lung parenchyma. Patients with the condition can present with a pneumothorax and sometimes they develop chylous pleural effusion. It is associated with tuberous sclerosis (approximately 40% of patients with tuberous sclerosis have LAM).

Pulmonary Langerhans cell histiocytosis occurs most commonly in smokers. Early in the disease it is seen as 3- to 10-mm nodules in the mid-upper zones; later in the process the nodules undergo cystic degeneration. The cysts are typically irregularly shaped and can coalesce to form 'bizarre'-shaped cysts. The lung parenchyma between cysts may demonstrate emphysematous change.

Birt-Hogg-Dubé syndrome is a genetic multisystem disease which is characterised by multiple lung cysts; these are predominantly in the lower zones with variable morphology and internal septation.

Lymphocytic interstitial pneumonia is associated with HIV and other connective tissue disorders such as Sjögren syndrome. Interstitial infiltrate causes findings of ground glass opacification, consolidation, centrilobular nodules and scattered pulmonary cysts.

*Pneumocystis jiroveci*is an infection of immunocompromised patients. The imaging finding in this fungal infection are typically of bilateral ground glass densities. Cysts can occur within the ground glass density, usually in the upper zones.

(The Final FRCR Complete Revision Notes Page 42)

26. (c) Löfgren syndrome

Löfgren syndrome is an acute form of sarcoidosis characterised by fevers, malaise, arthritis, lymph node enlargement and erythema nodosum.

Leukaemia can also cause similar symptoms along with erythema nodosum; however chronic lymphocytic leukaemia usually affects an older age group.

Löffler syndrome is another term for simple pulmonary eosinophilia and although sounding similar to Löfgren syndrome should not be confused with it. Patients are not usually particularly unwell, and chest radiograph should show transient infiltrates rather than being completely clear. Hilar lymph node enlargement is also not a feature.

Sapho syndrome is relatively rare and is a condition causing synovitis, acne, pustolosis, hyperostosis and osteitis. Skeletally, the sternoclavicular joint is most commonly involved.

Sever disease causes pain in the posterior foot due to calcaneal apophysitis.

(The Final FRCR Complete Revision Notes Page 95)

27. (d) Pericolic fat stranding

Pseudomembranous colitis, also called *Clostridioides difficile extradural soft tissue extension and extension* colitis, is commonly seen in patients following a course of antibiotics. It causes significant bowel wall thickening which may cause a 'thumbprint' appearance. Approximately 40% of cases can have ascites. It most commonly involves the entire colon including the rectum. Many radiological features of pseudomembranous colitis overlap with inflammatory bowel disease, and differentiation can be challenging. Wall thickening is typically more severe in pseudomembranous colitis and any hyperenhancement is centred on the mucosa due to the

predominantly mucosal inflammation caused by the condition. There is therefore minimal pericolic fat stranding in the adjacent tissues and so the presence of pericolic fat stranding in this case makes inflammatory bowel disease more likely.
(The Final FRCR Complete Revision Notes Page 182)

28. (d) Melanoma
Renal metastases are often small, bilateral and although peripherally sited are endophytic and do not breach the renal capsule, unlike renal cell carcinoma. Melanoma metastases are hypervascular and often appear slightly hyperdense to the renal parenchyma. Melanoma is also the most common cause of a splenic metastatic deposit.
Other primary sites of renal metastases are breast, lung and the gastrointestinal tract. Primary lymphoma is rare in the kidney due to a lack of lymphoid tissue and therefore secondary lymphoma, often non-Hodgkins, would be more likely. In this case the associated pulmonary nodules and the only mildly enlarged retroperitoneal and retrocrural lymph nodes make a metastatic malignancy more likely.
(The Final FRCR Complete Revision Notes Page 254)

29. (b) The tube tip should be projected approximately 1.5 cm proximal to the carina
Endotracheal tube placement in a neonate can be challenging and the aim is to site it in the mid trachea avoiding intubation of the right main bronchus or too proximal a placement above the thoracic inlet. There are various landmarks that can be used. Ideally, the tip should be approximately 1.5 cm above the level of the carina. The carina is usually around the level of T3/4. Other landmarks for the tube tip position mentioned in literature include the inferior clavicles and the T1 vertebral body.
(The Final FRCR Complete Revision Notes Page 332)

30. (d) Pilocytic astrocytoma
The radiological appearance, presentation and demographics are typical for pilocytic astrocytoma. Medulloblastoma typically arise from the midline rather than the cerebellar hemisphere, and are usually seen in younger patients (2–6 years). Ependymoma tends to fill the fourth ventricle and protrude out of the foramen of Luschka and Magendie. Cerebellar abscess has a different clinical presentation and does not have an enhancing nodule. Pleomorphic xanthoastrocytomas are almost invariably located supratentorially.
(The Final FRCR Complete Revision Notes Page 395)

31. (c) Haemochromatosis
Haemochromatosis typically causes reduced myocardial signal intensity on cardiac MRI. Patients often suffer with cardiac failure caused by the effects of iron deposition within the heart. A similar low signal appearance is seen in the hepatic parenchyma on liver MRI. Eventually iron deposition can lead to liver cirrhosis causing a small liver with a nodular contour. Musculoskeletal manifestations of haemochromatosis include a symmetrical arthropathy along with osteopenia. The heads of the second and third metacarpals are often squared with hook-like medial osteophytes.
Alcohol excess can lead to liver cirrhosis and cardiac failure due to dilated cardiomyopathy, but this would cause reduced contractility and dilatation of all cardiac chambers.
Haemosiderosis can cause similar liver MRI changes as haemochromatosis but it typically involves the liver, spleen and marrow rather than the heart.
On cardiac MRI, amyloidosis can cause low myocardial signal intensity but you may also expect to see other associated features, such as wall thickening, restricted diastolic filling and subendocardial delayed enhancement. The liver and radiographic skeletal changes would not be typical.
Cardiac sarcoidosis causes granuloma formation which lead to increased foci of T2 weighted signal which also hyper enhance.
(The Final FRCR Complete Revision Notes Pages 10, 15)

32. (a) Convex margin of the posterior vertebral body
The patient has two red flag symptoms for back pain – age >55 years and thoracic back pain. Bone marrow which is hypointense to disc or muscle on T1 and T2 weighted imaging is abnormal and suggestive of marrow infiltration due to sclerotic metastases. If a vertebral body fracture is not acute there may be no STIR hyperintensity. Some metastatic marrow deposits will be low on T1 but relatively high on T2 and STIR sequences; however, sclerotic deposits will often demonstrate low signal even on STIR imaging. In a male patient of this age, disseminated

prostate malignancy would be high on the list of differentials.

Features that suggest malignant over benign vertebral body collapse include convexity of the posterior vertebral body margin, extradural soft tissue extension and extension of abnormal marrow signal to the pedicles. In contrast, osteoporotic fractures are more likely to cause retropulsion, have normal marrow signal elsewhere, intervertebral vacuum phenomenon and multiple fractures. Post-contrast enhancement in a vertebral body fracture is non-specific.
(The Final FRCR Complete Revision Notes Page 101)

33. (d) Transarterial chemoembolisation (TACE) may be used for large, unresectable tumours.
Transplant remains the definitive, curative treatment for hepatocellular carcinoma (HCC). TACE is a non-curative, life prolonging treatment of HCC. It is indicated in large, unresectable tumours for patients with Child-Pugh scores A and B. Thermal ablation (radiofrequency ablation or microwave ablation) is indicated in small hepatic tumours not amenable to surgery, which is life prolonging but not curative. TACE can be used to reduce tumour volume prior to ablation. It can also be used post ablation to reduce recurrence.
(The Final FRCR Complete Revision Notes Page 212)

34. (a) Annular pancreas
An annular pancreas is when pancreatic tissue encircles the duodenum at D2 close to the ampulla of Vater. This can be a complete or incomplete ring. It can be diagnosed incidentally if asymptomatic but it can be symptomatic, causing duodenal obstruction. It is associated with other conditions such as oesophageal atresia, tracheo-oesophageal fistula and Down syndrome.
Pancreas divisum is the commonest congenital pancreatic abnormality caused by failure of ductal fusion leading to two ducts draining into the duodenum. MRCP and MRI pancreas is the most helpful test to diagnose the condition. It does not cause duodenal luminal narrowing.
A duodenal diverticulum would appear as an outpouching from the duodenal wall which may be filled with gas, fluid or debris; these are often asymptomatic. There can be intraluminal diverticulum which can cause obstruction, similar to a duodenal web.
Duodenal webs typically cause a 'windsock' appearance due to the membranous web projected into the duodenal lumen rather than an area of focal narrowing.
Duodenal atresia usually presents very early with bilious vomiting caused by complete obstruction just distal to the ampulla of Vater. There would be no distal bowel gas visible in this scenario and a 'double bubble' appearance on abdominal radiographs.
(The Final FRCR Complete Revision Notes Page 333)

35. (e) Wilson disease
Wilson disease can affect the liver, central nervous system and musculoskeletal system. The MRI changes are sometimes described as the 'giant panda' and 'cub of the giant panda' signs. This appearance is due to abnormal midbrain T2 hyperintensity. Abnormal copper deposition leads to high T2 signal in the tegmentum, caudate nuclei, thalami and putamina with sparing of the red nuclei and substantia nigra. Copper does not cause increased density on CT.
Similarly, central nervous system iron deposition in haemochromatosis does not lead to CT hyperdensity; however, there may be T2 hypointensity and susceptibility artefact on gradient echo sequences secondary to the paramagnetic effects of iron. The anterior pituitary, choroid plexus and pineal gland are all common sites of deposition.
Pantothenate kinase-associated neurodegeneration (previously called Hallervorden-Spatz syndrome) also causes brain iron accumulation leading to T2 hypointensity in the globus pallidi and substantia nigra with associated susceptibility artefact. The characteristic sign is referred to as 'eye of the tiger'.
Menke's disease is a multisystem disorder leading to copper deficiency. The imaging appearances may be secondary to intracranial haemorrhage caused by tortuous vessels or parenchymal changes with volume loss and T1 basal ganglia hyperintensity.
Creutzfeldt-Jakob disease (CJD) causes atrophy and characteristic T2 hyperintensity in the cortex, white matter, putamen, caudate and posterior thalamus leading to the 'hockey stick' and 'pulvinar' signs.
(The Final FRCR Complete Revision Notes Page 423)

36. (e) Pneumococcus
Causes of pneumonia depend on the age of the child. In school age children such as this

patient, the most common causes are *Mycoplasma pneumoniae*, influenza A and *Streptococcus pneumoniae*, also known as pneumococcus.

Pneumococcus causes a lobar pneumonia and is also a common cause of community-acquired pneumonia in adults. It can cause lower lobe opacification and air bronchograms. Cavitation and empyema is unusual. In children it is associated with round pneumonia.

Listeria and group B streptococcus are more common in neonates, along with *Escherichia coli* and cytomegalovirus. Group B streptococcus causes bilateral opacification and reduced lung volumes. Pleural effusions may be present.

Pre-school age children are more prone to infections with respiratory syncytial virus (RSV), *Haemophilus*, pneumococcus and chlamydia.

(The Final FRCR Complete Revision Notes Page 326)

37. (d) Marfan syndrome

Marfan syndrome is an autosomal dominant connective tissue disorder which can lead to cardiac failure. Other cardiovascular associations include a dilated aortic root, aortic aneurysm, coarctation and dissection. Patients also have an increased risk of spontaneous pneumothorax as well as emphysema and bullae formation. The condition is associated with both pectus excavatum and carinatum and scoliosis. Ocular complications include myopia, cataracts, glaucoma and lens dislocation.

Beals syndrome is also a connective tissue disorder which can have similar appearances to Marfan syndrome but without the cardiac or ocular manifestations.

Patients with homocystinuria can also experience lens dislocation, pectus excavatum and scoliosis. The condition also typically affects the central nervous system and patients have prothrombotic tendencies

Loeys-Dietz syndrome is a rare autosomal dominant connective tissue disorder presenting, amongst other features, with a triad of bifid uvula or cleft palate, hypertelorism and arterial tortuosity and aneurysm formation.

Multiple endocrine neoplasia type IIb can cause marfanoid appearances; however it is also associated with phaeochromocytomas, medullary thyroid cancer and mucosal neuromas.

(The Final FRCR Complete Revision Notes Pages 1, 114)

38. (e) Paget's disease

Paget's disease has various phases. The initial lytic phase leads to bone resorption followed by laying down of abnormal bone with coarsened trabeculae and then later sclerosis predominates. Paget's disease typically affects the skull, pelvis, spine and long bones. The skull lesions described in the question are in keeping with osteoporosis circumscripta and are usually well-defined without a sclerotic margin. The humeral lesion which is extending along the cortex is consistent with the 'blade of grass' sign which describes a lucent leading edge when Paget's affects long bones. During the lucent phase of Paget's disease there is often increased tracer uptake on nuclear medicine bone scan due to the osteoblastic activity.

Fibrous dysplasia typically causes a 'ground glass' appearance within the bones rather than lysis. With myeloma there would usually be more diffuse skull and skeletal lytic lesions causing a 'raindrop' appearance when affecting the skull. Metastatic disease is possible, although again, more diffuse lesions may be expected; the distal long bones are also not typically affected initially. When there is malignant vertebral body marrow infiltration the uptake on nuclear medicine bone scan would usually be focal rather than the diffuse uptake described. Similarly, the peripheral uptake in the skull lesions is typical for osteoporosis circumscripta. Langerhans cell histiocytosis can cause lytic skull lesions but is not typical in this age group and lesions also tend to have bevelled, sclerotic margins.

(The Final FRCR Complete Revision Notes Page 88)

39. (d) Central T2 hyperintense scar on MRI

Focal nodular hyperplasia (FNH) is a benign, hamartomatous malformation that is most common in young women. In 50% of cases there is a central scar which is T2 hyperintense and shows delayed enhancement. Unlike adenoma, FNH is composed of normal liver tissue containing Kupffer cells. Therefore, they will show increased uptake of $Tc^{99}m$ and hepatobiliary specific contrast agents in sulphur colloid and MRI scans respectively. FNH is also typically smaller (<5 cm) than an adenoma; the latter can be very large at presentation. Adenomas are lipid rich and therefore often demonstrate T1 hyperintensity, similarly if it has been complicated by acute haemorrhage there will be foci of high T1

signal. FNH is usually iso or hypointense on T1 sequences.
(The Final FRCR Complete Revision Notes Page 207)

40. (c) Papillary necrosis
The findings of radiolucent filling defects in the renal collecting system along with other radiological features of sickle cell disease – avascular necrosis of the femoral head and splenic calcification – is consistent with papillary necrosis. This often presents with flank pain and haematuria. It is usually bilateral except in ascending infection or renal vein thrombosis and causes include sickle cell disease, tuberculosis, NSAID use and diabetes.
Indinavir, associated with antiretroviral drugs used in HIV treatment, is one cause of radiolucent calculi; however there are no other features of this in the case.
Acute tubular necrosis can cause debris in the collecting system but the history is usually one of an ischaemic or nephrotoxic event preceding its development. Ultrasound can demonstrate enlarged echogenic kidneys and if contrast is administered for a CT or IVU there may be a persistent nephrogram with minimal or absent filling of the collecting system.
Pyonephrosis usually presents with fever. Imaging can demonstrate layered echogenic/high density debris and/or gas within the collecting system. There may be perinephric stranding and renal abscess.
The history in this case is not consistent with pyeloureteritis cystica which is associated with urinary tract infection and causes benign cysts in the renal pelvis and ureter.
(The Final FRCR Complete Revision Notes Page 256)

41. (c) Increased splenic enhancement
Hypoperfusion complex may be evident on CT scans for patients with hypovolaemic shock. Hyperdense adrenals and kidneys are due to increased enhancement and in the kidneys due to decreased renal excretion. In contrast to this, the liver and spleen can demonstrate reduced contrast enhancement. Both the aorta and inferior vena cava may be small calibre and there may be a ring of low density fluid surrounding the inferior vena cava. The bowel loops may be thickened with hyperenhancing mucosa; this most commonly affects the jejunum.
(The Final FRCR Complete Revision Notes Page 340)

42. (d) Herpes simplex encephalitis
Herpes simplex encephalitis is the most common cause of viral encephalitis. The typical features are bilateral temporal lobe involvement; however this can be asymmetrical, and involvement of the insular cortex, cingulate gyrus and frontal lobes is also common. There is frequently T2 and FLAIR hyperintensity involving the white matter and cortex and low T1 signal due to oedema. Areas of haemorrhage may develop, which will be high on T1 and low on T2 sequences. There is often restricted diffusion and gyral and leptomeningeal enhancement.
Encephalitis caused by other viruses, such as Epstein-Barr virus, can have similar imaging appearances; however, they are much less likely as HSV accounts for 90% of all viral encephalitis.
Autoimmune encephalitis is one differential; however, haemorrhage is more common in HSV encephalitis and sparing of the basal ganglia is also more suggestive of HSV.
Neurosyphilis is usually seen in association with HIV infection and can cause bacterial meningitis, encephalitis or arteritis leading to infarcts, often in the brainstem, basal ganglia and middle cerebral artery territory. HSV encephalitis is much more common and the distribution of signal changes in this case is typical for HSV encephalitis.
Middle cerebral territory infarcts are sometimes a differential for the changes associated with HSV encephalitis due to the territory involved; however, the bilateral abnormalities in this case and the sparing of the basal ganglia are less consistent with infarct.
Gliomatosis cerebri would be less likely in an acute presentation, especially with fever. The cerebral changes are often much more diffuse and confluent.
(The Final FRCR Complete Revision Notes Page 414)

43. (c) Pleural effusion
A wide spectrum of pleuropulmonary findings are seen in rheumatoid disease, the severity of which are not indicative of the arthritis severity. It occurs typically in patients who are positive for rheumatoid factor, and men are affected more commonly than women. The most frequent finding in the thorax in patients with rheumatoid arthritis is a pleural effusion. It is usually unilateral; however, it can be bilateral and small or moderate in size. Pleural thickening may also

be present. Patients are usually asymptomatic. Pulmonary (rheumatoid) nodules are usually well circumscribed; they may cavitate and can be multiple. Rheumatoid disease is also associated with pulmonary fibrosis, most commonly usual interstitial pneumonia but also non-specific interstitial pneumonia. Bronchiectasis and bronchiolitis obliterans are seen in a third of patients.
(The Final FRCR Complete Revision Notes Pages 52–53)

44. (b) No further action required
The features described are of osteitis condensans ilii, a benign appearance described typically in women who have had children but also seen in nulliparous females and males. Appearances affect the iliac side of the sacroiliac joint with subchondral sclerosis which is often triangular in shape. The sacroiliac joint space is preserved and normal in appearance. It is usually an incidental finding, although there are reports of it causing lower back pain.
In a case such as this where it is an incidental finding, no further action is required.
If there were features of sacroiliitis with changes affecting both sides of the sacroiliac joints and the joint itself, then review of other skeletal films and/or rheumatology referral may be indicated. An MRI or nuclear medicine bone scan would not be appropriate for this indication but can be helpful in detecting insufficiency fractures of the sacrum; however this would normally affect an older age group.
(The Final FRCR Complete Revision Notes Page 86)

45. (d) Pseudomyxoma peritonei
Pseudomyxoma peritonei is characterised by large volume of low attenuation, often loculated fluid. There may be peritoneal calcifications present and the fluid typically causes a scalloped appearance of the liver contour. The cause is thought to be secondary to a ruptured benign or malignant appendiceal or ovarian mucinous tumour.
Calcifications may be associated with tuberculosis; however, the ascites associated with tuberculosis tends to have a higher density.
The patient does not have any past medical history, such as previous peritoneal dialysis or a ventriculoperitoneal shunt, to suggest sclerosing peritonitis is likely, and the calcification associated with this tends to be extensive.
Peritoneal mesothelioma is rare and is not associated with large volume ascites. There is frequently evidence of pleural calcification as peritoneal calcification can be variable.
Enlarged lymph nodes would be expected with peritoneal lymphomatosis. There are also frequently splenic deposits and nodular peritoneal soft tissue thickening. Involvement may also extend both above and below the diaphragm.
(The Final FRCR Complete Revision Notes Page 191)

46. (b) Elevated Cho/NAA ratio
Table 2.4 displays some of the key factors that can be used to aid differentiation between tumour recurrence and chemoradiotherapy damage (pseudo progression).
In pseudo progression, ADC values usually increase as cell destruction occurs. ADC values are variable in progressing tumours and this is dependent on the tumour grade. This is therefore not a reliable way to differentiate between the two conditions. Lactate and lipid peaks are increased in both tumour progression and pseudo progression.
(The Final FRCR Complete Revision Notes Page 386)

Table 2.4: The Differentiation of Tumour Recurrence versus Pseudoprogression

	Pseudoprogression	Tumour Recurrence
MRI spectroscopy	↓Choline	↓NAA ↑Choline
CT perfusion	↓rCBV	↑rCBV
Thallium SPECT	↓	↑

Source: Modified from and reprinted with permission from V Helyar and A Shaw, *The Final FRCR: Complete Revision Notes*. CRC Press, Taylor & Francis Group, 2018, p. 386.

47. (e) Transient tachypnoea of the newborn
The history of the illness, with a baby born at term (>37 weeks' gestation) by caesarean section, onset within 6 hours following delivery and improvement after 2–3 days is suggestive of transient tachypnoea of the new born. The radiograph is also consistent with this due to normal lung volumes, perihilar air space opacification and pleural fluid which resolves with symptom resolution.
The history is not typical for meconium aspiration which is usually associated with a traumatic delivery. Meconium aspiration is most common in term or post-term infants and is associated with hyperinflation rather than normal lung volumes; however, other radiographic features do include perihilar changes and pleural effusions.
Beta-haemolytic streptococcal pneumonia more commonly affects premature infants. In contrast to this case, it is usually associated with reduced lung volumes and diffuse opacity. There may be pleural effusions.
Infant respiratory distress syndrome due to surfactant deficiency is also a condition affecting premature infants and is associated with reduced lung volumes. Pleural effusions are uncommon.
Patent ductus arteriosus (PDA) is most common in premature infants. The most common congenital heart defects are ventricular and atrial septal defects. Patent ductus arteriosus can be asymptomatic if small, but if large they present with signs of heart failure due to the left to right shunt. PDA is an acyanotic congenital cardiac anomaly and children may have signs of cardiomegaly and pulmonary oedema.
(The Final FRCR Complete Revision Notes Page 329)

48. (e) Right subdural collection
The right subdural collection has features of a subdural empyema with rim enhancement and restricted diffusion. This requires urgent surgical evacuation and is therefore the most urgent clinically relevant finding.
The collection adjacent to the left frontal lobe is thin and not causing significant mass effect. In the context of recent trauma, the areas of hypointensity on susceptibility weighted imaging at the grey–white matter interface and in the corpus callosum are consistent with diffuse axonal injury. It is important for the clinical team to be aware of this but it does not need to urgently be relayed to the them.
The left cerebellopontine angle lesion is consistent with an arachnoid cyst, which is a benign finding. Similarly, the cerebellar tonsil protrusion is within normal limits. At 3–5 mm below the foramen magnum this would be termed as benign tonsillar ectopia. Over 5 mm would correlate with a Chiari I malformation.
(The Final FRCR Complete Revision Notes Page 411)

49. (d) Abdominal ultrasound
This case describes alpha 1 antitrypsin deficiency. This is diagnosed with measurement of alpha 1 antitrypsin serum levels. Radiological features in the lungs include predominantly lower lobe emphysema and bronchiectasis in relatively young patients. The condition can also cause liver cirrhosis. Emphysema and cirrhosis are common causes of death. Therefore, abdominal ultrasound is the correct answer as the patient will likely have signs of liver disease and if chronic, may have features of portal hypertension with splenomegaly, varices and ascites. Other conditions associated with alpha 1 antitrypsin deficiency include asthma, pancreatitis and panniculitis.
(The Final FRCR Complete Revision Notes Page 17)

50. (e) Low T1 and low T2 signal in the sinus tarsi
The sinus tarsi is a tunnel between the calcaneus and talus which has important roles in foot stability and proprioception. It is a complex structure associated with the subtalar joint and several ligaments. It is usually filled with fat, which would be high on T1 and T2 weighted imaging. In sinus tarsi syndrome this is replaced with scar tissue, which is low both on T1 and T2 weighted imaging. Sinus tarsi syndrome can present with tenderness, pain on walking and instability. It can come on following ankle sprains, such as in this case, but it is also associated with inflammatory arthropathies.
A normal Böhler's angle is 20–40°. An angle <20° is suggestive of calcaneal fracture; however, it does not play a role in diagnosing sinus tarsi syndrome.
High STIR signal in the calcaneus is indicative of bone marrow oedema, which can have various causes.
(The Final FRCR Complete Revision Notes Page 97)

51. (d) Omental infarction

The differential lies between omental infarction and epiploic appendagitis. Epiploic appendagitis is most common in the rectosigmoid and ileocaecal regions; however, omental infarction is most likely adjacent to the ascending colon. The fact that this lesion is relatively large (>3 cm) is also more consistent with omental infarction. Both conditions cause high attenuation within the fat but epiploic appendagitis classically has additional features which may aid differentiation, including a hyperdense rim and a central hyperdense dot.

Diverticulitis and mesenteric vein thrombosis are both unlikely when the adjacent bowel has been described as normal. Desmoid tumours are rare and usually well-defined soft tissue masses, most commonly occurring in relation to the anterior abdominal wall, retroperitoneum or root of the mesentery.

(The Final FRCR Complete Revision Notes Page 190)

Pereira JM, Sirlin CB, Pinto PS et al. Disproportionate fat stranding: a helpful CT sign in patients with acute abdominal pain. RadioGraphics. 2004;24(3):703–715.

52. (e) 18F-FDG PET/CT and MRI pelvis

Royal College of Radiology and National Comprehensive Cancer Network guidelines suggest that PET/CT is indicated for locally advanced cervical cancer (≥FIGO stage Ib2 disease) considered for radical chemoradiotherapy. Based on the information provided in this case the patient has a FIGO Stage IIa1 tumour; therefore the most appropriate initial imaging from the available choices would be 18F-FDG PET/CT and MRI pelvis. Previously, CT and MRI were the modalities of choice, with PET/CT reserved for more challenging cases; however, recent studies have found that PET/CT can detect additional avid nodes which may change management, for example by extending the radiotherapy field to include the paraaortic region. US pelvis does not have a role in staging for cervical cancer.

(The Final FRCR Complete Revision Notes Page 271)

53. (d) Mesenchymal hamartoma

Mesenchymal hamartomas are benign. They are commonly multiloculated cystic lesions; some may contain vascular solid components and septae. They can have a very similar appearance to an infantile haemangioendothelioma; however unlike these, the aorta is normal calibre with a mesenchymal hamartoma.

Alpha-fetoprotein helps to differentiate between mesenchymal hamartoma and hepatoblastoma. Hepatoblastomas are also usually solid masses, although they may contain regions of haemorrhage and necrosis.

Wilms tumour, also known as nephroblastoma, can metastasise to the lungs, liver and lymph nodes. The normal appearance of the kidneys in this case makes metastases unlikely.

The diagnosis of hepatic adenoma is usually made in an older age group than this patient, classically in young females taking oral contraceptives. Their appearance can vary, but they are typically solid masses which may be heterogenous due to haemorrhage and fat.

(The Final FRCR Complete Revision Notes Page 344)

54. (a) Central neurocytoma

These are WHO grade II tumours with characteristic imaging appearances. They are typically seen in young adults. They appear as heterogenous intraventricular masses, typically attached to the septum pellucidum with a variable enhancement pattern. Calcification is common. Patients often present with headaches related to raised cerebrospinal fluid pressure.

Ependymomas are typically seen in the fourth ventricle and in younger patients. Intraventricular meningiomas would normally show more homogenous enhancement.

Subependymal giant cell astrocytomas (SEGAs) are usually seen in patients with tuberous sclerosis and show avid contrast enhancement. Choroid plexus papilloma is generally seen in children and show avid enhancement.

(The Final FRCR Complete Revision Notes Page 397)

55. (a) Bronchogenic cyst

Bronchogenic cysts are often solitary and asymptomatic. They typically have thin non-enhancing walls lined with respiratory epithelium and have a density similar to water, although this can be slightly higher depending on protein content. The subcarinal location is common but they can be anywhere adjacent to the trachea, and occasionally within the lungs themselves.

A lymph node does not have a wall. Usually there is cortex surrounding a fatty hilum, although abnormal nodes can become more rounded, necrotic and lose normal architecture. Unless necrotic, the density would usually be closer to soft tissue density and there may be enhancement following contrast administration.

Enteric cysts are uncommon, and compared to bronchogenic cysts have thick walls lined with gastrointestinal epithelium and are intimately related to the oesophagus. They can become symptomatic due to peptic ulceration, infection and haemorrhage.

Neurenteric cysts occur in the posterior rather than the middle mediastinum, between the oesophagus and spine, and are typically closely related to the spine. Similar to enteric cysts, they can be symptomatic, causing pain, and can be associated with vertebral anomalies.

Pericardial cysts are often asymptomatic lesions at the cardiophrenic angles (R > L) inseparable from the pericardium.

(The Final FRCR Complete Revision Notes Page 24)

56. (c) Kienböck disease

The description is that of avascular necrosis of the lunate bone. The usual age of onset in this condition is 20–40 years. The condition is associated with negative ulnar variance. Blount disease is avascular necrosis of the medial tibial condyle, usually affecting patients over 6 years age. Freiberg disease typically affects the head of the second metatarsal. Sometimes the third or fourth metatarsal may be affected. Köhler disease is avascular necrosis of the navicular in patients 3–10 years old, more common in boys. Preiser disease is non-traumatic osteonecrosis of the scaphoid.

(The Final FRCR Complete Revision Notes Page 82)

57. (c) Hepatic amyloidosis

Causes of increased liver attenuation include haemochromatosis, amiodarone use, thorotrastosis, iron overload, Wilson disease and haemosiderosis. The latter can occur due to haemolytic conditions such as thalassaemia or in conditions necessitating multiple blood transfusions. In contrast to this, causes of decreased liver attenuation include diffuse fatty infiltration, amyloidosis, hepatic venous congestion and steroid use. Glycogen storage disease can cause either increased or reduced attenuation.

Haemochromatosis and haemosiderosis have similar imaging appearances on CT and MRI but the distribution of changes varies slightly. MRI will demonstrate low signal with both conditions; however in haemochromatosis the hyperattenuation on CT and reduced signal intensity on MRI will be in the liver, pancreas and heart. In contrast to this, haemosiderosis causes hyperattenuation and reduced signal intensity in the liver and spleen.

(The Final FRCR Complete Revision Notes Page 197)

58. (d) Intraosseous lipoma

The features described are consistent with an intraosseous lipoma. This is a rare lesion, usually present in the metadiaphysis of long bones, particularly the intertrochanteric/subtrochanteric femur. Features on plain film are a lucent lesion with a thin sclerotic margin and a central calcified nidus. CT features are low density (–60 to –100HU). On MRI the lesion is high T1 with a low signal rim.

Chondromyxoid fibroma is a rare cartilaginous tumour which is a well-defined lucent lesion with a sclerotic rim. On MRI the lesions have a low signal on T1.

Although fibrous dysplasia can look like anything, the description of T1 high signal is more typical of a lipoma.

Intraosseous ganglion cyst has low T1 and high T2 signal on MRI.

Metastases would not be expected to have a sclerotic rim and would be low signal on T1.

(The Final FRCR Complete Revision Notes Pages 132–133, 143–144)

59. (c) IgA vasculitis (Henoch-Schönlein purpura)

IgA vasculitis often follows an upper respiratory tract infection. The condition is characterised by findings such as a rash on the extensor surfaces, arthralgia, glomerulonephritis, gastrointestinal bleeding and intussusception.

Granulomatosis with polyangiitis (formerly known as Wegener granulomatosis) can cause glomerulonephritis and haemoptysis but less commonly causes cutaneous or musculoskeletal manifestations.

Eosinophilic granulomatosis with polyangiitis (formerly known as Churg-Strauss) can also cause arthralgia and rashes but is not associated with the other findings in this case and would also be associated with asthma and sinusitis.

Systemic lupus erythematosus causes glomerulonephritis, musculoskeletal symptoms and a rash but it is usually a characteristic butterfly facial rash. Intussusception is not a feature, although there are commonly other gastrointestinal manifestations.

(The Final FRCR Complete Revision Notes Page 338)

60. (e) Tornwaldt cyst

Tornwaldt cysts are commonly asymptomatic, incidental findings on imaging of the head and neck. They are midline nasopharyngeal mucosal cysts and can have variable MRI signal depending on their protein content. On CT they can exhibit fluid density or be slightly hyperdense.

Ranula are cystic lesions that occur at the floor of the mouth in the sublingual space, although they can extend to the submandibular region (diving type).

Rathke cleft cysts are midline cysts but they occur intracranially adjacent to the pituitary gland in the sella.

Branchial cleft cysts are usually away from the midline and present as palpable neck masses occurring at a variety of locations, ranging from near the external auditory canal to adjacent to the thyroid gland.

Thyroglossal duct cysts cause palpable midline neck masses, most commonly in the paediatric population. They can be located anywhere along the course of the thyroglossal duct but they are most commonly infrahyoid.

(The Final FRCR Complete Revision Notes Page 430)

61. (b) Teratoma

The description is of a teratoma, a benign germ cell tumour. Teratomas are cystic and often have a fatty component. Calcification is common. A thickened soft tissue focus demonstrating enhancement would raise suspicion of malignancy.

Thymoma and thymic carcinoma are the most common neoplasms of the anterior mediastinum; however they are usually of soft tissue density. Although cystic and calcified foci are common, particularly in malignant types, fat density is not a feature.

Lymphoma is most commonly a well-defined homogeneous soft tissue mass. Cystic, calcific and fat densities are not usually seen.

Thymus hyperplasia can occur in response to stress, such as chemotherapy; however this is most likely soft tissue density.

Thymolipoma is a rare lesion composed of thymic tissue and adipose tissue, usually in equal portions. Calcification is rare, unlike in teratoma.

(The Final FRCR Complete Revision Notes Page 57)

62. (c) Haemarthrosis

Scurvy is caused by vitamin C deficiency which leads to abnormal collagen and bone development and a bleeding diathesis. Features include ground glass osteoporosis, sclerosis of the margins of the epiphysis (Wimberger sign), metaphyseal spurs, dense metaphyseal lines (lines of Frankel), Trummerfield zone (radiolucent zone on the diaphyseal line of the Frankel line), pencil-point cortical thinning, corner fractures, an exuberant periosteal reaction and haemarthrosis. Coarsened trabeculae are not features of the condition. Cloaca, involucrum and sequestrum are features of osteomyelitis.

(The Final FRCR Complete Revision Notes Pages 125–126, 87)

63. (c) IIIA

Cholangiocarcinoma can have varying appearances, forming a distinct mass, such as in this question, or having peri- or intraductal growth. In the mass-forming subtype, the typical CT appearances are of an iso- or hypodense mass with delayed centripetal enhancement. In peri- and intraductal cholangiocarcinoma they can cause narrowing of the bile ducts with distal dilatation. Cholangiocarcinoma most commonly affects the right hepatic lobe. They can be staged using the Bismuth classification, and the extent of bile duct involvement is key. This patient has abnormal signal associated with, and dilatation of, the right second-order ducts, which would make it IIIA.

(The Final FRCR Complete Revision Notes Page 200)

Table 2.5: Bismuth Classification of Cholangiocarcinoma

I	Common bile duct
II	Hilar and first-order ducts
IIIA	Hilar and extending into the second-order ducts of the right
IIIB	Hilar and extending into the second-order ducts on the left
IV	Hilar and extending into the second-order ducts bilaterally

Source: Reprinted with permission from V Helyar and A Shaw, *The Final FRCR: Complete Revision Notes.* CRC Press, Taylor & Francis Group, 2018, p. 200.

64. (a) Examination, imaging, biopsy
Triple assessment involves clinical examination, imaging and biopsy. In a patient of this age, it is likely the imaging will be an ultrasound; however sometimes other modalities are required, such as MRI, mammogram, contrast-enhanced mammography or tomosynthesis. The breast and axilla should always be assessed together. Most biopsies are ultrasound guided although sometimes stereotactic biopsy (guided by mammograms or tomosynthesis) is required. MDT discussion is routine following biopsy, particularly if malignant.
(The Final FRCR Complete Revision Notes Page 281)

65. (a) The posterior fossa has normal appearances
Aqueductal stenosis is the most common cause of congenital hydrocephalus. This is frequently detected on antenatal ultrasound scans. Neonatal cranial ultrasound scans can also be helpful. The key feature that helps differentiate aqueductal stenosis from Chiari or Dandy-Walker malformations is a normal appearing posterior fossa. Hydrocephalus affects the third and lateral ventricles and the fourth ventricle is normal. The absence of a T2 flow void at the level of the aqueduct is suggestive of the condition. The aqueduct may have a funnelled appearance and sometimes a web may be evident as an underlying cause. The most useful sequence for diagnosis is a sagittal acquisition.
(The Final FRCR Complete Revision Notes Page 288)

66. (d) Anterior communicating artery
The patient has presented with typical symptoms of subarachnoid haemorrhage: a sudden onset, and 'thunderclap' headache which can be associated with reduced GCS. The patient has polycystic kidney disease which is associated with intracranial aneurysms. The vast majority of cases of subarachnoid haemorrhage are due to a ruptured aneurysm. Other causes include trauma or an arteriovenous malformation. The most common sites for blood to be located in subarachnoid haemorrhage secondary to aneurysm rupture is around the circle of Willis or the Sylvian fissures. The anterior communicating artery is the most common site for intracranial aneurysm, and subarachnoid blood in the anterior interhemispheric fissure is a typical location. There is a 2% annual risk of rupture with a known aneurysm if there is no previous rupture.
(The Final FRCR Complete Revision Notes Page 376)

67. (d) Non-specific interstitial pneumonia (NSIP)
Sjögren syndrome is an autoimmune condition which affects the salivary glands and also has pulmonary associations. Whilst Sjögren syndrome is one of the only connective tissue diseases associated with lymphocytic interstitial pneumonitis (LIP), and the features described in the main stem could be in keeping with LIP. This condition is rare. The most common associated interstitial lung fibrosis is NSIP. This is demonstrated as predominantly ground glass change with reticular opacities and immediate subpleural sparing with traction dilatation of the small airways.
Usual interstitial pneumonitis may also be seen in Sjögren syndrome and should be considered if honeycomb destruction of the lung parenchyma is the main abnormality. Desquamative interstitial pneumonia is more common in men and strongly associated with smoking. It is not associated with Sjögren syndrome. Acute interstitial pneumonitis is an acute form of the interstitial pneumonias; however it is of unknown aetiology and not associated with Sjögren syndrome.
(The Final FRCR Complete Revision Notes Page 37)

68. (a) It always affects the mandible.
Cherubism was historically considered a subtype of fibrous dysplasia. It is inherited in an autosomal dominant pattern. It always affects the mandible, and presents with painless progressive swelling of the cheeks. The description provided in the question is a typical description of the radiographic features of the condition. Lesions usually extend from the molar teeth towards the midline. Mandibular involvement is most commonly bilateral but maxillary involvement is variable. It occurs less frequently and is less extensively involved. The condition does not occur without mandibular involvement. Dental abnormalities including incomplete development, root resorption and loss of teeth are common. It is not associated with ameloblastoma but histologically resembles a giant cell granuloma.
(The Final FRCR Complete Revision Notes Page 139)
Jain V and Sharma R. CT and MRI features of cherubism. Pediatric Radiology. 2006;36:1099–1104.

69. (e) Tailgut cyst
Tailgut cysts occur in the presacral space. They are frequently multilocular and can be simple, with high T2 and low T1 weighted signal on MRI, or they can be complicated by infection or haemorrhagic or mucinous components. Despite the history, the normal appearance of the ovaries and lack of high T1 signal on the fat-supressed sequence excludes an endometrioma. The intermediate T1 signal is suggestive of a mucinous component rather than the high T1 signal associated with fat which would be evident in a dermoid cyst. An anterior sacral meningocele would typically be associated with a sacral bone abnormality; however the bones in this case have normal appearances. A duplication cyst is another differential; however, they are usually unilocular.
Depending on the internal contents, these lesions are usually fluid or soft tissue density on CT. Malignant transformation is rare; however, these cysts are often removed surgically.
(The Final FRCR Complete Revision Notes Page 186)

70. (b) 500 µg of 1:1000 intramuscular adrenaline
Resuscitation Council UK has a clear algorithm for the management of anaphylaxis. Following diagnosis with an ABCDE approach and calling for help, the next step is adrenaline. For an adult the dose is 500 µg (0.5 mL) of 1:1000 intramuscular adrenaline. Intravenous adrenaline should only be used by clinicians experienced in administering it via this route. The dose of 1 mg of 1:10,0000 adrenaline is used during cardiopulmonary resuscitation. Following the dose of adrenaline, further steps such as high-flow oxygen, chlorphenamine, hydrocortisone and IV fluids should be administered as required. It is helpful if the algorithm is clearly displayed in all areas of the radiology department where contrast is administered and a pre-prepared anaphylaxis box is close at hand, along with resuscitation trolley, should it be required.
Resuscitation Council (UK). 2016. Emergency treatment of anaphylactic reactions: Guidelines for healthcare providers. https://www.resus.org.uk/anaphylaxis/emergency-treatment-of-anaphylactic-reactions/

71. (b) Main duct intraductal papillary mucinous neoplasm
Intraductal papillary mucinous neoplasm (IPMN) is a mucin-producing tumour that arises from the epithelium of the main pancreatic duct or a branch. The factors that suggest that this is a main duct IPMN are the dilatation of the pancreatic duct and pancreatic atrophy. These features are less common in branch duct IPMN. The enhancing solid nodule is suspicious for malignancy, which again is more common in main duct IPMN. Cystic lesions communicating directly with the main pancreatic duct suggest a branch duct IPMN. The mucinous secretions are high signal on T2 (aggregations of mucin can mimic the tumour itself and are low signal on T2).
Mucinous and serous cystadenoma do not communicate with the main pancreatic duct. Mucinous cystadenomas are more common in the pancreatic body and tail than the head, whereas serous cystadenomas have a more even distribution throughout the pancreas. Calcification can be a feature of both lesions; mucinous lesions tend to have calcification peripherally, whereas serous lesions have central calcification. The history is not typical for an insulinoma, which usually presents early due to hypoglycaemia.
(The Final FRCR Complete Revision Notes Page 232)

72 (b) Enhancing bilateral cerebellopontine angle masses
Neurofibromatosis (NF) 1 has an autosomal dominant inheritance pattern; however around half of cases are due to sporadic mutation. It is much more common than NF2. The central

nervous, musculoskeletal and renal systems are most commonly affected. Common central nervous system findings include optic nerve gliomas, sphenoid wing dysplasia, kyphoscoliosis and dural ectasia causing vertebral body scalloping. Focal areas of signal intensity (FASIs) are also a feature, and manifest as multiple cerebral and cerebellar high T2 and FLAIR foci. Bilateral acoustic neuromas are seen in NF2.

(The Final FRCR Complete Revision Notes Page 381)

73. (b) MacLeod syndrome

The finding is most likely due to MacLeod syndrome, also known as Swyer-James syndrome. It is often an incidental finding and is due to previous childhood infectious bronchiolitis. Radiographic findings are that of a hyperlucent lung with reduced lung markings and normal or small volume lung and hilum on the affected side. On HRCT there is also bronchiectasis and bronchial wall thickening.

Poland syndrome is a congenital unilateral absence of the pectoralis major and minor muscles which causes increased transradiancy of the hemithorax. There may also be associated chest wall deformity. This is within the differentials for this case; however, it is a comparatively rare condition and not associated with the paucity of vascular markings and small hilum.

Large pulmonary embolus may cause the imaging features of reduced lung markings. The 'Westermark' sign is a radiographic sign of focal increased lucency of the lung, thought to be secondary to occlusion of the pulmonary artery or due to vasoconstriction distal to the embolus. This sign is not commonly seen and the patient in the main stem is asymptomatic.

Hyperlucency due to rotation occurs in the same hemithorax as the direction of rotation and so this cannot account for the findings in this stem.

Pneumothorax is also an important consideration; however absent lung markings would be expected as well as presence of a lung edge.

(The Final FRCR Complete Revision Notes Pages 43, 49)

74. (a) Brown tumour

Brown tumours can be seen in primary or secondary hyperparathyroidism. They can mimic metastases and myeloma. Brown tumours are well-defined, lucent and expansile lesions commonly found in the jaw, rib or pelvis. There is no periosteal reaction. Following treatment they may become sclerotic or disappear. Subperiosteal bone resorption is pathognomonic for hyperparathyroidism and the distal clavicle is a common site.

Fibrous dysplasia can look like anything; however it would not be expected to resolve.

Haemangiomas are usually seen in the vertebrae and would have coarsened trabeculae.

Myeloma and metastases are important considerations; however the hormonal disorder and subperiosteal bone resorption favours a brown tumour.

(The Final FRCR Complete Revision Notes Page 132)

75. (c) Primary sclerosing cholangitis (PSC)

The description is typical for PSC. This condition typically affects males aged 20–40 years. It is an idiopathic, progressive, fibrosing inflammatory disorder of the biliary tree. Associated with ulcerative colitis (UC), Riedel thyroiditis, Sjögren syndrome, cystic fibrosis (CF) and retroperitoneal fibrosis. Imaging features include both intra- and extrahepatic duct strictures with alternating segments of dilatation and stenosis (the 'string of beads' appearance on MRCP). On ultrasound there is increased echogenicity of the portal triads. MRCP can demonstrate a 'pruned tree' appearance with obliteration of the peripheral ducts.

Primary biliary cirrhosis is the inflammatory destruction of peripheral bile ducts leading to cirrhosis. The majority of patients are female. It is associated with autoimmune disorders including rheumatoid arthritis, Sjögren syndrome, scleroderma and Hashimoto thyroiditis. The disease is limited to the intrahepatic bile ducts.

(The Final FRCR Complete Revision Notes Page 219)

76. (b) Adrenal haemorrhage

The appearances of the adrenal gland are most likely in keeping with haemorrhage, which can be seen following trauma. It can also be seen in association with shock or secondary to an underlying tumour. In the cases of shock, the haemorrhage is more likely to be bilateral. Bilateral haemorrhage can cause adrenal insufficiency, a life-threatening condition unless steroids are given. Haemorrhage can mature to a cystic lesion and become calcified.

Adrenal laceration occurs less commonly than adrenal haemorrhage, when it occurs the right adrenal gland is most commonly affected, due to compression of the gland between the liver and the spine.

Adrenal hyperplasia is diffuse thickening of the adrenal limbs, although it may be normal at the time of physiological stress.

Adrenal myelolipoma is a rare, benign adrenal tumour associated with punctate calcification. Low attenuation due to fat is diagnostic of this lesion.

(The Final FRCR Complete Revision Notes Page 268)

77. (a) Band heterotopia

Band heterotropia is a diffuse form of grey matter heterotopia almost exclusively affecting females. It is associated with seizures and developmental delay. On imaging, this condition is characterised by a band of grey matter located deep to and roughly paralleling the cortex.

Polymicrogyria is another form of cortical maldevelopment where there are numerous small gyri.

Schizencephaly is a rare cortical malformation that manifests as a grey matter–lined cleft extending from the ependyma to the pia matter.

Subependymal and subcortical heterotopia are more nodular types of heterotopia rather than the diffuse types (band and lissencephaly).

(The Final FRCR Complete Revision Notes Page 291)

78. (e) Wernicke encephalopathy

Wernicke encephalopathy is caused by thiamine (vitamin B1) deficiency and is typically seen in alcoholics or those who self-neglect. It presents with the classic triad of confusion, ataxia and ophthalmoplegia. Korsakoff psychosis is the chronic form of the condition and is characterised by confabulation and memory loss. MRI findings include symmetrical high signal on T2 and FLAIR sequences with post-contrast enhancement in the mammillary bodies, basal ganglia, paraventricular/medial thalamic regions, brain stem and periaqueductal grey matter. Korsakoff syndrome is associated with mammillary body atrophy and dilatation of the third ventricle.

Leigh syndrome can have similar imaging appearances but occurs in young children and the mammillary bodies are spared. Pontine glioma are also more common in children. Furthermore, the supra- and infratentorial abnormalities in this case are not consistent with this diagnosis. Osmotic demyelination is possible in patients with chronic alcohol misuse due to rapid correction of hyponatraemia; however, the radiological features are more consistent with Wernicke encephalopathy.

(The Final FRCR Complete Revision Notes Page 385)

79. (c) Nodule mass

Lung nodules are a common finding on CT chest imaging. The mixed ground glass nodule is a significant finding due to the high malignancy rate associated with them. A study published in the June 2018 *Clinical Radiology* journal by X-W Wang et al. considered features which may be useful in predicting invasive adenocarcinoma (ICA) compared to adenocarcinoma in-situ (AIS) and minimally invasive adenocarcinoma (MIA). There is emerging evidence to suggest that AIS and MIA may be able to undergo sublobar resection instead of lobectomy (an important consideration in the elderly or those with bilateral ground glass nodules), whereas IAC requires lobectomy. Thus presurgical assessment of the nodule is required. This study reports that the most powerful predictor of IAC over AIS or MIA is nodule mass. Mass can be calculated using computer-aided measurement, which considers nodule volume as well as CT attenuation value. Nodule volume and diameter were also found to be statistically significant predictor of IAC; however less powerful than mass, as they do not consider internal attenuation. Nodule location and multiplicity were not found to be significant predictors of IACs.

Wang XW, Chen WF, He WJ et al. CT features differentiating pre- and minimally invasive from invasive adenocarcinoma appearing as mixed ground glass nodule: mass is a potential imaging biomarker. Clinical Radiology. 2018;73(3) 549–554.

80. (a) The bony protrusion is directed away from the joint

An osteochondroma is a cartilage capped exostosis, classically directed away from the joint space. It most frequently affects the lower limbs. It is the most common benign bone tumour, seen between the ages of 2 and 60 years. Cartilage cap thickness of >2 cm on CT and >1 cm on

MRI is indicative of chondrosarcomatous change. This occurs in less than 1% of cases. Fracture of the stem is rare; the lesion is usually identified incidentally or with an enlarging painless lesion. Rarely they may be multiple, such as in diaphyseal aclasis, which is also known as hereditary multiple osteochondromatosis.
(The Final FRCR Complete Revision Notes Page 145)

81. (e) Signal dropout of the liver on out-of-phase MRI sequence.
Fatty liver disease is caused by accumulation of fat into hepatocytes. On ultrasound the renal cortex is hyporeflective compared to the adjacent liver. On CT a liver density of <40HU is specific but not sensitive. Density of >10HU less than the spleen on unenhanced CT is diagnostic. The spleen enhances earlier than the liver, so comparing densities in the arterial or early portal venous phases is unhelpful. Fatty liver shows reduced tracer uptake on $Tc^{99}m$ sulphur colloid scan. In- and out-of-phase imaging is best for diagnosis: there is loss of signal on out-of-phase imaging compared to in-phase imaging.
(The Final FRCR Complete Revision Notes Page 205)
Hamer OW, Aguirre DA, Casola G et al. Fatty liver: imaging patterns and pitfalls. RadioGraphics. 2006;26(6):1637–1653.

82. (c) Cardiac anomaly
Cytomegalovirus (CMV) is the most common intrauterine infection and intracranially can cause hydrocephalus, microcephaly, delayed myelination and cerebral calcification. The calcification tends to be periventricular and will be hyperechoic on a cranial ultrasound. More generally, it can cause intrauterine growth restriction and in the abdomen can cause hepatomegaly. There is overlap between many of the features in the congenital TORCH infections; however, CMV is not usually associated with congenital cardiac anomalies, whereas rubella frequently is.
(The Final FRCR Complete Revision Notes Page 290)

83. (b) Glioblastoma
The key features that make glioblastoma more likely are the central fluid signal suggesting necrosis, the complete rim of enhancement, mild restricted diffusion and markedly increased relative cerebral blood flow both in and around the lesion.
The patient has radiological features of multiple sclerosis (MS). The left temporal lobe lesion is different and the central fluid signal is concerning for necrosis and raises the possibility of a malignant lesion, infective process or tumefactive multiple sclerosis.
Lymphoma usually enhances homogenously (the exception is in patients with AIDS where there may be central necrosis and rim enhancement). The relative cerebral blood flow (rCBF) may be slightly raised with lymphoma but not to the same degree as a glioblastoma.
Differentiating ring enhancing lesions is important on an MRI brain. Tumefactive multiple sclerosis is an important differential in a patient with other signs of MS; however, unlike in this case, the rim of enhancement is usually incomplete and rCBF is usually reduced.
Intracranial abscesses would usually have restricted diffusion centrally and this is a useful differentiating factor between them and other pathologies. rCBF is also usually reduced compared to glioblastoma.
Metastases can have a similar appearance to glioblastoma; however the rCBF in the oedema surrounding the lesion is usually reduced.
(The Final FRCR Complete Revision Notes Pages 391, 419)

84. (c) Retinoblastoma
The location and MRI signal are characteristic of retinoblastoma. A calcified intraocular mass in a young child (<3 years) is a retinoblastoma until proven otherwise. Rhabdomyosarcoma, capillary and cavernous haemangiomas are extraocular tumours. Cavernous haemangiomas do not usually present until later adulthood. Furthermore, capillary and cavernous haemangiomas tend to show avid homogenous enhancement. Retrolental fibroplasia, also known as retinopathy of prematurity, is an ocular condition seen in the infant population which usually affects both eyes and can cause the globes to be small, calcification can also occur.
(The Final FRCR Complete Revision Notes Page 309)

85. (a) Allergic bronchopulmonary aspergillosis (ABPA)
This patient has typical features of ABPA. The 'finger-in-glove' appearance is caused by gross perihilar bronchiectatic airways filled with mucous. Late disease also has upper lobe fibrosis indicated by the elevated fissures and hila. ABPA is associated with asthma and cystic fibrosis. This

is a young patient with a central venous catheter indicating long-term drug therapy. In a cystic fibrosis patient this typically will be antibiotics. The upper lobe fibrosis is also typical of cystic fibrosis.

Drug-induced lung disease does not typically have these features and can be non-specific, varying depending on the drug therapy.

Invasive aspergillosis is associated with immunocompromised patients and CT features include poorly defined nodules with a ground glass halo representing haemorrhage.

Tracheobronchopathia osteochrondroplastica is a rare condition affecting the trachea and proximal airways where there are submucosal cartilaginous and osseous nodules which spare the posterior tracheal wall due to the lack of cartilage here.

Pulmonary manifestations of granulomatosis with polyangiitis (previously known as Wegener granulomatosis) include consolidation, ground glass opacification and pulmonary nodules. Larger nodules tend to cavitate and there is a lower lobe predominance.

(The Final FRCR Complete Revision Notes Pages 20, 23)

86. (d) Soap bubble

In aggressive disease, there is no time for the periosteum to consolidate. In benign processes there is time form new periosteum and so the periosteum is thickened and dense.

(The Final FRCR Complete Revision Notes Page 148)

Table 2.6: Characteristics of Benign and Malignant Periostitis

Benign (Never Malignant)	Aggressive (May Not Be Malignant)
Soap bubble	Codman's triangle (periosteum elevated)
Thick/dense	Lamellated
Wavy	Multilayered, 'onion skin'
	Sunray
	Spiculated, 'hair on end'

Source: Reprinted with permission from V Helyar and A Shaw, *The Final FRCR: Complete Revision Notes.* CRC Press, Taylor & Francis Group, 2018, p. 148.

87. (d) ^{99m}Tc-Na-pertechnetate scintigraphy

Meckel's diverticulum may be an incidental finding; however haemorrhage or small bowel obstruction are the most common causes of symptomatic presentations. Bleeding is often secondary to ulceration of ectopic gastric mucosa due to a persistent omphalomesenteric artery. It can be treated in the interventional radiology suite.

In the paediatric population 95% of diverticulum presenting with bleeding will contain ectopic gastric mucosa and scintigraphy is most sensitive in this population. CT angiogram is of limited value and also radiation dose would need to be considered in a paediatric patient. Identifying a diverticulum with ultrasound can be challenging and similar to small bowel fluoroscopy, and cannot confidently exclude the diagnosis. Angiography may be employed; however, it would not typically be a first-line investigation.

(The Final FRCR Complete Revision Notes Page 178)

88. (c) Septate uterus

Müllerian duct anomalies occur during foetal life and may not become apparent until the woman reaches childbearing age, with difficulty conceiving or recurrent miscarriage. All can be associated with renal anomalies and therefore it is important to always assess the kidneys too. The most common anomaly is an arcuate uterus which is considered a normal variant. There is mild indentation of the endometrium at the fundus. This is not thought to have an impact on the ability to conceive or maintain a pregnancy.

A septate uterus is caused by the incomplete resorption of the uterovaginal septum and the septum can be 'partial' or 'complete', extending to either the internal or external os. The external fundal contour of the uterus helps to differentiate a bicornuate from a septate uterus. A bicornuate uterus has a septum too; however, in contrast to a septate uterus it cannot be resected due to the risk of uterine perforation.

Uterus didelphys is complete duplication of the uterine horns leading to two separate uterine cavities and cervices. A unicornuate uterus is where there is just one uterine horn and fallopian tube and there may be a rudimentary horn on the contralateral side. Renal anomalies are most common with this subtype. Uterine agenesis is when the uterus has not formed at all and the upper two-thirds of the vagina will also be absent; however, the ovaries and fallopian tubes may or may not be present.

(The Final FRCR Complete Revision Notes Pages 276–277)

89. (e) Thin-walled dilated gallbladder

Kawasaki disease is a small or medium vessel vasculitis. Symptoms can include fever, rash, desquamation of the hands, a red tongue, conjunctivitis and lymph node enlargement. Coronary artery aneurysms can be encountered in some patients. A thin-walled dilated gallbladder is associated with the condition.

Abdominal aortic wall thickening would be associated with a large vessel vasculitis such as Takayasu arteritis. Renal artery microaneurysms are seen in a small and medium size vessel vasculitis such as polyarteritis nodosa.

Enlarged kidneys with loss of corticomedullary differentiation is suggestive of glomerulonephritis. This may be encountered with conditions such as Goodpasture syndrome.

(The Final FRCR Complete Revision Notes Page 342)

90. (e) Lhermitte-Duclos disease

This is a rare tumour of the cerebellum, associated with Cowden syndrome, which is likely hamartomatous in origin. It is a WHO grade I tumour. It has a classical 'tigroid', striated appearance on MRI, which has been described in the question.

A cerebellar infarct would be unusual in this age group and also typically demonstrates restricted diffusion. Acute demyelination, for example in multiple sclerosis, can affect the cerebellum, causing ataxia; however, other lesions would be likely, including supratentorially, around the lateral ventricles for example. Cerebellitis is more common in a younger group of patients, frequently as a post-infective condition leading to ataxia. Radiological manifestations include cortical FLAIR hyperintensity, restricted diffusion, oedema and cortical and leptomeningeal enhancement. Lymphoma also usually enhances and has restricted diffusion. Furthermore, primary CNS lymphoma is most commonly supratentorial.

(The Final FRCR Complete Revision Notes Page 390)

91. (d) Scleroderma

The description is typical for scleroderma, also known as systemic sclerosis. This is a connective tissue disease affecting multiple organs. In this condition the oesophagus is commonly involved and looks patulous.

The description of basal interstitial lung disease is common. The predominance of honeycombing is more in keeping with usual interstitial pneumonitis (UIP). Both UIP and non-specific interstitial pneumonitis can be seen in the condition.

Recurrent aspiration can cause infection, bronchiectasis and scarring.

Achalasia may cause oesophageal dilatation with hold-up of food debris; however, achalasia does not account for the UIP picture of fibrosis.

(The Final FRCR Complete Revision Notes Page 54)

92. (b) Chordoma

Chordoma is the most common primary malignancy of the sacrum. It affects other midline structures, including other spinal levels, the coccyx and the clivus. It is usually large at presentation and symptoms are due to local pressure effects. The high T1 signal foci represent haemorrhage and are relatively specific.

Chondrosarcoma is the most common malignant bone tumour in adults. It has a range of behaviour (slow growing to aggressive and metastasising), and is typically a large well-defined lytic lesion with endosteal scalloping and internal chondroid matrix.

Osteosarcoma is the most common malignant associated with encephaloceleprimary bone tumour in children and adolescents. It may also affect those aged 70–80 years if there is a history of Paget disease.

Sacrococcygeal teratoma is the most common solid tumour in neonates, usually presenting in the first few days of life.

(The Final FRCR Complete Revision Notes Page 134)

93. (d) Multiple, hypodense intramural nodules
Xanthogranulomatous cholecystitis, although uncommon, can look very similar to gallbladder cancer. It is an inflammatory condition characterised by multiple intramural nodules within a thickened gallbladder wall. All the other options in the question can be seen in both xanthogranulomatous cholecystitis and gallbladder cancer. The presence of hypoattenuating mural nodules is more suggestive of xanthogranulomatous cholecystitis. Given the similarities in the radiological features, a cholecystectomy is usually performed.
(The Final FRCR Complete Revision Notes Page 222)

94. (a) DWI
Table 2.7 helps to differentiate between cerebellopontine angle (CPA) mass characteristics. DWI is the most helpful sequence in confirming an epidermoid because it will demonstrate restricted diffusion, whereas a schwannoma and meningioma will not.
(The Final FRCR Complete Revision Notes Pages 405–407)

Table 2.7: Differentiating Features of Cerebellopontine Angle Masses

	Schwannoma	Meningioma	Epidermoid
Epicentre	Internal acoustic canal (IAC)	Dura	CPA
CT density	Iso	Hyper or iso	Hypo
Calcification	None	Frequent	Occasional
IAC	Wide	Normal or wide	Normal
Enhancement	++	++	None
Diffusion restriction	No	No	Yes

95. (b) Enlarged heart, plethoric lungs, left-sided aortic arch
Truncus arteriosus is due to a failure of the normal division of the primitive truncus arteriosus into the aorta and pulmonary artery. A single vessel leaves the heart giving rise to the pulmonary, coronary and systemic arteries. The condition causes cyanosis and cardiac failure. Chest radiograph commonly demonstrates cardiomegaly, pulmonary plethora and forked ribs. The aortic arch is right-sided in around a third of cases.
(The Final FRCR Complete Revision Notes Page 315)

96. (d) Subependymal giant cell astrocytoma
Tuberous sclerosis is an autosomal dominant disease which can present with seizures, development delay and, in around 75% of cases, a skin condition called adenoma sebaceum. Central nervous system features include subependymal hamartomas, cortical tubers, heterotopic grey matter islands and subependymal giant cell astrocytoma. Optic nerve gliomas and focal areas of signal intensity (FASIs) are associated with NF1. Subcortical calcification and prominent leptomeningeal enhancement is associated with Sturge-Weber syndrome.
(The Final FRCR Complete Revision Notes Page 383)

97. (b) Diaphragmatic rupture
Diaphragmatic rupture is often missed on trauma imaging and coronal and sagittal reformats can aid identification. The left hemidiaphragm is more commonly affected due to the protective effects of the adjacent liver on the right hemidiaphragm. The deviation of the nasogastric tube on the chest radiograph is commonly seen due to the stomach herniating through the defect into the left hemithorax. The left hemidiaphragm will be poorly defined or discontinuous. On CT, the 'collar' sign describes the constriction of the stomach or other viscera as they herniate through the defect. Sometimes the herniated viscera can also be seen dependently against the posterior ribs.

In aortic rupture there would normally be mediastinal widening and other signs such as a left apical cap and left pleural effusion.

Although this patient would be at risk from fat embolus due to the femoral fracture, the opacities associated with fat embolism tend to appear after around 48 hours, with normal initial radiographic appearances.

Radiographic appearances of tracheobronchial rupture would include pneumothorax and/or pneumomediastinum with the 'fallen lung' sign – the affected lung descends dependently within the chest due to the airway discontinuity.

Oesophageal rupture is usually iatrogenic rather than being seen in this sort of trauma scenario. Pneumomediastinum and left pleural effusion are classical features.

(The Final FRCR Complete Revision Notes Page 28)

98. (c) Rodent facies

Iron deficiency anaemia, severe enough that it is not able to support erythropoiesis, may occur for various reasons; some include deficient diet, impaired absorption in the GI tract and polycythaemia vera. The radiological findings in this condition include widening of the diploic spaces and thinning of the tables, as well as osteoporosis and hair-on-end appearance of the skull. They occur due to marrow expansion/marrow hyperplasia. Hair-on-end appearance represents marrow expansion through the outer cortex. The occiput is spared due to absence of red marrow at this site. Unlike in thalassaemia major, in iron deficiency anaemia the facial bones are usually not involved. Rodent facies refers to ventral displacement of the incisors due to marrow overgrowth in the maxillary sinus and causes dental malocclusion.

(The Final FRCR Complete Revision Notes Page 81)

99. (b) Mirizzi syndrome

Mirizzi syndrome occurs when there is extrinsic compression and obstruction of the common bile duct secondary to a gallstone in the cystic duct. Ultrasound shows dilatation of the common bile duct to the level of a stone that lies outside of the common bile duct in the cystic duct. The gallbladder wall is often thickened.

The gallbladder does have features of cholecystitis; however, the most accurate diagnosis is Mirizzi syndrome because this also explains the underlying cause. A gallbladder polyp will be within the gallbladder rather than in the ducts and will not demonstrate posterior acoustic shadowing. Adenomyomatosis is suspected when there are small hyperechoic foci in a frequently thickened gallbladder wall. A choledochocele does not match the description in this case, it is instead a focal dilatation of the intramural segment of the distal common bile duct within the duodenal wall.

(The Final FRCR Complete Revision Notes Page 216)

100. (b) Branching linear calcification extending from the right upper outer quadrant towards the nipple

Microcalcification is commonly detected on screening mammograms. It is useful to look at any available previous mammograms to assess whether there has been a change. The most concerning microcalcification is clustered, pleomorphic (varying in size and shape) or if it is in a ductal distribution with a branching linear pattern. The correct answer in this case describes this type of calcification, extending towards the nipple.

Bilateral scattered coarse calcification is commonly seen; the coarse appearance and bilateral distribution is reassuring. Calcification with a layered appearance on the MLO view is consistent with 'tea-cupping' and is seen in fibrocystic change. Coarse calcification may represent 'popcorn' calcification seen in fibroadenoma or eggshell calcification in fat necrosis. Tram-like calcification is consistent with vascular calcification.

(The Final FRCR Complete Revision Notes Page 282)

101. (c) Congenital lobar overinflation (CLO)

CLO usually presents in infancy with cyanosis and respiratory distress. It is thought to be caused by a 'ball valve'-type obstruction leading to overinflation of a lobe. It most commonly affects the left upper lobe. Initially radiographs may show an opacity in the affected region due to delayed clearing of lung fluid. Later, the lobe becomes hyperlucent with contralateral mediastinal shift.

Bronchial atresia can have similar appearances, but the absence of a mucous plug makes CLO the more likely option.

Bronchogenic cysts would not normally communicate with the bronchial tree, so would not be air-filled or lucent.

Congenital pulmonary airway malformation has cystic lucencies but the lung itself is not lucent.

Mucous impaction could explain the initial radiograph but not the follow-up one.
(The Final FRCR Complete Revision Notes Page 321)

102. (e) Progressive multifocal leukoencephalopathy

Progressive multifocal leukoencephalopathy is associated with immunocompromised states due to reactivation of the JC virus. The key distribution is in the white matter; it is asymmetrical and typically parieto-occipital and subcortical. There is T2 hyperintensity and T1 hypointensity, minimal, if any enhancement and no mass effect. There may be restricted diffusion at the leading edge of the changes.

In contrast to this, HIV encephalopathy is symmetrical and more typically frontal and focused on the periventricular white matter and centrum semi ovale. Cerebral atrophy is also a feature. Although there is similar T2 hyperintensity and no enhancement or mass effect, there are not usually the same T1 signal changes.

Cytomegalovirus encephalopathy causes T2 hyperintense brainstem and periventricular white matter abnormalities. These do not cause mass effect or enhancement unless there is ventriculitis, in which case there will be ependymal enhancement.

Posterior reversible encephalopathy syndrome classically also affects the parieto-occipital regions with minimal, if any enhancement or diffusion restriction; however, the history is the key factor and does not fit in this case.

Toxoplasmosis typically causes ring-enhancing lesions in the basal ganglia, thalamus and corticomedullary junction with mass effect.
(The Final FRCR Complete Revision Notes Page 416)

103. (e) Silicosis

The correct underlying diagnosis is silicosis. This is a pneumoconiosis found in those in sandblasting or mining industries, secondary to inhaled silica. The features of tiny calcified pulmonary nodules and calcified hila lymph nodes is indicative of this condition, complicated by progressive massive fibrosis (PMF). PMF occurs when the nodules coalesce and form large opacities in the upper zones with upper zone fibrosis.

Coal workers' pneumoconiosis (CWP) is secondary to inhalation of coal dust and can also produce calcified pulmonary nodules and hilar/mediastinal lymph node calcification; however eggshell calcification is more typical in silicosis. Silicosis is more likely than CWP to be complicated by PMF.

Caplan syndrome is CWP with features of rheumatoid arthritis.

Pulmonary alveolar microlithiasis is a rare idiopathic condition, in which diffuse, dense, miliary calcification is seen in both lungs, more conspicuous in the mid-lower zones.

Hypersensitivity pneumonitis, also known as extrinsic allergic alveolitis, is a response to inhaled antigen. In chronic cases it can cause fibrosis, typically in the upper zones. Centrilobular nodules seen in this condition are not typically calcified.
(The Final FRCR Complete Revision Notes Pages 45–47)

104. (e) Rhizomelic

Thanatophoric dysplasia is one of the lethal dwarfisms. Rhizomelia involves shortening of a proximal segment relative to a distal segment, for example the humerus or femur, as described in this case. Achondroplasia, thanatophoric dysplasia and chondrodysplasia punctata can be examples of this.

Mesomelia is the shortening of an intermediate segment (e.g. ulna and radius). This type of dwarfism is rare. Dyschondrosteosis is one example.

Acromelia is shortening of a distal segment (e.g. the hand). These conditions are also rare, and Jeune syndrome (also known as asphyxiating thoracic dysplasia) is one cause.

Micromelia is the shortening of an entire limb (e.g. humerus, radius, ulna and hand) and can be seen in some types of thanatophoric dysplasia and diastrophic dysplasia.

In metatropic dwarfism, there is a change of proportion of the trunk to the limbs over time secondary to developing kyphoscoliosis in childhood.
(The Final FRCR Complete Revision Notes Pages 110, 128–129)

105. (b) Antimesenteric border of the distal ileum

Meckel's diverticulum are most common in the terminal ileum on the antimesenteric border. The 'rule of 2s' suggests that they present in 2% of the population, 20% have ectopic gastric mucosa, they are 2 feet from the ileocaecal valve and usually around 2

inches long. If they present symptomatically, most commonly with haemorrhage or small-bowel obstruction, it is most likely to be in the first 2 years of life. Other presentations may include intussusception, Meckel's diverticulitis, perforation or neoplasm. Many patients remain asymptomatic, and the chance of them causing problems decreases with age.
(The Final FRCR Complete Revision Notes Page 178)

106. (d) Klippel-Feil syndrome
Klippel-Feil syndrome is a congenital abnormality of vertebral segmentation. Features include partial or complete fusion of C1 with the occiput, rib fusion, thumb anomalies (triphalangeal thumb, hypoplasia and polydactyly) and Sprengel deformity. Fusion of the posterior column of C2/3 is common and causes a restriction of neck movement.
Other causes of fusion of the cervical spine include ankylosing spondylitis and juvenile idiopathic arthritis.
Homocysteinuria is an autosomal recessive inherited defect which causes defects in collagen and elastin structure. Imaging features include osteoporosis, carpal bone abnormalities, scoliosis and biconcave vertebrae.
Features in Turner syndrome include squared lumbar vertebrae and kyphoscoliosis.
(The Final FRCR Complete Revision Notes Page 112)

107. (c) Enlarged right atrium
The chest radiograph can be normal in the early stages of an atrial septal defect. Common radiographic findings are related to increased pulmonary flow, for example enlarged pulmonary vessels, visible peripheral vasculature and upper zone vascular prominence. The right atrium and ventricle can enlarge whilst the left atrium and ventricle remain normal in size. The aortic arch is either small or normal in size.
(The Final FRCR Complete Revision Notes Page 312)

108. (d) Glioblastoma multiforme (GBM)
There is a short differential for masses that cross the midline via the corpus callosum. Primary cerebral lymphoma tends to demonstrate uniform enhancement and diffusion restriction because it is hypercellular. Tumefactive multiple sclerosis can have similar appearances to GBM but given it is an isolated lesion GBM is the more likely diagnosis. Furthermore, enhancement in tumefactive multiple sclerosis is usually described as an open, rather than a complete ring. Metastases and toxoplasmosis, whilst often ring enhancing, very rarely involve the corpus callosum and cross the midline.
(The Final FRCR Complete Revision Notes Page 391)

109. (d) Re-inflate the balloon proximal to the stenosis
The concern following sudden drop in blood pressure and tachycardia is one of rupture of the right common iliac artery causing significant pelvic haemorrhage. The most appropriate immediate management is to inflate the balloon just proximal to the stenosis which has just been dilated, and presumably the site of the haemorrhage. Once the patient is stabilised and the site confirmed with digital subtraction angiogram, then a covered stent could be deployed to cover the defect.
A CT angiogram of the lower limbs would take too long to organise and moving an anaesthetised patient to the CT scanner quickly could waste precious time. The cause can be both confirmed and treated in the interventional radiology suite, so it is more appropriate the patient stays where she is.
Embolisation coils are used to treat haemorrhage, but they would not be routinely used for this indication and there would be significant risk of distal ischaemia where there is not good collateralisation.
Removing the vascular access sheath, wire and balloon would be contraindicated as maintaining vascular access is essential to treat this complication.

110. (a) Anterior cruciate ligament tear
The imaging description on plain film is that of Osgood-Schlatter disease, which is caused by chronic microtrauma of the patellar tendon at the site of insertion of the tibial tuberosity, with subsequent osteochondritis of the tibial tuberosity. It affects active children between 10 and 15 years old. Options (b)–(e) are all features of the condition. Anterior

cruciate ligament tear is the most common knee ligamentous injury; however, it is not a feature of Osgood-Schlatter disease. It usually follows an episode of trauma and can be associated with injury to other ligamentous structures. It may be associated with avulsion of the tibial attachment.

(The Final FRCR Complete Revision Notes Page 117)

111. (c) Liposarcoma are the most common retroperitoneal sarcoma

Differentiating liposarcoma from a benign lipoma is not always possible; however, septations >2 mm thick or soft tissue components suggest sarcoma. Retroperitoneal leiomyosarcoma commonly metastasise to the liver and lung, particularly the intravascular subtype. Myxoid type liposarcoma is T2 hyperintense and shows delayed enhancement post contrast. Calcification occurs in approximately 25% of malignant fibrous histiocytomas. It is a relatively specific finding and rare in other types of retroperitoneal masses. Angiosarcoma are a very aggressive sarcoma and metastasises early.

(The Final FRCR Complete Revision Notes Page 192)

112. (c) Lymphocele

The lesion has features of a simple cystic structure which, along with the history of a well patient, would make abscess unlikely. A haematoma would typically have more complex features, possibly with internal echoes, septations and layering of debris.

Haematomas are also more likely in the immediate postoperative period and resolution would be expected after 3 years. A seroma could have similar appearances to the collection described in this case; however, this should also have regressed over a period of 3 years.

The main differential lies between urinoma and lymphocele. Lymphocele fits the description and they are the most common cause of a perirenal post-transplant collection. They can persist for a long time following renal transplant and may be asymptomatic or cause compression of surrounding structures. A urinoma is frequently secondary to anastomotic failure or ischaemia. They have fewer septations than haematomas and they frequently contour the renal outline due to the intimate relationship with the urinary tract.

(The Final FRCR Complete Revision Notes Pages 259–261)

113. (b) Venous drainage to pulmonary veins

Pulmonary sequestration tends to present in childhood and is more common in males. The extralobar subtype usually presents earlier than intralobar sequestration. The anomaly is a segment of lung with no communication to the pulmonary arteries or bronchial tree.

The most common type is intralobar. This is supplied from the descending thoracic aorta and drains via the pulmonary venous system. Intralobar sequestration is enclosed in visceral pleura. It does not have any associated conditions.

In contrast to this, extralobar sequestration is associated with other conditions such as duplication cysts and cardiac anomalies. The segment has its own pleura. The arterial supply is from the aorta or sometimes the splenic, intercostal or gastric arteries. The venous drainage is systemic and not via the pulmonary veins.

(The Final FRCR Complete Revision Notes Page 320)

114. (c) Diffuse, smooth dural enhancement

Intracranial hypotension is associated with postural headache, nausea, vertigo and vomiting. It can be spontaneous or secondary to procedures such as lumbar puncture or surgery. Radiological features can include acquired tonsillar ectopia, subdural effusions, a sagging brainstem, distension of the venous structures and pachymeningeal enhancement which is commonly diffuse and smooth.

(The Final FRCR Complete Revision Notes Page 388)

115. (a) Lymphoma

Although the imaging findings could be in keeping with sarcoidosis, the features of hilar and mediastinal lymph node enlargement, as well as the parenchymal infiltration would be in keeping with stage 3 sarcoidosis (according to the Siltzbach classification), which has not been given as an option.

Lymphoma is the most likely correct answer in this case. Hodgkin's lymphoma is more commonly a cause for enlarged lymph nodes than non-Hodgkin's lymphoma. The posterior mediastinum is not frequently involved; however it is an important site for recurrence of disease, as it may not be included in the radiotherapy field. The presence of nodular

Table 2.8: Siltzbach Staging of Sarcoidosis

1. Normal chest radiograph
2. Bilateral hilar lymph node enlargement
3. Bilateral hilar lymph node enlargement, parenchymal infiltration
4. Parenchymal infiltration
5. Parenchymal volume loss as a result of pulmonary fibrosis – 20% get to stage 4 with irreversible fibrosis

Source: Reprinted with permission from V Helyar and A Shaw, *The Final FRCR: Complete Revision Notes.* CRC Press, Taylor & Francis Group, 2018, p. 53.

interlobular septal thickening raises the possibility of lymphatic infiltration causing lymphangitis carcinomatosis, although this is rare.
(The Final FRCR Complete Revision Notes Page 53)

116. (b) External epicondyle
CRITOL is helpful in remembering the ossification centres of the elbow and the order in which they appear.
The patient in the case vignette would be expected to have the capitellum, radial head, internal epicondyle and possibly the trochlea. The olecranon and external epicondyle would not be expected in a 7 year old child. Careful scrutiny of the plain film is important; an ossification centre seen at the site of the trochlea, without the presence of internal epicondyle ossification centre, likely indicates avulsion of the internal epicondyle which is displaced inferiorly into the site where the trochlear ossification centre may be expected.
(The Final FRCR Complete Revision Notes Page 119)

Table 2.9: Ossification Centres of the Elbow and Age of their Appearance

Ossification Centre	Age of Appearance
Capitellum	1 year
Radial head	3 years
Internal epicondyle	5 years
Trochlea	7 years
Olecranon	9 years
External epicondyle	11 years

Source: Reprinted with permission from V Helyar and A Shaw, *The Final FRCR: Complete Revision Notes.* CRC Press, Taylor & Francis Group, 2018, p. 119.

117. (c) Hydatid cyst
This is caused by infection of the liver due to the parasite *Echinococcus granulosus*. It commonly occurs in the right lobe of the liver, and daughter cysts are typical. Eosinophilia is seen in many cases.
Amoebic abscesses also tend to occur people with a recent foreign travel history and classically affect the right lobe; however, they tend to have thick, hypoechoic nodular wall on ultrasound.
Pyogenic abscesses are most commonly due to ascending cholangitis from benign or obstructive biliary disease or from haematogenous seeding (e.g. from diverticulitis). On ultrasound they are usually poorly defined and may be septated with irregular walls.

Fungal abscesses typically occur in the immunosuppressed and are usually due to candidiasis. They have a classical 'wheel within wheel' appearance in the early stages due to a centrally necrotic nidus.

(The Final FRCR Complete Revision Notes Page 214)

118. (c) Displacement of the medulla and cerebellar vermis through the foramen magnum.

Chiari II malformations can have varying degrees of severity. There is a small posterior fossa with descent of structures through the foramen magnum along with a spinal myelomeningocele. It has various other associations including absence of the septum pellucidum, abnormality of the corpus callosum and polymicrogyria. The posterior fossa is small with inferior displacement of the cerebellar tonsils and vermis. There may be hydrocephalus and the fourth ventricle may be low lying.

Chiari I is when just the cerebellar tonsils are inferiorly displaced, and is commonly incidentally discovered on brain imaging.

Chiari III malformations are more unusual and are associated with encephaloceles.

(The Final FRCR Complete Revision Notes Page 289)

119. (b) Caudate lobe hypertrophy

Acute Budd-Chiari syndrome typically presents with abdominal pain, hepatomegaly and ascites. It is often secondary to thrombus in the suprahepatic vena cava or hepatic veins. The finding of hyperenhancement in the central liver on early phase post-contrast imaging with peripheral hyperenhancement on delayed images is called the 'flip-flop' pattern. Splenomegaly, absent hepatic veins and increased portal vein diameter are also features.

Hypertrophy of the caudate lobe is associated with the chronic form of the condition. It drains directly into the inferior vena cava and is therefore spared. It hypertrophies to compensate for the atrophy which can manifest in the other liver lobes. Gallbladder wall thickening is also commonly seen with chronic Budd-Chiari syndrome.

(The Final FRCR Complete Revision Notes Page 198)

120. (c) Neurocysticercosis

Neurocysticerosis is characterised by cysts at the grey–white matter junction and in the subarachnoid and intraventricular spaces. When intraventricular, they can affect the fourth ventricle and lead to hydrocephalus. The appearances of the cysts can vary depending on the life cycle of the larvae, and as they die can enhance. Breakdown of the cyst membrane leads to surrounding oedema. Calcification is seen in chronic cases.

Intracranial toxoplasmosis and cryptococcus infection are not common unless a patient is immunocompromised, and there is no history to suggest this. Toxoplasmosis does also cause ring-enhancing lesions and they can have a similar distribution, affecting the corticomedullary junction as well as the basal ganglia. Cryptococcus has non-specific imaging features, although one described feature is prominent perivascular spaces and ring-enhancing cryptococcomas.

Cerebral hydatid cysts often lie in the territory of the middle cerebral artery and are usually solitary. Enhancement and surrounding oedema is not typical unless there is superadded infection.

Another differential for these appearances is intracranial tuberculosis infection causing tuberculomas at the corticomedullary junction. These may also enhance peripherally and cause surrounding oedema. The other features of an intraventricular lesion and hydrocephalus are more consistent with neurocysticercosis.

(The Final FRCR Complete Revision Notes Page 415)

PAPER 3

1. A 64 year old female patient presents with shortness of breath on exertion. She smokes five cigarettes per day and her past medical history includes rheumatoid arthritis, hypertension, hypercholesterolaemia and atrial fibrillation. Initial bloods are normal apart from the arterial blood gas, which reveals a PaO_2 of 9.5 kPa (normal range 10.5–13.5 kPa) with a restrictive pattern on spirometry. High resolution CT chest demonstrates bilateral hyperdense consolidation which is predominantly peripheral, affecting the bases more than the apices with patchy ground glass opacification and reticulation.

   What is the most likely diagnosis?

   a. Amiodarone lung disease
   b. Eosinophilic granulomatosis with polyangiitis (Churg-Strauss syndrome)
   c. Simple pulmonary eosinophilia
   d. Non-specific interstitial pneumonia
   e. Gold induced lung toxicity

2. A 26 year old male presents to the GP with ongoing wrist pain that has not resolved with anti-inflammatory medications or physiotherapy. The GP requests a plain film. Amongst other findings, the report mentions positive ulnar variance and suggests further investigation with MRI to assess for complications.

   What is a likely complication of the condition described, which will be seen on the MRI?

   a. Avascular necrosis of the lunate bone
   b. Radioulnar convergence
   c. Scalloping of the distal radius by the ulna
   d. Tear of the triangular fibrocartilage complex
   e. Ulnar impingement syndrome

3. A 64 year old woman is referred by her GP for a CT abdomen pelvis indicated for weight loss and non-specific abdominal pain. The CT shows widening of the presacral space.

   Which of the following would NOT be within the differential for widening of the presacral space?

   a. Pelvic lipomatosis
   b. Chordoma
   c. Neurofibroma
   d. Dermoid cyst
   e. Mesenteric carcinomatosis

4. A 50 year old female has a CT abdomen and pelvis for unexplained abdominal pain following a normal ultrasound scan. This identifies a large cystic mass in the pancreatic tail with peripheral calcification. There are a couple of thin enhancing septations. There are no enlarged regional lymph nodes and no evidence of metastatic disease. An MRCP does not demonstrate a connection to the main pancreatic duct.

   What is the most likely diagnosis?

   a. Ductal adenocarcinoma
   b. Intraductal papillary mucinous neoplasm
   c. Mucinous cystic neoplasm
   d. Neuroendocrine tumour
   e. Serous microcystic adenoma

5. A 12 year old boy is referred for a chest radiograph. He has recurrent pulmonary infections and shortness of breath on exertion. The radiograph shows a small right lung with ipsilateral mediastinal shift. There is a curvilinear tubular opacity adjacent to the heart border.

   What is the most likely diagnosis?

   a. Partial anomalous pulmonary venous return
   b. Pulmonary sequestration
   c. Right middle lobe atelectasis

d. Tetralogy of Fallot
e. Unilateral absence of the pulmonary artery

6. An MRI whole spine of a 53 year old man reveals a solitary thoracic spinal cord lesion. It is intradural and has both an intramedullary and extramedullary component which is extending posteriorly. It extends inferiorly over 1–2 segments. It is well defined, low T1 signal and predominantly high T2 signal apart from very low T2 signal at its caudal margin. It has a small, rounded, enhancing soft tissue component and flow voids. There is high STIR signal in the surrounding cord.

   What is the most likely diagnosis?

   a. Arteriovenous malformation
   b. Astrocytoma
   c. Ependymoma
   d. Haemangioblastoma
   e. Meningioma

7. A 59 year old female presents with increasing shortness of breath and persistent cough. She has a 20 pack year smoking history. The GP requests a CT chest for further investigation. The CT shows volume loss in the lower lung zones. There is extensive honeycomb destruction of the lungs, predominantly in the dependent aspect of the lower zones but also at the lateral and anterior aspect of the mid and lower zones. The airways within the abnormal looking lung demonstrate traction dilatation. There is minimal ground glass opacification in both lungs. The upper and mid zones of the lung demonstrate mild background emphysematous change.

   What is the most likely diagnosis?

   a. Cryptogenic organising pneumonia
   b. Hypersensitivity pneumonitis
   c. Non-specific interstitial pneumonia
   d. Respiratory bronchiolitis-associated interstitial lung disease
   e. Usual interstitial pneumonia

8. A 56 year old male presents with neck pain following a fall. A CT cervical spine demonstrates a destructive lytic lesion in the right lamina of C4 which appears to encroach into the canal. A smaller lytic lesion is seen in the anterior aspect of the C7 vertebral body. The appearances are considered most likely in keeping with metastases.

   What is the most likely primary site of disease?

   a. Breast
   b. Bronchus
   c. Colon
   d. Kidney
   e. Prostate

9. A barium swallow study is performed on a 42 year old female patient on her third cycle of neoadjuvant chemotherapy for breast cancer with a plan to proceed to surgery and radiotherapy. The patient has been experiencing increasing odynophagia but no dysphagia, reflux or regurgitation.

   What appearances on the barium swallow study would be most likely in this clinical setting?

   a. Flask-shaped mucosal outpouchings
   b. Large areas of oesophageal ulceration
   c. Long, linear oesophageal filling defects
   d. Multiple, small, nodular oesophageal filling defects
   e. Smooth stricture in the mid-oesophagus

10. A 15 year old female presents the emergency department with a fall onto an outstretched hand. The referring clinician asks you to review the plain film wrist, which demonstrates bullet-shaped metacarpals, a wide radius and ulna and metacarpal irregularity but no fracture. The referrer explains there are features of dwarfism but no other history is provided.

You review previous imaging and see a plain film of the spine, which shows posterior vertebral body scalloping, platyspondyly and anterior central beaking of the vertebral bodies.

What is the most likely underlying aetiology?

a. Achondroplasia
b. Down syndrome
c. Hurler syndrome
d. Morquio syndrome
e. Pseudoachondroplasia

11. A 15 year old boy is under investigation for hypertension and polycythaemia. Renal ultrasound showed multiple bilateral renal cysts but nil else of note. He develops headaches and signs of cerebellar dysfunction and is referred for an MRI. This shows a large, T1 hypointense, T2 hyperintense lesion within the cerebellum. There is a centrally, avidly enhancing nodule. Multiple flow voids are seen within the periphery of the mass.

What is the most likely diagnosis?

a. Ependymoma
b. Haemangioblastoma
c. Medulloblastoma
d. Meningioma
e. Pilocytic astrocytoma

12. An adult passenger suffers a sudden acceleration-deceleration injury in a high-speed road traffic collision. He develops severe left-sided neck pain occipital headache, nausea and vertigo. He is suspected of having a left vertebral artery dissection.

What is the most likely location for this to occur?

a. At its origin from the subclavian artery
b. C2
c. C6
d. C7
e. Intracranial segment

13. A 24 year old female patient presents with a 2 day history of right flank pain and haematuria. The emergency department team are querying renal calculus. She has an abdominal ultrasound that incidentally finds at least three separate splenic structures in the left upper quadrant.

Which is most commonly associated with polysplenia?

a. Dextrocardia
b. Gallbladder agenesis
c. Bilateral bilobed lungs
d. Bilateral eparterial bronchi
e. Bilateral right atria

14. An 8 year old male has plain films to investigate acute right leg pain. In the proximal tibial diaphysis/metaphysis there is a well-defined central lucency with a thin sclerotic rim; the lesion is orientated along the long axis of the tibia and there is no periosteal reaction. In view of the patient's pain a CT is performed. This demonstrates the same features as the plain films as well as a cortical break which is considered in keeping with a fracture. A small bone fragment is also seen at the dependant aspect of the lesion.

What is the most likely diagnosis?

a. Chondroblastoma
b. Eosinophilic granuloma
c. Ewing sarcoma
d. Brodie abscess
e. Unicameral bone cyst

15. A 40 year old woman presents to her GP with right upper quadrant pain. An outpatient abdominal ultrasound is arranged. She is noted to have a 3-mm gallstone. The gallbladder

wall is thickened and there are multiple echogenic foci within the wall which demonstrate posterior acoustic shadowing.

What is the most likely differential?

a. Porcelain gallbladder
b. Emphysematous cholecystitis
c. Gallbladder carcinoma
d. Adenomyomatosis
e. Gallbladder polyp

16. A 32 year old female patient with no significant past medical history is brought into hospital with at least three abdominal stab wounds for which she has an arterial and portal venous phase CT abdomen pelvis. This demonstrates three sites of skin breach without evidence of deep extension or peritoneal breach. Incidental note is made of alternating dilatation and stenoses of the distal renal arteries bilaterally. The kidneys both enhance symmetrically and uniformly. There is no vascular calcification. Appearances elsewhere on the CT are normal. The patient continues to have normal observations on the ward. Following discharge she attends the renal outpatient clinic for follow-up and has normal serum renal function tests.

    What is the most appropriate management for this condition?

    a. Angioplasty
    b. Angioplasty plus stenting
    c. Continued follow-up
    d. No further management required
    e. Steroid treatment

17. A 13 year old boy with an underlying congenital syndrome undergoes an MRI brain. This demonstrates a lesion within the left cerebellar hemisphere with widened folia and a striated/tigroid appearance. The lesion is T1 hypointense and T2 hyperintense and does not enhance following contrast administration. No other lesions are identified. The child has a thyroid ultrasound recently which demonstrates a thyroid goitre.

    What underlying syndrome does the child likely have?

    a. Ataxia telangiectasia
    b. Cowden syndrome
    c. Neurofibromatosis type 1
    d. Sturge-Weber syndrome
    e. Tuberous sclerosis

18. You are asked to review an unenhanced CT head for a newly admitted 56 year old inpatient under the care of neurology. There is a 30-mm lesion in the right temporal lobe with significant surrounding oedema and effacement of the temporal horn of the right lateral ventricle. There is a similar, slightly smaller lesion in the left frontal lobe abutting the frontal horn of the left lateral ventricle. The team feel that cerebral abscess is more likely clinically than metastases; however, the patient suffers with claustrophobia and may only be able to tolerate a short time in the MRI scanner.

    Which of the below would you prioritise to help confirm the diagnosis of abscess?

    a. DWI + ADC map
    b. FLAIR
    c. MR perfusion
    d. Susceptibility weighted imaging
    e. T1 + gadolinium

19. A 64 year old inpatient with a history of atrial fibrillation is admitted with an acute exacerbation of shortness of breath. A chest radiograph is consistent with cardiac failure.

    What is the earliest radiographic feature of cardiac failure?

    a. Cardiomegaly
    b. Consolidation
    c. Interlobular septal thickening

d. Pleural effusion
e. Upper lobe diversion

20. A 77 year old female presents to the GP with right-sided hip pain. She has a plain film of the pelvis and right hip. There is cortical thickening of the proximal right femur and coarsening of the trabeculations. The visualised right femur itself appears mildly enlarged when compared to the left side, with evidence of bowing. There is the impression of ill-defined mixed lucent and sclerotic density at the greater trochanter and an aggressive periostitis with a hair-on-end periosteal reaction.

What is the most likely primary bone tumour?

a. Bizarre parosteal osteochondromatous proliferation
b. Haemangioma
c. Multiple myeloma
d. Osteoblastoma
e. Osteosarcoma

21. A 30 year old female with a background of medullary sponge kidney presents with right upper quadrant pain. On examination blood tests show elevated bilirubin levels. A liver ultrasound demonstrates multiple, dilated cystic structures converging towards the porta hepatis. The cysts communicate with the bile ducts. No peripheral biliary duct dilatation is identified. MRCP shows ectatic intrahepatic ducts extending into the periphery. The common bile duct is dilated but no strictures are seen.

What is the most likely diagnosis?

a. Primary sclerosing cholangitis
b. Polycystic liver disease
c. Choledochocele
d. Primary biliary cirrhosis
e. Caroli disease

22. A patient has a micturating cystogram following a renal ultrasound which diagnosed mild, bilateral hydronephrosis. Following contrast administration via a urinary catheter, there is reflux of contrast from the urinary bladder into both ureters, bilateral ureteric and renal pelvis dilatation and calyceal clubbing.

What vesicoureteral reflux grading would this patient have?

a. Grade I
b. Grade II
c. Grade III
d. Grade IV
e. Grade V

23. A CT abdomen pelvis for a 59 year old female patient with vomiting, abdominal pain and guarding is reported as small bowel obstruction secondary to an obstructed right obturator hernia.

Which anatomical landmarks are obturator hernias associated with?

a. Obturator externus and iliacus
b. Obturator externus and iliopsoas tendon
c. Obturator externus and pectineus
d. Obturator externus and piriformis
e. Obturator externus and pyramidalis

24. A 40 year old woman with known HIV presents with worsening confusion. Her partner reports she has been noncompliant with her antiretroviral medication. Her CD4 count is found to be <200 cells/mm^3 (500–1500 cells/mm^3). An MRI brain reveals bilateral basal ganglia lesions.

Which of these other imaging features also favours a diagnosis of toxoplasmosis over lymphoma?

a. Increased uptake on thallium SPECT

b. Intralesional haemorrhage
c. Solitary lesion
d. Subependymal distribution
e. Uniform enhancement

25. A 69 year old male patient with increasing shortness of breath is reviewed in the respiratory outpatient clinic following a GP referral. CT chest prior to the appointment demonstrates increased bilateral, predominantly lower lobe subpleural reticulation, interlobular septal thickening with associated bronchiectasis.

Which is the most likely underlying diagnosis?

a. Ankylosing spondylitis
b. Asbestosis
c. Chronic hypersensitivity pneumonitis
d. Silicosis
e. Sarcoidosis

26. A 6 year old male with a limp and left sided hip pain has plain films of the pelvis. AP and frog legged views are performed, and these are considered unremarkable. An ultrasound shows a joint effusion in the anterior recess with capsular distention of 3 mm. The synovium is not thickened. He had a viral illness for a week preceding the hip pain.

What is the most likely diagnosis?

a. Developmental dysplasia of the hip
b. Juvenile idiopathic arthritis
c. Septic arthritis
d. Slipped upper femoral epiphysis
e. Transient synovitis of the hip

27. A 60 year old female presents with weight loss and early satiety. She is found to have deranged serum liver function tests. A CT abdomen pelvis with contrast is performed. No pancreatic mass is identified but the 'double duct sign' is identified.

What is the most likely diagnosis?

a. Duplication cyst
b. Annular pancreas
c. Periampullary tumour
d. Pancreas divisum
e. Duodenal atresia

28. A 5 year old girl with recurrent urinary tract infection is investigated as an outpatient by the paediatric team with a urinary tract ultrasound. The appearances are highly suggestive of a right duplex kidney. There are normal appearances of the left kidney. There is no hydronephrosis. Appearances of the urinary bladder suggest a right sided ureterocoele. The patient has an excretory phase CT further investigate.

What is the most likely CT appearance?

a. Two right ureters converging just proximal to the urinary bladder
b. Two right ureters with upper moiety ureter inserting superolateral to lower moiety ureter
c. Two right ureters with upper moiety ureter inserting inferomedial to lower moiety ureter
d. Two right ureters with lower moiety ureter inserting superolateral to upper pole moiety
e. Two right ureters with lower moiety ureter inserting inferomedial to upper pole moiety

29. Following the delivery of a neonate who had an abnormal third trimester antenatal ultrasound scan, the neonatal intensive care team request a neonatal cranial ultrasound. There is evidence of hydrocephalus. In the region of the third ventricle there is an anechoic midline intracranial lesion with prominent flow on Doppler examination.

Which of the following imaging findings is most likely to be associated with this abnormality?

a. Absence of the corpus callosum
b. Cardiomegaly

c. Duodenojejunal flexure to the right of the midline
d. Radial hypoplasia
e. Spinal syrinx

30. A 30 year old man presents with hearing loss. Following review by the ear, nose and throat team, an MRI brain is performed. This shows bilateral masses at the cerebellopontine angle. The lesions have low to intermediate T2 weighted signal and intermediate T1 weighted signal. There is homogenous enhancement of both masses following gadolinium contrast. There are some peripheral, non-enhancing cystic lesions around the main mass. The lesions bulge in to the porus acousticus, which appears mildly expanded.

    What underlying syndrome does the man likely have?

    a. Ehlers-Danlos
    b. Neurofibromatosis 1
    c. Neurofibromatosis 2
    d. Tuberous sclerosis
    e. Von Hippel-Lindau

31. A 31 year homeless male patient attends the emergency department with haemoptysis, fever and shortness of breath. The team decide to do a CT pulmonary angiogram to exclude a pulmonary embolus, as well as look for another cause for the patient's symptoms. The CT does not demonstrate a pulmonary embolus; however there is a 5-cm thick-walled cavity in the left apex with surrounding consolidation, tree-in-bud nodularity and airway wall thickening. Further extensive tree-in-bud nodularity and consolidation is seen in the lingula.

    What is the most likely aetiology?

    a. Miliary tuberculosis
    b. Non-tuberculous mycobacterium infection
    c. Primary tuberculosis
    d. Post-primary tuberculosis
    e. Septic emboli

32. A 32 year old female has plain films and subsequent CT of the left hand for investigation of a firm lump on the dorsum. The images demonstrate a broad based, irregularly shaped, ossified, exophytic lesion arising from the dorsal aspect of the cortex of the metacarpal of the little finger. It projects into the adjacent soft tissue towards the joint. The lesion is not continuous with the medullary cavity and the cortex is intact. The lesion is thought to represent a benign tumour.

    What is the most likely diagnosis?

    a. Bizarre parosteal osteochondromatous proliferation
    b. Chondroblastoma
    c. Chondromyxoid fibroma
    d. Enchondroma
    e. Osteochondroma

33. An MRI small bowel is performed for a 39 year old female patient with abdominal pain and diarrhoea. This reveals small bowel fold thickening affecting the jejunum and ileum. There are several adjacent 11-mm short axis lymph nodes and a small amount of free fluid in the pelvis. The right lobe of the liver extends approximately 2 cm below the lower pole of the right kidney. The spleen measures 16 cm in craniocaudal extent. Both kidneys measure up to 10.5 cm in length. Patchy low T1 and T2 weighted signal is demonstrated in the imaged spine.

    What is the most likely unifying diagnosis?

    a. Amyloidosis
    b. Lymphoma
    c. Mastocytosis
    d. Tuberculosis
    e. Whipple disease

34. The paediatric team ask you to review a radiograph of a patient who is currently being kept as an inpatient due to concerns about non-accidental injury (NAI).

    Which of these is the commonest skeletal injury in NAI?

    a. Fracture of the distal clavicle
    b. Linear skull fracture
    c. Metaphyseal tibial fracture
    d. Posterior rib fracture
    e. Transverse humeral fracture

35. A 55 year old man is admitted with cognitive disturbance, ataxia and seizures. A CT head reveals anterior cerebellar vermian atrophy as well as more generalised cerebral volume loss which is excessive for the age of the patient. There is also subtle hypodensity in the corpus callosum. An MRI the following day finds that this area is T2 hyperintense with low signal on T1 sequences and primarily affecting the body and genu of the corpus callosum.

    What is the most likely diagnosis?

    a. Marchiafava-Bignami disease
    b. Methanol intoxication
    c. Multiple sclerosis
    d. Susac syndrome
    e. Wernicke's encephalopathy

36. A 1 day old preterm neonate is referred for a cranial ultrasound due to low Apgar scores following delivery and abnormal posturing. Hypoxic ischaemic injury is suspected.

    Which of the following sonographic findings is most likely?

    a. Cerebellar involvement
    b. Globally reduced Doppler signal
    c. Hypoechoic basal ganglia
    d. Normal study
    e. Widened Sylvian fissures

37. A 67 year old retired decorator presents to his GP following multiple episodes of chest pain during the past 2 weeks brought on by exertion. Past medical history includes hypertension and gallstones. The GP refers him to the rapid access chest pain clinic. As part of the investigations the patient has a cardiac MRI which demonstrates increased T2 weighted signal intensity in the mid anterior and septal walls, with delayed subendocardial hyperenhancement.

    What is the most likely diagnosis?

    a. Acute myocarditis
    b. Hibernating myocardium
    c. Myocardial infarct involving the left anterior descending artery
    d. Myocardial infarct involving the right coronary artery
    e. Myocardial stunning

38. A 7 year old female falls from a trampoline and develops wrist swelling. The parents take her to the emergency department and a plain film is performed. The imaging demonstrates buckling of the cortex; the cortex remains intact.

    What type of fracture is this?

    a. Greenstick fracture
    b. Lead pipe
    c. Plastic bowing
    d. Salter-Harris fracture
    e. Torus fracture

39. A 50 year old man has arthralgia, hyperpigmentation and new onset diabetes. His maternal grandfather had haemochromatosis.

    Which of the following liver MRI findings would help differentiate primary haemochromatosis from haemosiderosis?

a. Reduced signal on T1 and T2 weighted images in the liver and spleen
b. Reduced signal on T1 and T2 weighted images in the liver and bone marrow
c. Reduced signal on T1 and T2 weighted images in the liver and pancreas
d. Increased signal on T1 and T2 weighted images in the liver and spleen
e. Increased signal on T1 and T2 weighted images in the liver and pancreas

40. A trainee sonographer comes to you asking for advice about appearances on a transvaginal pelvic ultrasound examination of a 35 year old GP patient with intermittent lower abdominal pain. The sonographer could clearly see both ovaries. There are a couple of small (<10 mm), thin-walled, anechoic, avascular lesions associated with the right ovary. In the left ovary there is a 15 mm unilocular, anechoic cystic lesion which is thick walled with marked continuous peripheral vascularity. There is a trace of free fluid in the pouch of Douglas. The uterus is anteverted. The endometrium measures up to 8 mm.

Which of the following is most appropriate?

a. MRI pelvis
b. No follow-up
c. Recommend Ca-125 levels and gynaecology referral
d. Ultrasound pelvis in 6 weeks
e. Ultrasound pelvis in 3 months

41. A 10 year old child with a raised serum alpha-fetoprotein has an abdominal ultrasound. The liver has a coarse echotexture and reduced reflectivity. There is a 20-mm solid heterogenous lesion in the right hepatic lobe which is predominantly hypoechoic. There is no evidence of calcification. On MRI the lesion is T2 hyperintense and has mildly increased T1 signal. It enhances homogenously and rapidly following contrast. The lesion then becomes hypointense to the rest of the liver on portal venous phase images.

Which of the following is the most likely diagnosis?

a. Haemangioendothelioma
b. Hepatoblastoma
c. Hepatocellular carcinoma
d. Mesenchymal hamartoma
e. Regenerative nodule

42. A 20 year old woman presents with left sided complex partial seizures which are intractable to conventional antiepileptic medication. The neurologist suspects temporal lobe epilepsy and requests an MRI brain.

What sequence is best to identify mesial temporal sclerosis?

a. Axial FLAIR
b. Coronal T1 post contrast
c. Axial T2
d. Coronal FLAIR
e. Sagittal T1

43. A 44 year old male asthmatic has a high resolution CT chest due to worsening control of asthma symptoms. He is a smoker. The CT is mostly unremarkable, however the radiologist reports there is a 4-mm well-defined nodule in the right middle lobe, with no evidence of calcification.

What is the most appropriate onward management in view of this nodule?

a. CT of the abdomen and pelvis to look for primary site of malignancy
b. Follow-up CT chest in 3 months
c. Follow-up CT chest in 12 months
d. PET/CT scan
e. No further CT follow-up

44. A 31 year old male has an MRI for further investigation of a lucent lesion at the distal left femur which has a narrow zone of transition, mild bone expansion and a well-defined margin. The MRI report suggests that the lesion is most likely in keeping with a giant cell tumour.

Which of the following radiographic features is most likely to be present?

a. Multiple tumours
b. The lesion abuts the physis
c. Non-sclerotic margin
d. Matrix calcification
e. The tumour is centred on the medullary cavity

45. Following a road traffic collision a 12 year old cyclist is brought into hospital by ambulance intubated and ventilated. A trauma CT is performed. Thoracic imaging reveals a right sided pneumothorax, bilateral rib fractures and a fractured right proximal humerus. The abdominopelvic imaging demonstrates abdominal free fluid with retroperitoneal free gas. There is a short segment of duodenal mural thickening with disruption of the wall and adjacent free gas locules.

Where in the duodenum is the rupture most likely to be sited?

a. At the level of the ampulla of Vater
b. At the level of the ligament of Treitz
c. D1–2
d. D2–3
e. D3–4

46. A 15 year old boy with epistaxis is reviewed by the ear nose and throat (ENT) team. There is a red/blue mass visible on nasoendoscopy and an MRI head confirms a diagnosis of juvenile angiofibroma. The ENT team request radiological guided embolisation prior to surgical management.

Which artery is the most likely feeding vessel?

a. Ascending pharyngeal
b. Facial
c. Internal maxillary
d. Lingual
e. Superficial temporal

47. A 16 year old boy is referred for a MR angiogram for suspected aortic coarctation. He has a left sided aortic arch. The coarctation lies distal to the brachiocephalic trunk but proximal to the origin of the left subclavian artery.

What rib notching pattern would be most likely?

a. Bilateral first and second ribs
b. Bilateral third to ninth ribs
c. Left third to ninth ribs
d. Right first and second ribs
e. Right third to ninth ribs

48. A 7 year old girl presents with ataxia, diplopia and facial droop. On clinical examination she is found to have cranial nerve VI and VII palsies. A CT brain shows a mass enlarging the pons and flattening the floor of the fourth ventricle. There is resultant mild hydrocephalus. MRI brain reveals the lesion has low T1 and heterogeneously high T2 signal relative to cortical grey matter. There is minimal enhancement and the affected area does not restrict on diffusion weighted imaging.

What is the most likely diagnosis?

a. Acute demyelinating encephalomyelitis
b. Diffuse brainstem glioma
c. Medulloblastoma
d. Osmotic demyelination
e. Rhombencephalitis

49. The respiratory team request a CT chest for a 64 year old female patient presenting with increased shortness of breath on exertion. The patient has a 20 pack-year history and has previously been exposed to asbestos. Past medical history includes hypertension and pancreatitis, for which she has had two intensive care admissions. Previous imaging requests

state that on one of these admissions she developed acute respiratory distress syndrome (ARDS).

Where would you be most likely to see the long term pulmonary changes associated with her previous ARDS?

a. Anteriorly
b. Apical regions
c. At the lung bases
d. Perihilar region
e. Posteriorly

50. A 60 year old male patient has an unenhanced CT urinary tract for left sided renal colic. There is a 3-mm left renal calculus. Incidentally, a bone lesion is identified within the T12 vertebral body; the lesion is lucent with coarse vertical trabeculations and a 'polka-dot' appearance on axial slices. There is no soft tissue component, the cortex is intact and there is no periosteal reaction.

What is the most appropriate next investigation for the bone lesion?

a. FDG PET-CT scan
b. Follow-up CT scan in 6 months
c. Further assessment with whole spine MRI
d. No further investigation required
e. SPECT study

51. A 16 year old female patient has a urinary tract ultrasound following several urinary tract infections. This shows the right kidney is atrophic and the left kidney is normal in appearance. Previous ultrasound from when the patient was younger demonstrated a large right kidney. There is no hydronephrosis and the renal hilum is normal; however, there are multiple anechoic right renal lesions varying in size. These are separated by hyperechoic linear tissue without increased vascularity.

What is the most likely underlying diagnosis?

a. Autosomal recessive polycystic kidney disease
b. Juvenile nephronophthisis
c. Mesoblastic nephroma
d. Multicystic dysplastic kidney
e. Cystic nephroma

52. A 32 year old male with a background of multiple endocrine neoplasia type 1 undergoes surveillance imaging. He has been previously diagnosed with a parathyroid adenoma and pancreatic gastrinoma.

Which of these radiological findings is most likely to be present in this patient?

a. Hypoechoic thyroid nodule with tiny hyperechoic foci on ultrasound
b. A markedly T2 hyperintense right adrenal nodule
c. Polypoid caecal lesion on CT colonoscopy
d. Minimally enhancing pituitary lesion on MRI brain
e. An avidly enhancing right hilar mass

53. Twins are born by caesarean section at 34 weeks' gestation. They are treated with surfactant replacement therapy at birth and require treatment on the neonatal intensive care unit. One of the twins develops signs of respiratory distress syndrome, and a chest radiograph at day 5 post birth reveals small lung volumes and multiple bilateral lucencies. The thymic lobes are displaced laterally and surrounded by air. The trachea and mediastinum are central.
The endotracheal tube and vascular catheters are positioned appropriately, with the tip of the umbilical artery catheter at the level of T8.

Which of the following statements is most accurate?

a. An umbilical artery catheter tip should be sited between T10 and L3
b. Bronchopulmonary dysplasia is associated with meconium aspiration
c. Surfactant deficiency is associated with increased lung volumes

d. The patient has radiographic features of pneumothorax
e. This likely represents pulmonary interstitial emphysema

54. A 4 year old boy with hypotonia and occasional seizures is under the care of neurology. A CT brain reveals subtle low density of the subcortical white matter and on a subsequent MRI brain there is associated T1 hypointensity, FLAIR hyperintensity and restricted diffusion. The appearances are symmetrical and diffuse. There is no abnormal enhancement following contrast administration. The internal capsule and caudate nucleus are spared and the cerebellum has normal appearances. MR spectroscopy reveals a high *N*-acetyl-aspartate to creatine ratio.

What is the most likely diagnosis?

a. Adrenoleukodystrophy
b. Alexander disease
c. Canavan disease
d. Krabbe disease
e. Pelizaeus-Merzbacher disease

55. A 73 year old male presents with chest pain to the emergency department and has a CT aortogram to look for dissection. The aorta is mildly unfolded with no evidence of dissection. There is a 5.5-cm mass at the right upper lobe with evidence of local rib erosion. There is also an 11-mm nodule in the right lower lobe, a right sided pleural effusion and a pericardial effusion. A subcarinal lymph node is 2 cm in short axis dimension. Furthermore, there are two ill-defined low attenuation lesions in the liver.

Which of the following is most important when considering the M stage for this patient in the TNM staging?

a. Local rib erosion
b. Pleural effusion
c. Pericardial effusion
d. Presence of liver lesions
e. Size of the main tumour

56. A 22 year old male has plain films of the left femur for investigation of pain. There is an abnormal appearance of the metadiaphyseal region. The bone has a permeative appearance with a wide zone of transition and lamellated periosteal reaction.

What is the most likely site of metastases for Ewing's sarcoma?

a. Brain
b. Bone
c. Lung
d. Liver
e. Lymph nodes

57. A contrast-enhanced CT abdomen and pelvis is performed for a 57 year old man. The request states non-specific abdominal pain, unintended weight loss and fatigue with a history of hypertension, hypercholesterolaemia and excess alcohol intake. The CT reveals multiple low attenuation liver lesions and enlarged upper abdominal and para aortic lymph nodes. Apart from a couple of Bozniak II renal cysts measuring up to 30 mm, the other solid upper abdominal viscera have normal appearances. The stomach appears diffusely thickened, with a small lumen and perigastric fat stranding. There is moderate volume ascites with several superficial peritoneal soft tissue nodules. The colon is normal calibre without obvious primary lesion.

A subsequent CT chest demonstrates several bilateral lower lobe lung nodules measuring up to 8 mm. The patient undergoes a gastroscopy and biopsy which come back negative.

What would you suggest that the team request?

a. Colonoscopy
b. CT guided lung biopsy
c. Repeat gastroscopy and biopsy
d. Ultrasound guided liver biopsy
e. Ultrasound guided peritoneal biopsy

58. A 12 year old boy has a plain film of the pelvis for investigation of 8 weeks' history of left sided hip pain. Radiographs demonstrate joint space widening on the left when compared to the right. On ultrasound there is bulging of the anterior joint capsule and >3 mm distance between the bony femoral neck and joint capsule. He is thought to have juvenile idiopathic arthritis.

    Which of the following statement is most accurate in this condition?

    a. Bone changes occur early
    b. Most are seronegative
    c. Periostitis is considered atypical
    d. The hip joint is the most common site for the monoarticular variant
    e. There is often late closure of the growth plates

59. A baby is admitted to the neonatal intensive care unit with respiratory distress. Following an abnormal chest radiograph, an arterial phase CT is performed. There is a right lower lobe mass. This contains multiple air-fluid levels. There is a clear connection between the mass and the right bronchial tree. The mass does not have a systemic vascular supply.

    What does this mass most likely represent

    a. Bronchogenic cyst
    b. Congenital lobar over inflation
    c. Congenital pulmonary airway malformation
    d. Diaphragmatic hernia
    e. Intralobar pulmonary sequestration

60. A 60 year old man is found unconscious at home. Following ambulance transfer to hospital, a CT head is requested. This shows bilateral hypodensity affecting the globus pallidi bilaterally. On MRI the same area shows high signal on T2 weighted imaging and restricted diffusion.

    Which of the following is the cause of his findings?

    a. Asphyxiation
    b. Carbon monoxide poisoning
    c. Hypoglycaemia
    d. Lead poisoning
    e. Methanol poisoning

61. A 49 year old male patient with no fixed abode is admitted with a 3 day history of increasing abdominal pain. CT abdomen and pelvis demonstrates an infrarenal saccular dilatation of the abdominal aorta measuring up to 45 mm in maximum diameter with para-aortic soft tissue stranding. Adjacent para-aortic and aortocaval lymph nodes measure up to 11 mm in short axis.

    What is the most likely causative organism?

    a. Actinomycosis
    b. Cryptococcosis
    c. Histoplasmosis
    d. Salmonella
    e. *Treponema pallidum*

62. A 19 year old male who is usually fit and active has plain films of the right knee for ongoing knee pain. The radiograph demonstrates subtle flattening of the lateral surface of the medial femoral condyle with a loose osteochondral fragment. He has an MRI for investigation of suspected osteochondritis dissecans.

    Which finding is most likely to be seen on MRI?

    a. Blooming artefact on gradient echo sequence
    b. Cartilaginous defect on T1
    c. Fat-fluid level within joint effusion
    d. Low signal material within the defect on T2
    e. Synovial proliferation

63. A 56 year old male presents with acute epigastric pain. He is found to have a grossly elevated amylase level and leucocytosis. He is admitted under the general surgeons for conservative

management. However, after several days he becomes febrile and septic and a CT abdomen pelvis confirms severe pancreatitis with associated complications. The radiology report gives a severity score based on the CT severity index incorporating the Balthazar score.

Which of the following imaging features would be included in the Balthazar score?

a. Associated intestinal ileus
b. Background features of liver cirrhosis
c. Peripancreatic inflammation
d. Splenic vein thrombosis
e. The underlying cause of pancreatitis

64. A renal transplant patient is 4 days post-surgery and the transplant team request an ultrasound Doppler due to increased tenderness in the right iliac fossa, decreased urine output and haematuria. It is a single artery, vein and ureter organ from an adult cadaveric donor. The unobstructed transplant measures 15 cm in bipolar length and there is a trace of perinephric fluid. Corticomedullary differentiation appears normal. There is generalised Doppler vascularity evident within the kidney. The arcuate arterial traces at the upper, lower and middle poles demonstrate a sharp upstroke and a resistive index of 0.71. The renal artery and vein are difficult to visualise but the main renal artery demonstrates reverse flow in diastole. The urinary bladder has normal appearances.

What is the most likely diagnosis?

a. Pseudoaneurysm
b. Rejection
c. Renal artery stenosis
d. Renal artery thrombosis
e. Renal vein thrombosis

65. A neonate fails to pass meconium. A water-soluble contrast enema identifies dilated loops of proximal colon with a transition point at the splenic flexure. Contrast outlines retained meconium in a normal calibre descending colon. The rectum is normal calibre.

Given the above findings, which of the following conditions is most likely?

a. Hirschsprung disease
b. Ileal atresia
c. Meconium ileus
d. Meconium plug syndrome
e. Zuelzer-Wilson syndrome

66. You are reporting an MRI brain for a neurology outpatient with a history of epilepsy. There is unilateral partial opacification of the left maxillary sinus by a rounded lesion. The opacity demonstrates high T2 signal and intermediate T1 signal without restricted diffusion or enhancement. The maxillary ostia are symmetrical. On a CT brain from 2 months previously there is a similar appearance with a hypodense lesion in a partially aerated left maxillary sinus.

What does this mass most likely represent?

a. Allergic fungal sinusitis
b. Antrochoanal polyp
c. Mucocele
d. Mucous retention cyst
e. Papilloma

67. A 33 year old female presents with left sided chest pain and shortness of breath. She has a chest radiograph in the emergency department which shows a left sided pleural effusion. She is under outpatient follow-up with the rheumatology team for systemic lupus erythematosus (SLE). She has a CT pulmonary angiogram as the team are concerned that she is at increased risk of pulmonary embolus. This shows no evidence of pulmonary embolus; however, there are radiological features consistent with her underlying diagnosis.

What is the most common radiological chest finding associated with SLE?

a. Interstitial lung disease

b. Pericardial thickening
c. Pleural effusion
d. Pneumonia
e. Pulmonary haemorrhage

68. A 3 year old girl is brought to the emergency department following a fall. The consultant looking after the child requests a CT head. The patient, who is known to have an autosomal-dominant inherited abnormality, has blue tinting of the sclera and suffers with recurrent fractures. Previous plain films of the lower limbs demonstrate poor bone density, evidence of previous fractures with callus formation, and a 'shepherd's crook' deformity of the femur.

What are the most likely findings on CT head?

a. Greater than 10 wormian bones
b. Ground-glass appearance of the sphenoid wing
c. Optic nerve atrophy
d. Subdural haematoma
e. Widening of the diploic space

69. A patient is discussed at the upper gastrointestinal multidisciplinary team meeting. They presented with dysphagia and weight loss. A barium swallow revealed mid-oesophageal mucosal irregularity and endoscopic biopsies confirm moderately differentiated oesophageal squamous cell carcinoma. Staging imaging is required to aid management.

What is the most appropriate staging imaging?

a. Contrast enhanced CT chest abdomen and pelvis
b. Endoscopic ultrasound
c. Endoscopic ultrasound and 18F-FDG PET/CT
d. Endoscopic ultrasound and contrast enhanced CT chest, abdomen and pelvis
e. Thoracic MRI and contrast enhanced CT chest, abdomen and pelvis

70. A 6 year old boy with developmental delay is referred to the paediatric neurologists for an MRI brain due to recurrent seizures. This reveals multiple subependymal nodules which return high T1 and intermediate T2 signal. Previous ultrasound of the abdomen demonstrated bilateral echogenic renal masses.

Based on the above findings, what other feature is most likely on the MRI head?

a. Cystic lesion in right cerebellum containing an enhancing solid nodule
b. Homogenous intermediate signal durally based lesion adjacent to the right frontal lobe
c. Intraventricular markedly enhancing lobulated mass
d. Multiple foci of FLAIR hyperintensity in the cortical and subcortical regions
e. Several foci of T2 hyperintensity in the deep white matter bilaterally

71. A 54 year old man presents with nausea, weight loss and abdominal pain. The surgeons refer him for a contrast-enhanced CT abdomen and pelvis. This demonstrates a well-defined, heterogenous mass at the mesenteric root. The mass envelops the vessels, but the terminal ileum and large bowel are unaffected. The vessels are surrounded by a circumferential low-attenuation area of adipose.

What is the most likely diagnosis?

a. Radiation enteritis
b. Mesenteric panniculitis
c. Tuberculosis
d. Carcinoid
e. Mesenteric lipoma

72. A 42 year old man is referred for a CT head due to partial complex seizures. The CT shows a large, well defined mass involving the left frontal cortex and white matter. It erodes the inner table of the skull. The mass shows diffuse, amorphous calcification. There is little mass effect. Following contrast administration there is heterogenous enhancement.

What is the most likely diagnosis?

a. Astrocytoma

b. Ependymoma
c. Glioblastoma multiforme
d. Meningioma
e. Oligodendroglioma

73. A 49 year old female patient is admitted under the gynaecologists with pain, fever and nausea 3 days following uterine artery embolisation performed for menorrhagia caused by multiple uterine fibroids. A CT abdomen and pelvis scan is requested which demonstrates density of −1000HU in a couple of fibroids with a small amount of pelvic free fluid. On transvaginal ultrasound scan multiple intramural and submucosal fibroids are again demonstrated and the uterus appears bulky. There is small volume free fluid in the pouch of Douglas; the endometrium is partially effaced by the fibroids but the thickness is approximately 8 mm at the fundus and the ovaries have functional appearances.

What is the most likely diagnosis?

a. Endometritis
b. Fibroid torsion
c. Infection within the fibroids
d. Post-embolisation syndrome
e. Uterine necrosis

74. A 44 year old female patient attends the orthopaedic outpatient clinic with a fracture of her right distal radius following a fall onto an outstretched hand. The orthopaedic registrar asks you to review the plain films. There is a well-defined, expansile, lytic lesion at the site of the fracture which has thinned the cortex. Other findings include generalised sclerosis and subperiosteal resorption along the radial aspect of the middle phalanges. MRI of the wrist confirms a cystic and solid lesion with fluid-fluid levels and enhancement of the solid components.

What other imaging finding would most likely correlate with these appearances?

a. A focus of tracer uptake in the region of the thyroid on a Tc-99m pertechnetate scan
b. Diffusely increased thyroid tracer uptake on a Tc-99m pertechnetate scan
c. Multiple low attenuation liver lesions on CT abdomen pelvis
d. Renal cortical thickness of 5 mm on abdominal ultrasound
e. Cortical irregularity with adjacent sclerosis at the medial aspect of the proximal femur

75. A 28 year old male patient, under the care of the gastroenterology team, has been admitted with an exacerbation of ulcerative colitis. After 48 hours in hospital he is stable but has some increased abdominal discomfort. You are asked to review his contrast-enhanced CT abdomen and pelvis. This demonstrates mural thickening and pericolic fat stranding affecting the entire colon and rectum. There is a rim of lower attenuation in the wall of the colon with a Hounsfield unit of −95 and minimal faecal residue in the colon. There is a tiny amount of peritoneal free fluid but no free gas. The colon measures up to 50 mm in diameter. Mesenteric lymph nodes measure up to 11 mm in short axis.

What is the most appropriate recommendation to the clinical team?

a. Abdominal radiograph in 24 hours
b. Barium enema in 24 hours
c. Colonoscopy within 48–72 hours
d. Repeat CT abdomen pelvis in 48 hours
e. Urgent surgical referral

76. A 23 year old builder is seen in the emergency department following a fall from scaffolding. CT chest abdomen pelvis demonstrates several right rib fractures and a small amount of free fluid in the pelvis. The patient has haematuria and blood at the urethral meatus. The urology team request retrograde urethrography. This demonstrates extravasation of contrast into the retropubic space, but continuity of the urethra is maintained.

Where is the urethral injury most likely to be sited?

a. Above the urogenital diaphragm
b. Below the urogenital diaphragm
c. Bladder dome

d. Bulbous urethra
e. Penile urethra

77. A 5 year old child undergoes a barium swallow for dysphagia. This shows an anterior indentation over the oesophagus just above the level of the carina.

What is the most likely cause for this appearance?

a. Aberrant left pulmonary artery
b. Aberrant right subclavian artery
c. Double aortic arch
d. Enlarged left atrium
e. Right sided aortic arch

78. A 53 year old female patient with metastatic breast cancer has a CT head to assess for intracranial metastases. This demonstrates no evidence of intracranial disease; however, there is a solitary enhancing right parotid lesion within the deep lobe. It is not amenable to ultrasound-guided biopsy. An MRI head is suggested.

Which MRI sequence would be most helpful in confirming that this is a pleomorphic adenoma?

a. Fat supressed T1
b. Gradient echo
c. Post contrast T1
d. T1
e. T2

79. An emergency department junior doctor requests a CT pulmonary angiogram to look for a pulmonary embolus in a 52 year old patient who is complaining of acute onset pleuritic chest pain and shortness of breath. The patient is tachycardic with heart rate of 120 bpm; the Wells score is 4.5. They have had a normal chest radiograph. You agree to a CTPA; however the pulmonary artery opacification achieved is inadequate. The main pulmonary artery is noted to be wider than the ascending aorta and the proximal arteries are also dilated; the peripheral vessels are reduced in calibre. There is a mosaic appearance to the lung parenchyma.

What is the most appropriate next step?

a. Advise further investigation with CT abdomen pelvis to look for underlying malignancy
b. Advise further investigation with myocardial perfusion study
c. Advise referral to the respiratory team
d. Perform expiratory phase CT chest
e. Perform a ventilation-perfusion (VQ) scan

80. A 45 year old male has a plain film of the knee for investigation of ongoing knee pain. This shows evidence of degenerative change and genu varus. There is also cortical hyperostosis affecting the diaphysis of the lateral aspect of the tibia, which is described as dripping candle wax in appearance.

What is the most likely diagnosis?

a. Caffey disease
b. Focal scleroderma
c. Melorheostosis
d. Osteopoikilosis
e. Pyknodysostosis

81. A 65 year old male who has a background of chronic alcohol abuse presents to the emergency department with an upper gastrointestinal bleed. He undergoes endoscopy which confirms oesophageal varices. These are injected and the patient improves. An abdominal ultrasound is subsequently arranged.

Which of the following ultrasound findings is UNLIKELY to be identified in this patient?

a. Ascites
b. Gallbladder wall thickening
c. Hepatopetal portal venous flow

d. Portal venous flow of 8 cm/sec
e. Splenomegaly

82. A 4 year old female patient has splenomegaly, gallstones and bilateral enlarged kidneys on an abdominal ultrasound scan. A previous chest radiograph from the year before demonstrates consolidation; this is no longer present on the current radiograph.

Which of the following findings may also be present in a patient with this condition?

a. Anterior inferior vertebral body beaking
b. H-shaped vertebrae
c. Posterior vertebral scalloping
d. Ribbon ribs
e. Narrowed interpedicular distance

83. A 19 year old male presents with headache, and on examination he is found to have paralysis of upward gaze. CT head reveals dilatation of the lateral ventricles. There is a well-defined, hyperdense mass in the posterior aspect of the third ventricle. The mass has some central calcification present. On MRI the mass is isointense to grey matter on both T1 and T2 sequences with cystic high T2 signal foci. The mass enhances avidly on T1 post contrast sequence but there is no evidence of blooming on susceptibility weighted imaging. A further similar 2-cm mass is also seen in the midline within the suprasellar region.

What is the most likely diagnosis?

a. Pineoblastoma
b. Pineocytoma
c. Pineal germinoma
d. Pineal yolk sac carcinoma
e. Pineal teratoma

84. A child is born at term with severe neurological compromise. An MRI brain reveals a cystic space in the brain in the right frontoparietal region. The fluid in the lesion supresses on FLAIR sequences but does not demonstrate restricted diffusion. The lesion lacks septations, communicates with the ventricles and is lined by white matter.

What does this abnormality likely represent?

a. Closed-lip schizencephaly
b. Hydrancephaly
c. Neuroglial cyst
d. Open-lipped schizencephaly
e. Porencephaly

85. A 57 year old female patient is referred for a CT chest by the respiratory clinicians. There is bronchial wall thickening with the airways having a similar diameter to the adjacent vessels at the lung peripheries and there is patchy ground glass opacification. The pleural spaces are clear. There are no size-significant hilar or mediastinal lymph nodes. Further images acquired following expiration demonstrate areas of lung which are comparatively low attenuation compared to the rest of the lungs. You note that the vessels are also smaller in the more lucent areas.

What is the most likely diagnosis?

a. Acute interstitial pneumonia
b. Alveolar proteinosis
c. Chronic eosinophilic pneumonia
d. Chronic hypersensitivity pneumonitis
e. Obliterative bronchiolitis

86. You report the plain film of a 29 year old male who has ongoing knee pain. The imaging shows enlargement of the physis, juxta-articular osteoporosis, erosion of the articular surface with subchondral cysts. There is a squared patella and widening of the intercondylar notch. There is no previous imaging available and no details of relevant medical history provided.

Which underlying diagnosis would you suspect in this patient?

a. Haemophilia
b. Homocysteinuria
c. Juvenile rheumatoid arthritis
d. Pigmented villonodular synovitis
e. Primary synovial chondromatosis

87. The clinical team ask your opinion on the best form of imaging for a 49 year old male with a family history of multiple endocrine neoplasia. He has symptoms of diarrhoea, abdominal pain and reflux. The patient has also presented twice during the past year to his GP with episodes of haematemesis.

What test would you recommend to the team?

a. Barium meal
b. CT chest, abdomen pelvis with arterial and portal venous phase contrast
c. 18F-FDG PET/CT
d. MRI brain
e. MRI small bowel

88. A 57 year old male patient is investigated for painless haematuria. Past medical history includes hypertension and type 2 diabetes, for which he is on oral medication. On ultrasound the kidneys are unobstructed but eccentrically positioned lower than normal with poor visualisation of the lower poles. There are normal appearances of the urinary bladder. CT urogram is completed and confirms a horseshoe kidney. There are several small filling defects in the renal pelvises and proximal ureters; these have a density of 10HU on the non-contrast sequence and then 15HU following contrast administration.

What is the most likely diagnosis?

a. Leukoplakia
b. Multiple calculi
c. Pyeloureteritis cystica
d. Transitional cell carcinoma
e. Tuberculous urethritis

89. You are asked to review imaging for a 2 month old child with bilious vomiting. An ultrasound and then an upper gastrointestinal contrast study have been completed. Both sets of imaging confirm malrotation.

Which of the following findings is NOT consistent with this conclusion?

a. Cephalad positioning of the caecum
b. Duodenojejunal flexure is at the level of the duodenal bulb
c. Duodenojejunal junction lies to the right of the right vertebral body pedicle
d. Superior mesenteric vein lies to the left of the superior mesenteric artery
e. Whirlpool appearance of the mesenteric vessels

90. An 18F-FDG PET/CT for a 71 year old patient seen in outpatients with decline in memory and cognitive function reveals changes suggestive of Alzheimer disease. The clinician feels that is in keeping with the clinical findings.

Which of these patterns of reduced tracer uptake is consistent with this conclusion?

a. Anterior and medial temporal lobes
b. Basal ganglia and posterior frontoparietal lobes
c. Corpus striatum
d. Occipital cortex and cerebellum
e. Precuneus, posterior cingulate cortex, posterior temporoparietal lobes

91. A 60 year old female presents to her GP with a cough and fever. She has a chest radiograph which reports consolidation in the left lower zone. A follow-up plain film following treatment is suggested. She returns to the department with ongoing symptoms for a repeat radiograph 6 weeks later. The left lower zone consolidation has resolved; however, there is new opacification in the left mid zone. The GP organises an unenhanced CT chest which is performed a couple of months after initial presentation. There is ground glass opacification at

the periphery of the left mid zone which is surrounded by dense crescentic opacification. Further patchy consolidation is seen in the periphery of the right lower lobe.

What is the most likely diagnosis?

a. Adenocarcinoma in situ
b. Cryptogenic organising pneumonia
c. Invasive fungal infection
d. Pulmonary haemorrhage
e. Pulmonary infarct

92. A 6 year old female suffers an inversion injury of her ankle on a trampoline. She is taken to the emergency department and plain films are performed. There is subtle slip of the distal fibula epiphysis.

What type of Salter-Harris fracture is this?

a. Type I
b. Type II
c. Type III
d. Type IV
e. Type V

93. A 42 year old woman undergoes a liver transplant for primary biliary cirrhosis. She is reviewed in the transplant clinic 2 weeks after discharge and undergoes a routine surveillance ultrasound.

Which of the following statements regarding this patient's liver transplant ultrasound is correct?

a. A perihepatic haematoma is an unexpected finding
b. A tardus parvus Doppler waveform is normal in the early post-transplant period
c. Biliary strictures are an uncommon early complication
d. Hepatic vein thrombosis is the most common vascular complication
e. The gallbladder may be mildly oedematous

94. A 23 year old female with no past medical history except taking the oral contraceptive pill presents with headache and a tonic clonic seizure. An unenhanced CT head shows a small parenchymal haemorrhage in the subcortical region of the right temporal lobe which does not conform to a vascular territory. There is associated sulcal effacement.

What is the next best investigation?

a. CT intracranial angiogram
b. Catheter angiogram
c. MR venogram
d. Intracranial Doppler
e. Lumbar puncture

95. A neonate is noted to be cyanotic from birth. A frontal chest radiograph is performed which shows a grossly dilated heart and right atrium with elevated apex. The lungs are oligaemic.

What is the most likely diagnosis?

a. Aortic coarctation
b. Ebstein anomaly
c. Tetralogy of Fallot
d. Total anomalous pulmonary venous return (TAPVR)
e. Transposition of the great arteries

96. A 49 year old male patient has had his care transferred to the local ear, nose and throat team after relocating to the area. He has a history of thyroid cancer for which he has undergone total thyroidectomy 18 months previously. At the time of the ultrasound the patient is not sure about the type of thyroid cancer he had and the referral letter is not available. The scan demonstrates a 9-mm left level III lymph node with microcalcification. Early pathological assessment confirms malignant cells.

Which underlying malignancy is most likely?

a. Anaplastic thyroid carcinoma
b. Follicular thyroid carcinoma
c. Lymphoma
d. Medullary thyroid carcinoma
e. Papillary thyroid carcinoma

97. A 73 year old female patient is seen in the respiratory outpatient clinic with increasing shortness of breath over the past year. Subsequent CT chest shows right lower lobe volume loss with an enhancing, pleurally based lesion forming an obtuse angle with the pleura. Looking back at a previous CT 3 years ago, this has not increased in size. The vessels and bronchi seen extending from the right hilum towards the mass appear crowded and distorted. There is evidence of increased subpleural reticular markings in the lower lobes bilaterally.

What additional feature would confirm the diagnosis?

a. Cavitation
b. Intralesional fat
c. Pleural thickening and calcification
d. Right hilum lymph node enlargement
e. Water-lily sign

98. A 45 year old male is reviewed in the orthopaedic clinic with knee pain causing restricted range of movement. On examination the pain is localised to the retropatellar region and crepitation is noted on passive and active movement.

Which of the below is most consistent with patella baja?

a. An Insall-Salvati ratio of 0.6
b. It is associated with chondromalacia patellae
c. Requires sagittal MRI knee for diagnosis
d. The condition is frequently an incidental finding
e. The condition describes an abnormally high riding patella

99. A 26 year old male is investigated for recurrent pancreatitis with an MRCP. This identifies pancreas divisum.

Which of the following is most likely in this patient's imaging?

a. Choledochal cysts are also likely to be present
b. The major papilla drains the dorsal duct
c. There is likely to be a connection between the dorsal and ventral ducts
d. The minor papilla drains the pancreatic body and tail
e. The duct of Santorini drains the pancreatic head

100. A 57 year old woman with predominantly fatty breasts is recalled from screening for an area of new clustered microcalcification in the right breast. The radiographer asks whether you need any additional mammographic imaging prior to ultrasound.

Which of the following is the most appropriate initial further investigation?

a. Contrast-enhanced mammograms
b. Ecklund technique
c. Magnification views
d. Paddle view
e. Tomosynthesis

101. A 12 month old boy is referred to the paediatricians for abnormal head circumference. A skull radiograph confirms premature fusion of the coronal suture with frontal bossing. Both sides of the head are affected causing the skull to appear short and wide.

What type of craniosynostosis is described?

a. Brachycephaly
b. Oxycephaly
c. Plagiocephaly

d. Scaphocephaly
e. Trigonocephaly

102. A 10 year old boy presents with a reduced GCS. An urgent CT brain reveals a large mixed solid and cystic suprasellar lesion causing hydrocephalus. The mass contains calcification. A subsequent MRI demonstrates that the lesion has heterogeneously high T2 signal. The solid components of the mass enhance avidly on T1 post contrast imaging.

What is the most likely diagnosis?

a. Craniopharyngioma
b. Intracranial teratoma
c. Meningioma
d. Pituitary macroadenoma
e. Rathke cleft cyst

103. A 53 year old male has ongoing cough and shortness of breath following a lung transplant 18 months earlier. He has a CT chest as part of his workup to look for complications. He has suffered intermittent infective episodes since the transplant, which have required treatment with antiviral therapy. He is increasingly symptomatic and the clinicians are concerned about chronic rejection. The CT scan shows hyperinflated lungs, bronchiectasis and airway wall thickening with mosaicism, worse in the lower zones.

What is the most likely diagnosis?

a. Acute transplant rejection
b. Bronchiolitis obliterans
c. Cytomegalovirus infection
d. Post-transplant lymphoproliferative disease
e. Reperfusion syndrome

104. A 15 year old male with back pain, who has a diagnosis of Scheuermann's disease, has an MRI of the whole spine.

When reviewing the imaging, which of the following is most accurate?

a. The kyphosis is <35°
b. Less than three vertebral bodies are affected
c. The lumbar spine is most likely affected
d. There is preservation of the disc spaces
e. Schmorl nodes are one of the most common features

105. A 54 year old patient with chronic hepatitis B infection and a high body mass index has an abdominal ultrasound to monitor her liver. Her previous scan was 12 months previously. The most recent ultrasound shows no sonographic evidence of cirrhosis; however, there is an indeterminate hypoechoic area in the left lobe. Further liver imaging is advised.

With regard to liver MRI, which of the below is correct regarding normal liver appearances?

Table 3.1:

	MRI T1 Signal	MRI T2 Signal	MRI In- and Out-of-Phase Sequences
a	Spleen < liver	Spleen < liver	No change between sequences
b	Spleen > liver	Spleen < liver	Reduced on out-of-phase sequence
c	Spleen < liver	Spleen > liver	No change between sequences
d	Spleen < liver	Spleen > liver	Reduced on out-of-phase sequence
e	Spleen > liver	Spleen < spleen	No change between sequences

106. A 12 year old male with repeated fractures attends the emergency department following a fall. He has a plain film of the left femur which demonstrates increased bone density of the medulla, a 'bone-in-bone' appearance, Erlenmeyer flask deformity and evidence of previous healed fracture but no acute fracture seen.

What is the most likely underlying diagnosis?

a. Fibrous dysplasia
b. Lead poisoning
c. Melorheostosis
d. Osteopetrosis
e. Pkynodysostosis

107. A 7 year old boy undergoes an MRI brain. This shows a dilated, high-riding third ventricle which appears to communicate with the interhemispheric cistern. The lateral ventricles appear widely spaced with small frontal horns. The interhemispheric fissure is also widened.

Given this description, what is the most likely diagnosis?

a. Cavum septum pellucidum
b. Cavum vergae
c. Cavum velum interpositum
d. Corpus callosum agenesis
e. Interhemispheric arachnoid cyst

108. A 48 year old patient has had surgical resection for a right frontal lobe glioblastoma, followed by radiotherapy and chemotherapy. The MRI brain following treatment demonstrates a lesion in the right frontal lobe with FLAIR hyperintensity and mass effect. The clinical team are concerned about tumour recurrence. Following further imaging, including MRI spectroscopy and MR perfusion studies, the multidisciplinary team conclude that it most likely represents cerebral radiation necrosis.

Which of the following characteristics of the areas of FLAIR hyperintensity in the right frontal lobe fit with this diagnosis?

Table 3.2:

	Enhancement	MRI Spectroscopy Choline Level	Relative Cerebral Blood Flow (rCBF)
a	Present	Low	Low
b	Absent	High	Low
c	Present	High	High
d	Absent	Low	High
e	Absent	High	Low

109. A 42 year old female patient is referred to the respiratory team for persistent cough and recurrent chest infections. A chest radiograph that the GP requested 6 weeks ago reveals right lower lobe atelectasis. The patient attends for CT chest which identifies a well-defined 15-mm soft tissue lesion containing calcification. This is centred on the right hilar region with associated right lower lobe consolidation. There are a couple of 10-mm right hilar lymph nodes and a subcarinal lymph node. The patient is referred for lung multidisciplinary team (MDT) meeting discussion.

What further imaging would be appropriate to recommend to the MDT prior to surgery?

a. 18F FDG PET/CT
b. 18F DOPA PET/CT
c. Gallium 68 PET/CT
d. Liver MRI
e. Repeat CT chest in 6 months

110. A 21 year old female with a known chromosomal abnormality has a fall onto an outstretched hand and attends the emergency department, where a plain film is performed to assess for scaphoid fracture. She has had previous investigations which described a Madelung deformity.

Which of the following is most likely to be seen on plain film?

a. Medial radial curvature
b. Shortening of the second and fifth middle phalanx
c. Shortening of the third and fourth metacarpal
d. Short radius with a triangularised distal epiphysis
e. Ulnar impingement

111. A 54 year old man has biopsy proven adenocarcinoma of the body of pancreas following an endoscopic ultrasound. He undergoes a staging CT chest, abdomen and pelvis prior to MDT discussion.

Which of the following findings WOULD NOT be a contraindication to surgical resection?

a. Invasion of the duodenum
b. Tumour involves 60% of the circumference of the superior mesenteric vein
c. Tumour is in contact with more than half of the superior mesenteric artery
d. Enlarged lower para-aortic lymph nodes
e. Invasion of the adrenal gland

112. A 63 year old male patient is discussed at the urology multidisciplinary team (MDT) meeting. He has a T1a N0 renal cell carcinoma diagnosed on a CT colonoscopy requested for iron deficiency anaemia. The mass is located at the right upper pole of an unobstructed horseshoe kidney, which is positioned in the midline at approximately the level of L3/4. The kidney otherwise has normal appearances. Serum renal function tests are normal. Completion staging CT chest showed no thoracic metastatic disease. The MDT discusses partial nephrectomy as a treatment option.

Which additional information is particularly helpful in this clinical scenario?

a. 18F-FDG PET/CT to exclude occult metastases
b. Delayed phase CT urogram to exclude pelviureteric filling defects
c. Renal arterial anatomy assessment with CT angiogram
d. Split renal function with DTPA nuclear medicine study
e. Micturating cystourethrogram to assess for urinary reflux

113. A 6 year old child with known scoliosis is referred for an MRI spine due to progressive bilateral lower limb leg weakness and sensory loss. The T2 weighted sagittal sequence shows an abnormally widened dural space from T10 to L2. The T2 weighted coronal shows increased interpedicular distance, cord widening and splitting at this level. Axial T2 weighted sequences demonstrate a thin hypointense septum between the cord.

What is the most likely diagnosis?

a. Diastematomyelia
b. Diplomyelia
c. Myelomeningocele
d. Syringomyelia
e. Tethered cord

114. A 70 year old woman presents with a two day history of left sided weakness. A CT brain shows acute intracerebral haematoma within the right frontal lobe with surrounding oedema. The patient goes on to have an MRI brain the same day.

What is the most likely signal characteristic of the haematoma on MRI?

Table 3.3:

	T1	T2
a	Low	Low
b	High	High
c	High	Low
d	Isointense	Low
e	Isointense	High

115. A 29 year old female has a CT scan of the chest. This shows an incidental finding of lobulated soft tissue within the anterior mediastinum which is thought to represent a thymic abnormality. She undergoes an MRI scan to further characterise this lesion.

Which of the following sequences is most useful to assess for thymic hyperplasia?

a. Diffusion weighted imaging
b. In- and out-of-phase imaging
c. Post-contrast fat saturated T1 imaging
d. T1 weighted imaging
e. T2 weighted imaging

116. A 36 year old woman is referred for an MRI brain due to tinnitus and vertigo. This demonstrates a mass at the left cerebellopontine angle.

Which of the following radiological features is most suggestive of a vestibular schwannoma compared to a meningioma?

a. Blooming artefact due to calcification on gradient echo sequence
b. Expansion of the internal acoustic canal
c. Hypointensity on T2 weighted imaging
d. Obtuse angle with the dura
e. Restricted diffusion

117. A 36 year old cyclist is involved in a collision with a car. In the emergency department he is hypotensive. On examination there is guarding in the left upper quadrant. A split bolus, trauma protocol CT chest abdomen and pelvis is performed. This demonstrates left-sided rib fractures. There is hyperdense (50HU) free fluid in the splenic bed. Within the upper pole of the spleen there is a linear area of hypoenhancement that measures 4 cm. No contrast extravasation or blush is identified.

According to The American Association for the Surgery of Trauma (AAST) grading scale, what is the grade of splenic injury?

a. Grade I
b. Grade II
c. Grade III
d. Grade IV
e. Grade V

118. A cranial ultrasound is performed on a premature neonate. Germinal matrix haemorrhage is identified.

Which of the following radiological findings indicates the worst prognosis?

a. Hyperechoic foci in the peritrigonal area
b. Intraparenchymal haemorrhage
c. Intraventricular haemorrhage
d. Intraventricular haemorrhage with ventricular dilatation
e. Subependymal haemorrhage

119. A 42 year old woman with a history of Sjögren syndrome presents with acute abdominal pain. On examination she is tender with guarding in the epigastric region. Blood tests show highly elevated serum amylase level. She undergoes a CT abdomen pelvis with contrast. This shows a diffusely enlarged pancreas with a surrounding hypoattenuating rim. There is minimal peripancreatic stranding and no pseudocyst formation or necrosis. An autoimmune pancreatitis is considered to be most likely clinically.

Which of the following biochemical test results are most likely to be associated with these imaging features?

a. Elevated serum IgG4
b. Elevated serum Ca 19-9
c. Elevated serum chromogranin A
d. Elevated chromogranin B
e. Elevated serum alpha-fetoprotein

120. You are asked to review the MRI brain protocol for cases of suspected multiple sclerosis at your institution.

Which of the following sequences is best for assessing for posterior fossa involvement?

a. DWI and ADC map
b. FLAIR
c. Gradient echo
d. T1 post gadolinium
e. T2 spin echo

ANSWERS 3

1. (a) Amiodarone lung disease

This woman has a history of atrial fibrillation, for which amiodarone is often used. Amiodarone lung disease commonly presents with shortness of breath on exertion caused by hypoxia. The hyperdense consolidation is typical and the distribution is often asymmetrical and peripheral. It can occur 1–12 months following a treatment course of ≥6 months. Other features include a hyperdense liver and heart.

Eosinophilic granulomatosis with polyangiitis can cause peripheral consolidation however, it causes serum eosinophilia and this patient's blood tests are normal. It also tends to present in a younger age group than this patient, around the third to fourth decade. Patients often present with asthma but can also suffer with sinusitis, diarrhoea and arthralgia.

Simple pulmonary eosinophilia would also cause serum eosinophilia and although can cause peripheral fleeting ground glass opacification would not cause a restrictive pattern on spirometry.

Usual interstitial pneumonia is more commonly associated with rheumatoid arthritis compared to non-specific interstitial pneumonia (NSIP). NSIP can cause predominantly basal and subpleural ground glass opacification. Hyperdense consolidation is not a feature.

The treatment of rheumatoid arthritis with gold has reduced over the years due to the introduction of newer agents, and gold-induced lung toxicity is uncommon and would not cause the hyperdense consolidation typical of amiodarone lung disease.

(The Final FRCR Complete Revision Notes Page 18)

2. (d) Tear of the triangular fibrocartilage complex

Positive ulnar variance is a condition in which the ulnar-carpal articulation is more distal than the radial-carpal articulation. The condition causes pain and can result in ulnar impaction syndrome. Ulnar impaction syndrome occurs due to degenerative changes and causes thinning of the triangular fibrocartilage, which is then more easily torn.

This is a separate entity to ulnar impingement syndrome, which occurs due to a shortened ulnar (negative ulnar variance). In ulnar impingement syndrome, radioulnar convergence causes impingement of the distal ulnar on the distal radius, proximal to the sigmoid notch. After a prolonged period of time, subchondral sclerosis and scalloping of the distal radius at the distal radio-ulnar joint may be seen.

Avascular necrosis of the lunate bone, also known as Kienböck disease, is more associated with negative ulnar variance.

(The Final FRCR Complete Revision Notes Page 81)

3. (e) Mesenteric carcinomatosis

The pre-sacral space is measured between the sacrum and the mid-rectum. Up to 15 mm is normal.

(The Final FRCR Complete Revision Notes Page 189)

TABLE 3.4: Causes of Widening of the Pre-Sacral Space

Bowel	Inflammatory Bowel Disease or Tumour
Fat	Previous surgery or radiotherapy, pelvic lipomatosis/fibrosis, developmental cysts such as dermoid/epidermoid/duplication cysts
Sacral disease	Chordoma, teratoma, meningocele, neurofibroma or osteomyelitis

Source: Hain KS, Pickhardt PJ, Lubner MG et al. Presacral masses: multimodality imaging of a multidisciplinary space. *RadioGraphics*. 2013;33(4):1145–1167.

4. (c) Mucinous cystic neoplasm

There are certain features that can help to differentiate between pancreatic tumours. The description of this lesion fits with a mucinous cystic neoplasm: The patient is middle-aged and the mass is large and cystic, containing only a couple of cysts, and it is located in the pancreatic tail. There is peripheral calcification and no connection with the pancreatic duct.

Serous microcystic adenoma classically affects elderly, usually female, patients. In contrast to mucinous cystic neoplasms, they favour the pancreatic head. They are made up of innumerable small cysts, and calcification tends to be centrally located. They also do not have a connection to the main pancreatic duct.

Ductal adenocarcinoma is the most common type of pancreatic cancer and is solid and usually hypodense compared to the adjacent enhancing pancreas. Due to non-specific symptoms and subsequent late presentation, regional lymph node enlargement and metastases are not unusual findings.

Intraductal papillary mucinous neoplasms are thin-walled cysts which have a connection with the pancreatic duct. They can be split into branch or main duct lesions. Branch duct lesions often resemble a bunch of grapes and the main duct subtype causes pancreatic duct dilatation. Neither usually contain calcification.

Neuroendocrine tumours of the pancreas are also called islet cell tumours, and insulinomas are most common. They are also usually solid tumours and hypervascular.

(The Final FRCR Complete Revision Notes Page 229)

5. (a) Partial anomalous pulmonary venous return (PAPVR)

Scimitar or hypogenetic lung syndrome is a form of PAPVR. It is characterised by a hypoplastic right lung with an anomalous vein that drains the abnormal right lung segment into the systemic venous system. Most commonly, the anomalous vein drains into the inferior vena cava giving rise to the curvilinear tubular opacity described on radiographs. However, it can also drain into other structures including the right atrium, hepatic veins or portal vein. Its arterial supply can be variable.

The description in this case is typical for scimitar syndrome; however, pulmonary sequestration also has alternative vascular supply with both intra- and extralobar types deriving their arterial supply from the systemic arteries. Intralobar sequestration has a pulmonary venous drainage, whereas extralobar drains into the systemic veins. Neither have a connection with the bronchial tree.

Unilateral absence of the pulmonary artery is characterised by a small affected lung with oligaemia and contralateral lung compensatory over inflation. However, the tubular opacity adjacent to the right heart border is not consistent with this diagnosis.

Tetralogy of Fallot is not associated with the findings in this case. The typical finding is a boot-shaped heart, pulmonary oligaemia, and a right-sided aortic arch may be present.

Right middle lobe atelectasis may look similar with opacity adjacent to the right heart border, but the other findings are more consistent with scimitar syndrome.

(The Final FRCR Complete Revision Notes Page 315)

6. (d) Haemangioblastoma

Haemangioblastoma are most common in the thoracic and cervical spine. They are usually intramedullary and can have an extramedullary component. Characteristic features include a well-defined mass which is cystic containing an enhancing solid nodule. Flow voids can be evident in larger lesions and there can be a haemosiderin cap which manifests as very low T2 signal, as described in this case at the lesion's caudal aspect.

Arteriovenous malformations will also demonstrate flow voids and potentially high T2 cord signal in the cord due to oedema, as well as prominent feeding or draining vessels. However, the cystic and soft tissue component of the mass is not typical.

The main two differentials for intramedullary cord lesions include ependymoma and astrocytoma. Ependymomas are similar in that they can exhibit a haemosiderin cap and are usually well-defined. However, they most commonly affect the cervical spine and are also frequently described in the filum terminale. They tend to affect three to four segments.

Astrocytomas are most common in the paediatric population and more frequently occur in the thoracic spine. In contrast to the lesion in this case, they are usually ill-defined and more infiltrative. They also usually extend over more than four segments.

Meningiomas are solid lesions which are usually extramedullary, unlike the lesion in this case. They can sometimes be low on T1 and T2 if they are calcified.

(The Final FRCR Complete Revision Notes Page 450)

7. (e) Usual interstitial pneumonia (UIP)

The CT description provided is that of a fibrotic lung process and is typical of a UIP pattern of disease. A UIP pattern of disease is associated with predominantly honeycomb destruction of the lung which has an apicobasal gradient and tends to be peripheral.

Ground glass opacification is the predominant finding in non-specific interstitial pneumonia. The imaging findings of chronic hypersensitivity pneumonitis can overlap significantly with UIP pattern. However, the fibrosis distribution is more typically basal and peripheral in UIP, whereas in hypersensitivity pneumonitis the fibrotic change is less likely to be peripheral and is typically upper zones, although all zones can be affected. Hypersensitivity pneumonitis may also be associated with mosaicism secondary to air trapping.

The predominant imaging finding in cryptogenic organising pneumonia is ground glass change and dense consolidation. Respiratory bronchiolitis–associated interstitial lung disease represents a spectrum of disease associated with smokers. The findings on CT chest are more typically centred on the airways with airway wall thickening and evidence of air trapping. There may be small centrilobular nodules which represent occlusion of the small airways.

(The Final FRCR Complete Revision Notes Page 37)

8. (b) Bronchus

Bone metastases favour the axial skeleton rather than the appendicular skeleton due to the presence of red marrow. The most common malignancy associated with bone metastases is carcinoma of the bronchus. Colon cancer is another cause of lytic bone metastasis. Renal and thyroid malignancies may be associated with lytic, expansile lesions. Breast cancer is a common cause of lytic, mixed lytic/sclerotic and sclerotic bone metastases; however this is much less common in male patients.

(The Final FRCR Complete Revision Notes Page 143)

9. (c) Long, linear oesophageal filling defects

The patient is likely immunocompromised due to the chemotherapy regimen and therefore opportunistic infections such as candida, herpes simplex and cytomegalovirus (CMV) should be considered. Candida oesophagitis is the most common infectious cause, and findings include long linear plaque-like lesions, ulceration and pseudomembrane formation. CMV (and HIV) cause massive ulcers, whereas herpes simplex oesophagitis tends to lead to multiple small ulcers.

Flask-shaped mucosal outpouchings are typical for pseudo diverticulosis of the oesophagus caused by the mucous glands filling with contrast. It is associated with reflux, strictures and oesophagitis.

Multiple small nodular oesophageal filling defects are seen in glycogenic acanthosis, a condition associated with the elderly due to glycogen deposition.

Smooth oesophageal strictures infer benign causes such as previous caustic ingestion, radiation, Barrett oesophagus and skin diseases with oesophageal manifestations, such as epidermolysis bullosa and pemphigoid. A likely cause in a breast oncology patient would be radiation; however, this patient is currently only having neoadjuvant chemotherapy.

(The Final FRCR Complete Revision Notes Page 158)

10. (d) Morquio syndrome

Morquio syndrome is the most common mucopolysaccharidosis, associated with multiple skeletal abnormalities and presenting within the first 18 months of life. There are several features seen on spinal radiographs; central beaking of the anterior vertebral bodies is relatively specific. Other features include platyspondyly, posterior vertebral body scalloping, exaggeration of the lumbar lordosis and atlantoaxial subluxation due to odontoid hypoplasia. Appendicular skeleton findings include lateral sloping of the tibial plateau, genu valgus, bullet-shaped metacarpals and short, wide tubular bones with metaphyseal irregularity. The other conditions provided as options are examples of anteroinferior vertebral body beaking.

(The Final FRCR Complete Revision Notes Page 114)

11. (b) Haemangioblastoma
The child has von Hippel-Lindau syndrome. This is an autosomal dominant syndrome giving rise to multiple tumours, both benign and malignant. It is associated with renal cysts, angiomyolipoma and renal cell carcinoma. Other associations include pancreatic cysts and cancer and phaeochromocytoma.
Haemangioblastomas can occur in the brain or spinal cord and are part of the diagnostic criteria.
Pilocytic astrocytoma can have very similar appearances but given the visceral stigmata, haemangioblastoma is more likely. Medulloblastoma, meningioma and ependymoma have more solid appearances.
(The Final FRCR Complete Revision Notes Pages 306–307)

12. (c) C6
The vertebral artery is more commonly affected at C6 (at the entry to the foramen transversarium) and C1 (at the foramen magnum). On unenhanced CT it can appear as a hyperdense vessel filled with thrombus or crescentic peripheral high attenuation due to mural thrombus. On CT angiogram there may be subtle narrowing of the lumen on the affected side; rarely is a dissection flap seen. MRI is more sensitive, particularly T1 fat saturated sequences.
(The Final FRCR Complete Revision Notes Page 369)

13. (c) Bilateral bilobed lungs
Heterotaxy syndromes are frequently diagnosed in utero, especially if there are cardiac defects, but polysplenia can be diagnosed later than asplenia because the associated congenital heart defects are less severe. Females are more commonly affected than males.
Other features associated with polysplenia include bilateral bilobed lungs, bilateral left atria, a midline liver and bilateral bronchi which arise inferior to the level of the pulmonary artery (hyparterial).
There are numerous associated conditions including small bowel malrotation, gallbladder agenesis, biliary atresia, dextrocardia, inferior vena cava and portal vein anomalies and renal agenesis or cysts. The pancreas can be shorter than normal or have a semi-annular configuration, and there is also an association with tracheo-oesophageal fistula.
(The Final FRCR Complete Revision Notes Page 6)

14. (e) Unicameral bone cyst
The description is that of a unicameral or simple bone cyst. The small bone fragment represents the 'fallen fragment' sign which occurs in association with a fracture.
Chondroblastoma is a rare tumour, occurring before growth plate fusion. It usually demonstrates chondroid matrix mineralisation.
Eosinophilic granuloma is also a condition mostly seen in children. It usually has a 'punched-out' appearance. On CT there is soft tissue seen within the area of bone lysis (compared to the fluid content of a bone cyst).
Ewing sarcoma is a malignant lesion, associated with a wide zone of transition, periostitis and a soft tissue component.
Brodie abscess is typically a lucency surrounded by dense sclerosis, a thin lucent channel may also extend towards the growth plate.
(The Final FRCR Complete Revision Notes Page 149)

15. (d) Adenomyomatosis
Adenomyomatosis is found more commonly in females and has a strong association with gallstones. The classical appearance on ultrasound is of cholesterol-filled Rokitansky-Aschoff sinuses which appear as hyperechoic foci in a thickened gallbladder wall. On MRI the 'string of beads sign' refers to the characteristic curvilinear multiple rounded T2 hyperintense intraluminal cavities. Gallbladder carcinoma is the main differential.
(The Final FRCR Complete Revision Notes Pages 195–196)
Boscak AR, Al-Hawary M, Ramsburgh SR. Best cases from the AFIP: adenomyomatosis of the gallbladder. RadioGraphics. 2006;26(3):941–946.

16. (c) Continued follow-up
The case describes fibromuscular dysplasia with the typical appearances of alternating stenoses and dilatation of the renal arteries. This more commonly affects women between the ages of 30 and 50 years and often presents with hypertension. Although the renal arteries are

most commonly affected, other sites such as the vertebral, iliac, coeliac and extracranial internal carotid arteries can also be involved. Therefore symptoms including headache, stroke, angina or mesenteric ischaemia are possible, depending on the site of involvement.

If asymptomatic, patients are kept under observation but if presenting symptomatically the condition is amenable to angioplasty and responds well. Stenting is rarely required.

Patients with fibromuscular dysplasia have weakened vascular walls and can encounter complications, including dissection and aneurysm formation.

(The Final FRCR Complete Revision Notes Page 252)

17. (b) Cowden syndrome

The lesion described is typical for Lhermitte-Duclos disease (also known as dysplastic cerebellar gangliocytoma) which is associated with Cowden syndrome. Other features include thyroid goitres, skin lesions and gastrointestinal polyps. Although Cowden syndrome and dysplastic cerebellar gangliocytoma are rare, the answer to this question can also be deduced from knowledge of the other, more common conditions.

Ataxia telangiectasia leads to cerebellar atrophy and on imaging low T2 signal foci likely represent haemosiderin deposition secondary to bleeds from abnormal telangiectatic vessels.

Neurofibromatosis 1, Sturge-Weber syndrome and tuberous sclerosis have multiple central nervous system manifestations, none of which are present in this case. Cerebellar tumours and thyroid goitres are not typical features.

(The Final FRCR Complete Revision Notes Page 292)

18. (a) DWI + ADC map

It can be difficult to determine the underlying cause of intra-axial lesions on imaging, particularly when differentiating abscess from a malignant process. Abscesses are commonly low on T1, high on T2 and FLAIR sequences with significant adjacent oedema and mass effect. The ring of enhancement is often described as thinner compared to malignancy; however, the sequence that can be most helpful in differentiating the two is DWI and ADC map. The presence of central diffusion restriction favours abscess over a necrotic tumour.

The 'dual rim' sign may be seen in cases of intracranial abscesses. It is an outer hypointense rim and inner hyperintense rim. This may be appreciated best on T2 and susceptibility weighted imaging.

MR perfusion may be helpful as the relative cerebral blood flow (rCBF) in the surrounding oedema of an abscess is usually reduced compared to tumour oedema.

(The Final FRCR Complete Revision Notes Pages 411–412)

19. (e) Upper lobe diversion

Pulmonary oedema is commonly due to cardiac failure or fluid overload. The earliest feature is upper lobe diversion. Following this, interstitial oedema develops, causing ground glass opacification and interlobular septal thickening. Alveolar oedema will develop if the condition continues to progress and this manifests as consolidation. Cardiomegaly may be present and can be assessed by measuring the cardiothoracic ratio.

(The Final FRCR Complete Revision Notes Page 52)

20. (e) Osteosarcoma

There are features of Paget disease, a bone disorder due to excessive bone remodelling, indicated by enlarged bone with coarse trabeculae and cortical thickening. The presence of periostitis with a 'hair-on-end' or 'sunburst' periosteal reaction is indicative an aggressive bone lesion, consistent with development of a secondary osteosarcoma, a complication of Paget disease. Osteosarcoma is most common in children and adolescents, with a second peak in 70–80 year olds.

Bizarre parosteal osteochondromatous proliferation is characterised by heterotopic ossification arising from cortical bone.

Haemangiomas are benign bone lesions, which can manifest as coarsened trabeculae. The bone cortex is not usually affected and there is no aggressive periostitis.

Multiple myeloma is the most common primary bone tumour in adults. This may manifest as a plasmacytoma, a solitary expansile soft tissue bone lesion or as well-demarcated, punched-out radiolucent lesions without a sclerotic border.

Osteoblastoma is a benign lesion, without aggressive features, presenting between 20 and 30 years.

(The Final FRCR Complete Revision Notes Page 148)

21. (e) Caroli disease
Caroli disease is an autosomal recessive disease that is associated with medullary sponge kidney and renal cysts. Patients most often present in the second and third decades of life with recurrent cholangitis. Caroli disease is a type V choledochal cyst according to the Todani classification. The absence of strictures on MRCP excludes primary sclerosing cholangitis and primary biliary cirrhosis as diagnoses. In polycystic liver disease the cysts do not communicate with the biliary tree. A choledochocele is defined as a dilation of the duodenal part of the common bile duct.
(The Final FRCR Complete Revision Notes Pages 199, 202)

22. (d) Grade IV
Vesicoureteral reflux is graded from I to V, with V being most severe.
Grade I: Reflux into non-dilated ureters
Grade II: Reflux reaches the renal pelvis but there is no ureteric dilatation
Grade III: Mild dilatation but no calyceal clubbing
Grade IV: Moderate dilatation with calyceal clubbing
Grade V: Severe dilatation with ureteral tortuosity
(The Final FRCR Complete Revision Notes Page 257)

23. (c) Obturator externus and pectineus
Obturator hernias are more common in older women or in patients with conditions such as chronic obstructive pulmonary disease or ascites, due to chronically raised intrabdominal pressure. They are usually asymptomatic unless they contain obstructed bowel. The bowel will pass through the obturator foramen and lie superficial to obturator externus and deep and inferior to pectineus. This is in contrast to inguinal hernias, which lie superomedial to the pubic tubercle, femoral hernias which lie inferolateral to the pubic tubercle and Spigelian hernias which lie in the inferior abdominal wall. Other abdominal hernias to consider when reporting bowel obstruction include lumbar hernias and paraumbilical hernias, as well as hernias following surgery, such as incisional and port site hernias. Internal hernias may also lead to bowel obstruction but are often more challenging to identify. However, they should be suspected if there are crowded loops of obstructed bowel in an abnormal location.
(The Final FRCR Complete Revision Notes Page 174)

24. (b) Intralesional haemorrhage
Toxoplasmosis and lymphoma are most frequently occurring intracerebral lesions in patients with HIV/AIDS. As treatment is substantially different, differentiating the two conditions is important. CNS lymphoma shows subependymal spread and is often solitary whereas toxoplasmosis tends to have multiple lesions typically involving the basal ganglia. Lymphoma usually demonstrates uniform enhancement whereas toxoplasmosis typically has ring enhancement. Haemorrhage can be seen in toxoplasmosis but is uncommon in lymphoma. Thallium SPECT shows increased uptake in lymphoma and decreased uptake in toxoplasmosis.
(The Final FRCR Complete Revision Notes Pages 393, 417)

25. (b) Asbestosis
The case describes features of pulmonary fibrosis affecting the lower lobes. Of the available answers, asbestosis is the only one typically associated with lower lobe fibrosis. It can be very difficult to differentiate asbestosis and idiopathic pulmonary fibrosis and often the clinical history is critical. However, it is an important diagnosis to make, as patients can be awarded compensation if they have had previous occupational asbestos exposure. Other features that can be associated with asbestosis include honeycombing, pleural plaques and pleural effusions. Lymph node enlargement is not typical. Other causes of lower lobe fibrosis include systemic inflammatory conditions, such as scleroderma and rheumatoid arthritis, and drug reactions, for example secondary to amiodarone, methotrexate or bleomycin.
The other available answers typically cause upper lobe fibrosis. Other causes of upper lobe fibrosis include cystic fibrosis, Langerhans cell histiocytosis, radiation-induced fibrosis and tuberculosis.
(The Final FRCR Complete Revision Notes Pages 19–20)

26. (e) Transient synovitis of the hip
This is the most common cause of limp in children aged 5–10 years. It is of uncertain aetiology, possibly related to viral illness, infection, previous trauma or allergy. Features on

ultrasound are that of a joint effusion in the anterior recess without synovial thickening, which resolves after 10–15 days.

Developmental dysplasia of the hip is often undetected until adulthood; however, children with risk factors (including breech delivery, oligohydramnios, family history) are now screened. Ultrasound is the test of choice in infants less than 6 months old. On radiographs there may be an abnormal acetabular angle, it should measure less than 22° in children older than 1 year of age.

Juvenile rheumatoid arthritis is associated with synovial hypertrophy and effusion.

Septic arthritis is an important consideration; radiographs may be normal in the very acute phase. There may be juxta-articular osteoporosis due to hyperaemia, narrowing of the joint space due to cartilage destruction, as well as destruction of the subchondral bone on both sides of a joint. Spontaneous resolution would not be expected.

Slipped upper femoral epiphysis is most commonly seen in those 10–16 years of age. Early slippage is best seen on lateral or frog lateral views and the epiphysis may be reduced in height due to slippage.

(The Final FRCR Complete Revision Notes Pages 108–109)

27. (c) Periampullary tumour

Periampullary tumours tend to be small and are often not seen with imaging. On CT they can appear as a low-density mass centred on the ampulla. Alternatively, the 'double duct sign' (dilated common bile duct and pancreatic duct), with no detectable pancreatic head mass, can be the only finding. On MRCP there is an abrupt cutoff of the distal common bile duct.

An annular pancreas encircles the duodenum and is associated with Down syndrome.

Pancreas divisum is commonly an incidental finding of two different pancreatic ducts draining dorsal and ventral parts of the pancreas. It can predispose patients to pancreatitis.

Duodenal atresia is associated with the 'double bubble' sign and presents in neonates with bilious vomiting.

(The Final FRCR Complete Revision Notes Page 230)

28. (c) Two ureters with upper moiety ureter inserting inferomedial to lower moiety ureter

A duplex kidney does not necessarily imply a complete ureteric duplication; however, with the ultrasound appearances of ureterocele there is suspicion of an ectopic insertion of the upper moiety ureter.

Incomplete duplication is when the ureters converge above the level of the bladder and often this can exist with a degree of 'yo-yo' reflux from one ureter into the other. When there is complete duplication the upper pole moiety often obstructs due to the presence of a ureterocele. This can cause the 'drooping lily' sign due to hydronephrosis and lack of filling of the upper pole moiety and subsequent displacement of the opacifying lower pole moiety.

The upper moiety ureter inserts ectopically, often into the urinary bladder, but this can insert into the urethra, vagina or seminal vesicles, potentially causing continuous wetting in older children. The lower moeity ureter inserts normally but is prone to reflux. The Weigert-Meyer rule states that the upper moiety ureter inserts inferomedial to the lower moiety ureter.

(The Final FRCR Complete Revision Notes Pages 264–265)

29. (b) Cardiomegaly

The case describes a vein of Galen malformation. These are often diagnosed in third trimester antenatal scans as a vascular anechoic structure close to the third ventricle. They cause a left-to-right shunt and therefore lead to high-output cardiac failure leading to cardiomegaly, pulmonary oedema and widening of the superior mediastinum.

The other conditions are not associated with vein of Galen malformations but may be associated with other congenital abnormalities.

(The Final FRCR Complete Revision Notes Page 306)

30. (c) Neurofibromatosis (NF) 2

NF2 usually presents in young adults. Half of cases are spontaneous and half of cases are inherited through an autosomal dominant pattern of inheritance. The condition causes multiple central nervous system tumours including bilateral acoustic neuromas (as described in this case) which are pathognomonic of the condition. NF2 is also associated with ependymomas, meningiomas and schwannomas. These can occur on spinal roots or cranial nerves.

(The Final FRCR Complete Revision Notes Page 382)

31. (d) Post-primary tuberculosis
The description in the case vignette is most consistent with post-primary tuberculosis (TB), typically found in the apices (this represents reactivation of previously healed primary TB). The presence of tree-in-bud nodularity and consolidation in the lingula is indicative of endobronchial spread of infection and highly suggestive of active infection. Primary TB is typically seen as consolidation in the middle/lower lobe with ipsilateral nodal enlargement and effusion. Cavitation is more common in post-primary TB compared to primary TB.
Miliary TB represents haematogenous spread of the infection, and the finding on imaging is that of miliary nodules (1–3 mm).
Non-tuberculous mycobacterium infection can present with a variety of imaging features, some of which are similar to TB; however this is not as common.
Septic emboli can be a cause for lung cavities; however the presence of bronchiolitis would not necessarily be expected. Cavities may also be multiple and tend to have a predilection for the lower zones.
(The Final FRCR Complete Revision Notes Pagse 55–57)

32. (a) Bizarre parosteal osteochondromatous proliferation
The description is typical for bizarre parosteal osteochondromatous proliferation, also known as a Nora lesion, an osteochondroma-like lesion. This consists of heterotopic ossification which arises from the cortical bone.
Unlike an osteochondroma, the lesion is not angulated away from the joint and there is no medullary continuity.
A chondroblastoma is a well-defined lytic lesion within the epiphysis or apophysis of a long bone with internal chondroid mineralisation.
A chondromyxoid fibroma is typically a well-defined lucent lesion in the metaphysis with a sclerotic rim.
An enchondroma is a well-defined lucent lesion within the medullary cavity of the metaphysis, commonly seen in the metacarpals and long bones.
(The Final FRCR Complete Revision Notes Page 146)

33. (c) Mastocytosis
Causes of thickened mucosal small bowel folds include mastocytosis, amyloidosis, Whipple disease, radiotherapy and graft-versus-host disease. In this case the hepatosplenomegaly, lymph node enlargement and bone sclerosis all fit with mastocytosis. Mastocytosis can also cause ascites; however, a small amount of free pelvic fluid is common in women of reproductive age.
Thickened mucosal folds caused by amyloidosis are most commonly seen in the duodenum, with the stomach being the second most frequently affected site.
Whipple disease is caused by a bacterial infection and as well as the thickened valvulae conniventes, any associated lymph node enlargement typically demonstrates central low density (due to fat). The other findings in this case would not be typical.
Tuberculosis (TB) is a cause of hepatosplenomegaly; however the combination of other findings is not typical. If TB affects the bowel it is frequently the ileocaecal region.
Lymphoma can affect the bowel, causing wall thickening, lymph node enlargement and hepatosplenomegaly. Often the bowel lumen appears dilated due to involvement of the myenteric plexus.
(The Final FRCR Complete Revision Notes Page 178)

34. (e) Transverse humeral fracture
The most specific injuries for non-accidental injury (NAI) include metaphyseal fractures and fractures of the distal clavicle, posterior ribs, sternum, spinous processes and scapula. Moderately specific fractures include fractures of differing ages, bilateral injuries, spiral humeral fractures, complex skull fractures and vertebral fractures or subluxations. Fractures such as those at the mid-clavicle, linear skull fractures and greenstick fractures have low specificity for NAI. However, the most common fractures are transverse long bone fractures.
(The Final FRCR Complete Revision Notes Pages 330–332)

35. (a) Marchiafava-Bignami disease
The imaging has features of chronic excess alcohol intake with generalised volume loss and atrophy of the anterior cerebellar vermis. The abnormal MRI signal in the corpus callosum is

indicative of Marchiafava-Bignami disease. In the acute stage of the disease there is oedema and over time this progresses to necrosis and atrophy. It often starts in the body of the corpus callosum and progresses to the genu and splenium. Treatment is with B vitamins.

Susac syndrome has a preference for the corpus callosum with lesions affecting the body and splenium. There tend to be multiple small lesions which resemble 'snowballs' on T2 sequences. The other radiological features of excess alcohol intake in this case make Marchiafava-Bignami more likely. The clinical history in Susac syndrome is usually one consistent with brain, retinal and vestibulocochlear involvement.

Multiple sclerosis is a differential for hyperintense T2 lesions; however the distribution is different and typically affects areas including the inferior aspect of the corpus callosum, internal capsule, optic tracts and periventricular white matter.

Methanol intoxication affects the putamina causing haemorrhage and necrosis.

Wernicke encephalopathy can also cause haemorrhage and necrosis; however it typically affects the mamillary bodies, periaqueductal grey matter, posteromedial thalami and tectal plate.

(The Final FRCR Complete Revision Notes Page 418)

36. (d) Normal study

The abnormalities associated with hypoxic ischaemic injury in neonates depend on the gestational age. Frequently cranial ultrasounds are normal within the first 2 days. Hyperechoic changes are then commonly encountered. In a term baby the deep grey matter structures are affected; however, in a preterm baby it is more typically the periventricular white matter. In older children (>2 years) there can be a reversal of normal grey–white matter appearances and a 'white cerebellum' due to cerebellar sparing in diffuse cerebral oedema.

(The Final FRCR Complete Revision Notes Page 298)

37. (c) Myocardial infarct involving the left anterior descending artery

The left anterior descending artery and its branches supply the anterolateral and apical walls of the left ventricle and the interventricular septum. The high T2 weighted signal in this region is secondary to oedema suggesting a relatively acute insult, and the delayed hyperenhancement is typical in infarcted myocardium and tends to be subendocardial or full thickness.

Myocardial stunning and hibernation often have similar imaging findings. Stunning is caused following a transient period of ischaemia, whereas hibernation is thought to be related to more chronic ischaemia where the myocardial cells adapt to reduced perfusion by hibernating and reducing metabolic activity. Both these conditions lead to impaired function, manifesting as reduced contractility. Stunned myocardium tends to have preserved perfusion whereas it can be reduced in myocardial hibernation.

Acute myocarditis may demonstrate increased myocardial T2 weighted signal however other findings such as a focal area of wall motion abnormality would also be expected. Enhancement in myocarditis tends to involve the epicardium and be early rather than the delayed subendocardial enhancement described in this case.

(The Final FRCR Complete Revision Notes Page 11)

38. (e) Torus fracture

The features describe a buckle or torus fracture which occurs due to compression injury, for example falling on an outstretched hand. In a greenstick fracture, there is a cortical break on one side of the bone; the cortex on the other side remains intact, this is an unstable fracture. A lead pipe fracture is characterised by a torus fracture on one side of the bone and a greenstick fracture on the other side of the bone. In a plastic bowing fracture, there is no discernible cortical compression or break; however the bone appears deformed or bent. A Salter-Harris fracture is a fracture of the physis, which is divided into types 1–5.

(The Final FRCR Complete Revision Notes Page 110)

39. (c) Reduced signal on T1 and T2 weighted images in the liver and pancreas.

Haemochromatosis is the deposition of iron in the body and haemosiderosis is haemosiderin deposition. Haemochromatosis is an autosomal recessive condition leading to hepatomegaly, arthralgia, diabetes, skin hyperpigmentation and cardiac failure. On MRI there is reduced signal in the liver, pancreas and heart.

Haemosiderosis is associated with multiple blood transfusions. In contrast to haemochromatosis, there is reduced MRI signal in the liver and spleen.

(The Final FRCR Complete Revision Notes Pages 210–211)

40. (b) No follow-up

The appearances are consistent with a corpus luteum cyst, they occur in premenopausal women following the release of an ovum and usually involute and resolve if fertilisation does not occur. There are described as thick walled with intense peripheral 'ring of fire' vascularity. Sometimes this vascularity can be described in association with ectopic pregnancies; however, these are usually extra-adnexal and not within the ovary. The anechoic, avascular lesions on the contralateral ovary likely represent follicles and are physiological.

In premenopausal women simple ovarian cysts <5 cm do not require follow-up. If they are larger than this, then follow-up in at least 6 weeks (at a different phase in the menstrual cycle) is suggested. In postmenopausal women, follow-up of cysts >3 cm is suggested. If there are any concerns about vascular solid components, then an MRI pelvis can help to characterise further. Ca-125 and gynaecology referral may also be indicated; however Ca-125 is non-specific and can be raised in lots of benign conditions.

(The Final FRCR Complete Revision Notes Page 276)

41. (c) Hepatocellular carcinoma

The patient has features of liver disease. This finding and the imaging characteristics of the lesion are consistent with hepatocellular carcinoma (HCC), which is the second most common malignant paediatric liver lesion. They have the same radiological features as HCC in adults with arterial phase enhancement followed by portal venous phase washout. In contrast to this, regenerative nodules do not display this type of enhancement and are typically hypointense on T2 weighted imaging.

Hepatoblastoma is more common in a younger age group – typically children less than 5 years old. Similar to hepatocellular carcinoma, they are associated with raised alpha-fetoprotein; however the radiological features differ. Hepatoblastomas are usually T1 hypointense with heterogenous enhancement.

Haemangioendothelioma and mesenchymal hamartomas have similar appearances to each other and are usually quite large lesions comprising solid and cystic elements with internal vascularity. The finding of reduced calibre aorta distal to the coeliac trunk is indicative of a haemangioendothelioma.

(The Final FRCR Complete Revision Notes Page 339)

42. (d) Coronal FLAIR

Temporal lobe epilepsy is a common cause of complex partial seizures and is associated with mesial temporal or hippocampal sclerosis. MRI findings which suggest the diagnosis are hippocampal T2 signal hyperintensity and volume loss. The mesial temporal lobes are best assessed on coronal acquisitions and T2 or FLAIR sequences are most helpful. Nuclear medicine can also have a role with SPECT and PET studies demonstrating hyperperfusion immediately following a seizure. It can be important to identify as the ictal focus can be treated surgically if seizures continue despite anti-epileptic medication.

(The Final FRCR Complete Revision Notes Page 383)

43. (e) No further CT follow-up

The British Thoracic Society provide guidelines for the management of incidentally detected intrapulmonary nodules, that is nodules discovered in patients who do not have active or past history of malignancy.

The most recent guidelines released in 2015 state that nodules <4 mm and those which are obviously benign do not require further follow-up. Typical perifissural/subpleural nodules which are homogeneously solid, lentiform or triangular within 1 cm of the pleural surface and <10 mm in diameter also do not need further follow-up.

Solid 5–6 mm nodules should be followed up with 1 year CT.

Solid 6–7 mm nodules should have follow-up in 3 months.

Unlike the 2013 guidelines, risk stratification is advised for nodules ≥8 mm using the Brock calculator which considers patient factors as well as nodule characteristics. There are separate algorithms for solid and sub-solid nodules.

(The Final FRCR Complete Revision Notes Page 31)

Callister MEJ, Baldwin DR, Akram AR et al. British Thoracic Society Guidelines for the investigation and management of pulmonary nodules. Thorax. 2015;70(2):ii1–ii54.

44. (c) Non-sclerotic margin

Giant cell tumours are benign tumours, usually occurring between 20 and 50 years old. They typically occur when the growth plates are fused, are eccentric in location (although it can be difficult to tell if they are large). They abut the articular surface and have a well-defined non-sclerotic margin. There is no internal matrix mineralisation. They are usually seen in the long bones, most commonly the femur, and they can occur with Paget disease. Malignant transformation can rarely occur (less than 1%).

(The Final FRCR Complete Revision Notes Page 141)

45. (d) D2–3

Duodenal trauma is most likely to affect the retroperitoneal D2–3 segments, as they are relatively fixed. Deceleration injuries in particular are associated with duodenal trauma. Duodenal rupture is suggested if there is retroperitoneal free gas, wall thickening, discontinuity of the wall, adjacent free fluid and fat stranding. This requires surgical management and may be associated with other intra-abdominal injuries.

In the context of trauma, duodenal wall thickening and a heterogenous soft tissue attenuation mass adjacent to the duodenum without any evidence of perforation would be in keeping with a duodenal haematoma. This is usually managed conservatively unless there is evidence of active haemorrhage. The distinction between haematoma and rupture can be challenging especially with other concomitant trauma findings.

The D1 segment of the duodenum is least likely to be affected. The ligament of Treitz at the duodenojejunal flexure is another possible site of injury due to the fixation the ligament provides.

(The Final FRCR Complete Revision Notes Page 166)

46. (c) Internal maxillary

Juvenile angiofibromas are benign lesions which typically present with epistaxis in adolescent males. Characteristic imaging findings include widening of the pterygopalatine fossa, erosion of the medial pterygoid plate and anterior bowing of the posterior wall of the maxillary sinus. They can spread through the skull base and typically enhance homogenously and avidly. Biopsy is contraindicated due to their high vascularity. Preoperative embolisation can be helpful prior to surgical management. These lesions are most commonly supplied by the internal maxillary artery, a branch of the external carotid artery.

(The Final FRCR Complete Revision Notes Page 427)

47. (e) Right third to ninth ribs

Rib notching occurs secondary to dilated intercostal collateral vessels which allow blood to bypass the coarctation and reach the descending aorta. The first and second ribs do not become notched because the first and second posterior intercostal arteries arise from the costocervical trunk, a branch of the subclavian artery. They therefore do not communicate with the aorta and so are not involved in collateral formation. Rib notching commonly affects the third to ninth ribs bilaterally due to the coarctation being distal to both subclavian arteries. If there is unilateral right rib notching, as in this case, then the coarctation lies distal to the brachiocephalic trunk but proximal to the origin of the left subclavian artery, or there may be a right sided aortic arch with aberrant left subclavian artery which is distal to the coarctation.

(The Final FRCR Complete Revision Notes Page 312)

48. (b) Diffuse brainstem glioma

The history and description of the mass are typical for diffuse brainstem glioma.

Acute demyelinating encephalomalacia (ADEM) and rhombencephalitis usually have a different history with features such as fever or recent infectious illness or vaccination. Both conditions can affect the brainstem but lesions usually have some enhancement or restricted diffusion.

Osmotic demyelination is also not typical with this history and the condition is commonly secondary to iatrogenic correction of hyponatraemia. The MRI features are also not typical and restricted diffusion is an early feature.

Medulloblastomas are classically related to the roof of the fourth ventricle rather than the floor. Unlike this lesion, they diffusely enhance and demonstrate restricted diffusion.

(The Final FRCR Complete Revision Notes Page 389)

49. (a) Anteriorly

Acute respiratory distress syndrome (ARDS) is caused by diffuse alveolar damage leading to bilateral pulmonary oedema with normal hydrostatic pressures, that is non-cardiogenic oedema. Typically this causes patchy, peripheral consolidation rather than the perihilar oedema seen in cardiac and renal failure. Cardiomegaly and prominent pulmonary vessels

would not be expected, and pleural effusions and interstitial lines are also less frequent than in cardiac or renal failure, although some patients may have a mix of underlying pathologies. Often on CTs of ITU patients with ARDS, the ground glass consolidation is more marked in the dependent region of the lungs, which protects this region from barotrauma caused by ventilation. Hence the long-term fibrotic changes associated with the condition are typically anteriorly distributed, although many patients do not demonstrate any significant chronic pulmonary changes.
(The Final FRCR Complete Revision Notes Page 16)

50. (d) No further investigation required
The description is that of a haemangioma. This is a benign vascular malformation; the vertebral bodies and skull are commonly affected. The trabeculae appear coarse, causing a 'polka-dot' appearance on axial slices. The differential diagnosis is Paget disease. The cortex is spared in a haemangioma compared to Paget disease where it is thickened and sclerosis is more apparent. On MRI the lesion would be high signal on T1 and T2 imaging; however the CT images are adequate to make the diagnosis. The lesions are usually incidental and asymptomatic. In atypical rare cases, symptoms may occur due to soft tissue extension or haemorrhage.
(The Final FRCR Complete Revision Notes Page 142)

51. (d) Multicystic dysplastic kidney
Multicystic dysplastic kidney (MCDK) in infancy can demonstrate multiple cysts of varying sizes with intervening hyperechoic fibrous tissue and very little normal parenchyma. The kidney appears enlarged due to the multiple cysts. This condition is caused by ureteral obstruction in utero which stops normal nephron formation. The condition can be asymptomatic, going unrecognised and causing an atrophic kidney later in life. The condition is typically unilateral; bilateral involvement is fatal.
Autosomal recessive kidney disease also causes large kidneys but is bilateral and symmetrical with small 1- to 2-mm cysts. It can also cause hepatosplenomegaly.
Juvenile nephronopthisis causes normal or small kidneys cysts, atrophy and fibrosis. There is reduction in corticomedullary differentiation and multiple <15 mm cysts later in the disease process.
Mesoblastic nephroma is a solid lesion but sometimes there can be areas of cystic degeneration or necrosis within it.
Multilocular cystic nephroma, or simply cystic nephroma, also has imaging features of multiple cysts with fibrosis; however, it tends to be a discrete renal mass rather than affecting the whole kidney and is often described as herniating into the renal hilum. There can also be Doppler flow seen in the septations of these lesions.
(The Final FRCR Complete Revision Notes Page 254)

52. (d) Minimally enhancing pituitary lesion on MRI brain
Multiple endocrine neoplasia (MEN) 1 predisposes patients to pancreatic tumours, parathyroid adenoma and pituitary adenoma. This patient is therefore most likely to have a minimally enhancing pituitary lesion on MRI brain.
A hypoechoic ill-defined thyroid nodule is suggestive of thyroid carcinoma and medullary thyroid carcinoma in particular is associated with MEN 2. Medullary thyroid carcinoma frequently contains microcalcification.
Phaeochromocytomas cause markedly T2 hyperintense adrenal lesions, referred to as the 'light bulb' sign. They are commonly part of MEN 2. MEN 2B is also associated with gastrointestinal and cutaneous neuromas, marfanoid habitus and prognathism.
(The Final FRCR Complete Revision Notes Page 230)

53. (e) This likely represents pulmonary interstitial emphysema
The child has features of pulmonary interstitial emphysema (PIE). This typically develops in premature infants with severe surfactant deficiency causing respiratory distress syndrome. Surfactant deficiency is associated with reduced lung volumes. Artificial ventilation can cause air to track into the interstitial space causing pneumothoraces. Air can also track centrally and cause pneumomediastinum. The appearance of the thymus in this case is consistent with pneumomediastinum, with surrounding air and displacement of the thymic lobes laterally. Both pneumothorax and pneumomediastinum are important complications to recognise and

inform the clinical team about promptly.

The main differential is bronchopulmonary dysplasia, which is an acquired condition, also associated with ventilated premature infants. It usually occurs more gradually than PIE. PIE also tends to occur within the first week, whereas bronchopulmonary dysplasia occurs slightly later. Bronchopulmonary dysplasia is not associated with meconium aspiration, which usually affects post-term babies.

The umbilical artery catheter tip can either be positioned 'high' (above T10) or low (below T3) to avoid the major aortic branches.

(The Final FRCR Complete Revision Notes Page 328)

54. (c) Canavan disease

Canavan disease causes subcortical white matter abnormality with involvement of the deep grey matter. The caudate, corpus callosum and internal capsule may be spared. There is associated restricted diffusion but no enhancement. The characteristic feature is elevated *N*-acetyl-aspartate (NAA).

Adrenoleukodystrophy is X-linked, affecting young male patients. It classically has a posterior distribution affecting the occipitoparietal region, particularly the periventricular area. There is involvement of the splenium of the corpus callosum. Peripheral enhancement is frequently seen.

Alexander disease has a predominantly anterior distribution which progresses posteriorly and becomes more diffuse during the course of the disease. It causes abnormal white matter T2 hyperintensity and enhancement. NAA is normal.

Pelizaeus-Merzbacher is also X-linked and causes subcortical white matter abnormalities. There is usually cerebellar atrophy. Importantly, the perivascular regions are usually spared, which leads to 'tigroid' appearance, similar to metachromatic leukodystrophy. NAA is usually reduced.

Krabbe disease favours a more periventricular distribution and causes abnormal MRI signal in a more central and posterior position. It also leads to optic nerve hypertrophy.

(The Final FRCR Complete Revision Notes Page 421)

55. (d) Presence of liver lesions

Lung cancer is one of the most common cause of cancer deaths worldwide. It is broadly divided into non-small cell lung cancer (NSCLC; 85%) and small-cell lung cancer. Whilst the RCR has published guidance that the TNM staging will not be specifically tested in the Final FRCR Part A, demonstration of understanding and knowledge of the evaluation of common malignancies is required. In lung cancer, the size of the main tumour and invasion of local structures contributes to the T stage. The feature that will most assist with M staging is the presence of two liver lesions which have imaging features in keeping with metastases; these have a higher M stage (M1c) than the presence of a pleural or pericardial effusion (M1a).

(The Final FRCR Complete Revision Notes Pages 39–41)

56. (c) Lung

The most common site for Ewing sarcoma to metastasise to is the lungs. Bone is the next most common site of metastases. Metastases to lymph nodes, liver and brain are less common. The presence of distant metastases significantly affects prognosis.

(The Final FRCR Complete Revision Notes Page 137)

57. (e) Ultrasound guided peritoneal biopsy

Appearances of the stomach are difficult to assess on CT; however, the diffuse thickening and small lumen along with perigastric fat stranding, ascites and upper abdominal lymphadenopathy is highly suspicious of malignancy, specifically linitis plastica. Linitis plastica can have multiple causes including malignancy, inflammation and infection. The most common cause is scirrhous adenocarcinoma of the stomach. This often causes submucosal infiltration and hence endoscopic biopsies are frequently negative; therefore a repeat may not yield any further information.

The lung nodules are relatively small for biopsy and the lower lobe location can also make biopsy more challenging due to diaphragmatic respiratory motion. US guided liver biopsy could be considered; however with moderate ascites this would be relatively contraindicated due to risk of haemorrhage, and drainage should be considered first. The peritoneal nodules are superficial and may be amenable to ultrasound guided biopsy. Colonoscopy would not be helpful in this scenario.

(The Final FRCR Complete Revision Notes Pages 168–169)

58. (b) Most are seronegative

The imaging description is that of a joint effusion, causes of which include septic arthritis, transient synovitis and juvenile idiopathic arthritis. Juvenile idiopathic arthritis presents in patients less than 16 years old with a duration greater than 6 weeks. Most are seronegative; raised erythrocyte sedimentation rate and anaemia may be present. The knee joint is the most common site for the monoarticular variant. Periostitis is considered typical and is most common in the metacarpal and metatarsal bones. There is often premature closure of the growth plates/accelerated skeletal maturation. Unlike in rheumatoid arthritis, bone changes occur late and there is more ankylosis and widening of the metaphysis.

(The Final FRCR Complete Revision Notes Pages 111–112)

59. (c) Congenital pulmonary airway malformation (CPAM)

CPAM, previously known as congenital cystic adenomatoid malformation, is a hamartomatous lesion of the lung most commonly causing a mass composed of multiple large cysts (type I). Detected either antenatally or in neonates with respiratory distress, these lesions initially are fluid filled and then, due to their connection with the bronchial tree, fill with air. Their appearance therefore changes to contain air-fluid levels. types II and III are less common, type II are multiple smaller cysts and type III has microscopic cysts and therefore the lesions appear solid.

A bronchogenic cyst has no connection with the bronchial tree and therefore would not typically contain air-fluid levels (unless complicated, e.g. by infection).

As the name suggests, congenital lobar overinflation (CLO) causes significant hyperinflation of a lung lobe. Although fluid may be in the lung initially following birth, there is no cystic component in CLO. It also most commonly affects the left upper and right middle lobes, whereas CPAM has no lobar predilection.

Diaphragmatic hernias may contain air-fluid levels if they contain bowel loops and, if large, they can lead to respiratory distress. However, large diaphragmatic hernias are usually left-sided Bochdalek hernias and not right sided, as in this case.

Pulmonary sequestration can present with a multiloculated cystic mass; however, it is most common in the left lower lobe and has a systemic arterial supply which the lesion in this case does not have. The vascular drainage of pulmonary sequestration helps to differentiate between the intra or extra lobar subtypes.

(The Final FRCR Complete Revision Notes Page 321)

60. (b) Carbon monoxide poisoning

Carbon monoxide poisoning typically affects the globus pallidi causing hypodensity on CT. On MRI there is T1 hypointensity and T2 and FLAIR hyperintensity with restricted diffusion. The caudate, putamen and thalamus can also be involved.

Methanol poisoning classically affects the putamen causing putaminal necrosis. It can also lead to retinal and optic disc necrosis and generalised cerebral oedema.

The distribution also differs in hypoglycaemic encephalopathy which causes signal abnormality in the posterior limb of the internal capsules, basal ganglia, hippocampi and cerebral cortex.

Anoxic brain injury would likely cause more widespread changes involving other grey matter structures such as the cortex, thalami and cerebellum and leading to diffuse cerebral oedema and effacement of the cerebrospinal fluid spaces.

Lead poisoning is unusual, and the history is usually one of prolonged excessive exposure leading to neurological decline, psychiatric symptoms and anaemia. Cyanide and manganese poisoning can particularly affect the globus pallidi; however, both of these diagnoses would be far more unusual than carbon monoxide poisoning.

(The Final FRCR Complete Revision Notes Pages 380–381)

61. (d) Salmonella

The case describes a mycotic aortic aneurysm. These are usually saccular, and features include interruption of arterial wall calcification, adjacent inflammatory changes and lymphadenopathy. There can be extension into the adjacent vertebrae and retroperitoneal collections. The most likely causative organisms are *Staphylococcus aureus* and salmonella.

Treponema pallidum is associated with syphilis. Aortic aneurysms in syphilis can have similar periaortic inflammation and also tend to be saccular; however, they more typically affect the ascending aorta.

Actinomycosis, cryptococcosis and histoplasmosis are not associated with aortic aneurysms. Actinomycosis causes homogenous, often lobar, pulmonary opacification with a propensity for cavitation and associated pleural thickening and effusions. Crytococcosis is a fungus which can cause both lung and central nervous system infection. Histoplasmosis is another fungus which can manifest in both the lungs and mediastinum causing pulmonary nodules, calcified hilar and mediastinal lymph nodes and fibrosing mediastinitis.

(The Final FRCR Complete Revision Notes Page 1)

62. (b) Cartilaginous defect on T1

Osteochondritis dissecans is an osteochondral fracture of the articular epiphysis thought most likely due to trauma and ischaemia. It is more common in males and most commonly affects the knee, talar dome, tibia, patella and femoral head. Features on plain film include flattening and cortical irregularity of the articular surface and a detached loose osteochondral defect may also be visible. On MRI a cartilaginous defect may be seen on T1, the defect may demonstrate high T2 signal in keeping with fluid and there may also be high signal seen within the articular cartilage.

Synovial proliferation is a feature of pigmented villonodular synovitis, which may also show blooming on gradient echo imaging due to haemosiderin deposition. A fat-fluid level may be seen in an acute intra-articular fracture, not typically seen in osteochondritis dissecans.

(The Final FRCR Complete Revision Notes Page 119)

63. (c) Peripancreatic inflammation

The CT severity index (CTSI) is based on the Balthazar score and the extent of pancreatic necrosis.

In order to calculate the CTSI, the pancreas is scored based on its appearance from 0 to 4, with 0 been least severe and 4 the being most severe. The five categories are:

- Normal appearance
- Focal/diffuse enlargement
- Peripancreatic inflammation
- Single peripancreatic fluid collection
- >2 collections ± retroperitoneal gas

Following this, points are awarded for the amount of pancreatic necrosis. No necrosis gains 0 additional points, <30% scores 2 points, 30–50% scores 4 points and >50% gains 6 points.

Therefore, the maximum CTSI score is 10. A score of >7 is associated with 20% mortality.

A modified CTSI was released in 2014 which also takes into account extrapancreatic complications such as pleural effusions and vascular complications.

(The Final FRCR Complete Revision Notes Pages 233–235)

Balthazar EJ. Acute pancreatitis: assessment of severity with clinical and CT evaluation. Radiology. 2002;223(3):603–613.

64. (e) Renal vein thrombosis

There is reverse flow in diastole on the arterial trace which is consistent with renal vein thrombosis; flow should always be flowing forwards even in diastole. The typical presentation is with tenderness and decreased urine output in the first week following transplant. The kidney can appear swollen and can be hypoechoic on ultrasound. The renal vessels can be difficult to clearly visualise immediately following transplant depending on position and body habitus. If the renal vein could be visualised and assessed with Doppler, there would be no venous flow.

Renal artery thrombosis is also an early complication but thankfully quite rare. There would be no vascularity on the ultrasound Doppler, and diagnosis is imperative as it requires prompt return to theatre to try and salvage the graft.

Pseudoaneurysm formation, rejection and renal artery stenosis are late complications. Pseudoaneurysms usually form as a result of biopsy, not due to the transplant surgery itself. On Doppler ultrasound there will be a focus of abnormal colour flow with very turbid flow.

Rejection is also a late complication. Typically the kidney is enlarged with large renal pyramids and reduced corticomedullary differentiation. The resistive index tends to be high and there can be mild pelvicalyceal dilatation.

Features of renal artery stenosis on ultrasound Doppler include increased resistive indices (>0.7) and a parvus-tardus wave form, in contrast to the sharp upstroke seen in a normal

transplant trace. It usually occurs at the site of the anastomosis.
(The Final FRCR Complete Revision Notes Pages 259–261)

65. (d) Meconium plug syndrome
Meconium plug syndrome is the most common cause of failure to pass meconium, but unlike Hirschsprung disease it resolves without requiring surgical intervention. A contrast enema will demonstrate a dilated proximal colon and contrast outlining impacted meconium in the descending colon. Unlike Hirschsprung disease, the rectum is normal calibre.
The finding of a microcolon indicates it has not developed normally in-utero due to intestinal pathology such as atresia or meconium ileus. Meconium ileus is associated with cystic fibrosis. Radiological findings include dilated distal small bowel loops with filling defects in the distal ileum and proximal large bowel due to meconium. There is associated microcolon affecting the entire colon.
Findings indicative of ileal atresia include microcolon and dilated proximal small bowel loops.
Zuelzer-Wilson syndrome is also known as total colonic aganglionosis. It is similar to Hirschsprung disease but more severe and affects the entire colon rather than just a segment.
(The Final FRCR Complete Revision Notes Page 345)

66. (d) Mucous retention cyst
Mucous retention cysts are commonly seen in the maxillary sinus but can occur in other paranasal sinuses. They are commonly incidental findings. They typically have intermediate T1 and high T2 signal. They occur within partially aerated sinuses, in contrast to mucoceles, which are found in a non-aerated sinus.
Antrochoanal polyps frequently arise from the maxillary sinus but protrude into the nasal cavity via a widened maxillary ostium. They can have similar MRI signal but usually demonstrate peripheral enhancement. Similarly, a papilloma usually demonstrates heterogenous avid enhancement. Papillomas are frequently described as having a cerebriform appearance due to alternating high and low signal.
On CT, allergic fungal sinusitis typically appears as central hyperdensity surrounded by hypodense oedematous mucosa filling a sinus. This inflamed, oedematous mucosa is therefore T2 hyperintense and enhances. There may be bony expansion, thinning and erosion.
(The Final FRCR Complete Revision Notes Pages 426–429)

67. (c) Pleural effusion
Systemic lupus erythematous (SLE) is a multisystem collagen vascular disease which commonly affects the lungs. It is more commonly seen in women and can have a variety of manifestations. The presence of pleuritis is one of the many features which can be used in the diagnostic criteria. The most common thoracic finding in SLE is the presence of a pleural effusion (50% are bilateral) which are usually small and consisting of an exudate. Pericarditis is also with the diagnostic criteria for SLE, and is present in 17–50% of patients. It may be seen on CT chest as pericardial thickening and pericardial effusion. Patients commonly develop pulmonary disease in the form of pneumonia, pulmonary haemorrhage and acute lupus pneumonitis (diagnosis of exclusion). Patients are at significantly increased risk of developing pneumonia due to immunological deficiency, as well as immunotherapy treatment. Interstitial lung disease can be seen in SLE, however it is not the most common feature (only 3% of patients) and is less commonly seen in SLE than in other collagen vascular diseases.
(The Final FRCR Complete Revision Notes Page 55)
Lalani TA, Kanne JP, Hatfield GA et al. Imaging findings in systemic lupus erythematosus. RadioGraphics. 2004;24(4):1069–1086.

68. (a) Greater than 10 wormian bones
The patient in the case vignette has osteogenesis imperfecta (OI). This is rare disorder due to a defect in type 1 collagen formation which causes brittle bones with a tendency to fracture. Typical radiographic features of the appendicular skeleton include poor bone density, bone deformity (e.g. shepherd's crook deformity) and evidence of previous fractures. The presence of >10 wormian bones may be seen in OI. An important differential diagnosis is non-accidental injury. Subdural haematoma and optic nerve atrophy are not associated with OI. Ground glass appearance of the sphenoid wing may be seen in fibrous dysplasia. Widening of the diploe is seen in sickle cell anaemia and thalassaemia.
(The Final FRCR Complete Revision Notes Pages 120–121)

69. (c) Endoscopic ultrasound and 18F-FDG PET/CT

Oesophageal cancer is very FDG avid. Ideally it is locally staged with endoscopic ultrasound which differentiates T1 (limited to mucosa) from T2 (involving muscularis propria) disease and also assesses local lymph nodes. Locoregional and distant staging can be achieved with 18F-FDG PET/CT and this is more accurate than CT alone. PET/CT is also helpful in disease follow-up as it can help to distinguish between recurrence and fibrosis. Similarly, PET/CT is more accurate than PET alone. Thoracic MRI cannot differentiate between T1 and T2 disease and therefore other modalities are preferred.

(The Final FRCR Complete Revision Notes Pages 177–178)

70. (d) Multiple foci of FLAIR hyperintensity in the cortical and subcortical regions

The patient has features of tuberous sclerosis with subependymal nodules and renal angiomyolipomas. Other findings associated with tuberous sclerosis include white matter abnormalities, subependymal giant cell astrocystomas and cortical tubers. Tubers manifest as small areas of FLAIR and T2 hyperintensity in the cortical and subcortical regions.

The cystic cerebellar lesion with the enhancing soft tissue nodule is suggestive of either a haemangioblastoma or pilocytic astrocytoma. The intraventricular lobulated enhancing mass is consistent with a choroid plexus papilloma. Both haemangioblastoma and choroid plexus papillomas are associated with von Hippel-Lindau.

The homogenous durally based lesion is consistent with a meningioma in Neurofibromatosis (NF) 2 and the T2 hyperintense deep white matter lesions are typical for focal areas of signal intensity (FASI) which are seen in NF1.

(The Final FRCR Complete Revision Notes Pages 305–306)

71. (b) Mesenteric panniculitis

This is a rare, chronic inflammation of small bowel mesenteric fat. Typically on CT it manifests as a well-defined mesenteric root mass with a 'misty' appearance and surrounding fat halo. Classically it envelops but does not distort the mesenteric vessels and does not involve the bowel. It has a predilection for the jejunal mesentery. The finding of a low-attenuation fat halo surrounding the vessels is highly suggestive of mesenteric panniculitis.

Carcinoid tumours can present with similar symptoms but they are centred on the bowel, most commonly the terminal ileum. However, they can cause significant desmoplastic reaction in the adjacent mesentery.

Radiation enteritis is not possible without significant medical history and usually causes mural thickening and luminal narrowing. The bowel in this case is unaffected.

Tuberculosis usually affects the terminal ileum and caecum rather than the mesenteric root and can also cause characteristic low attenuation lymph node enlargement.

Mesenteric lipoma are unusual and would be uniformly fat attenuation rather than the heterogenous misty appearance associated with mesenteric panniculitis.

(The Final FRCR Complete Revision Notes Page 190)

72. (e) Oligodendroglioma

The location and appearance is consistent with an oligodendroglioma. These most commonly occur between 30 and 50 years of age. They are commonly located in the frontal lobe and the majority contain calcification. Enhancement is very variable and they can erode adjacent bone; both are features which can help to differentiate them from meningiomas. Meningiomas homogenously enhance and can cause adjacent hyperostosis but not erosion.

Astrocytomas can have variable appearances depending on their grade, from low grade pilocytic astrocytomas in children, to high grade anaplastic astrocytomas and glioblastoma multiforme (GBM). Unlike this lesion, they usually cause mass effect, and calcification is uncommon. Adjacent bone erosion is also not a typical feature. GBM is aggressive and infiltrative with significant adjacent oedema and enhancement.

The location of this lesion is not typical for an ependymoma. They arise from glial cells lining the ventricles or spinal canal. In children they are usually infratentorial affecting the fourth ventricle, but they can be supratentorial in adults.

(The Final FRCR Complete Revision Notes Page 395)

73. (d) Post-embolisation syndrome

Post-embolisation syndrome is thought to be an immune-mediated response that can occur following chemoembolisation, for example in liver lesions or following arterial embolisation procedures such as uterine artery embolisation. Symptoms include fever, nausea and pain and they usually peak around 48 hours post procedure and then improve within a week. Gas within a recently embolised lesion is relatively common and this does not necessarily infer infection.

With endometritis, the endometrium would be thickened with other findings including fluid and/or gas in the endometrial cavity and increased vascularity.

Fibroid torsion is uncommon and is associated with pedunculated subserosal fibroids. It can present with pain; however uterine artery embolisation does not predispose to this and the most likely diagnosis in this case remains post-embolisation syndrome.

Non-target organ ischaemia can occur as a complication following any embolisation procedure but the most common organs affected by this are the ovaries rather than the uterus. Normal uterine tissue tolerates the ischaemia induced by uterine artery embolisation compared to fibroids.

(The Final FRCR Complete Revision Notes Page 14)

74. (d) Renal cortical thickness of 5 mm on abdominal ultrasound

The question describes a pathological fracture through a Brown tumour of the distal radius. These are lytic expansile lesions which are similar to giant cell tumours histologically and can contain fluid-fluid levels on MRI. The other findings of osteosclerosis and subperiosteal resorption of the phalanges are typical for hyperparathyroidism.

Brown tumours are historically most commonly attributed to primary hyperparathyroidism, of which the most frequent cause is a parathyroid adenoma. This could be detected with a nuclear medicine 99-Tc-MIBI scan which should reveal the parathyroid adenoma. A pertechnetate thyroid scan investigating for a parathyroid adenoma (e.g. in answer A) would detect a region of decreased tracer uptake compared to the thyroid, rather than increased uptake.

In recent times, secondary hyperparathyroidism has become more common, and the most frequent cause of the secondary form of the condition is chronic renal failure, which would manifest with renal cortical thinning. Other causes of secondary hyperparathyroidism include vitamin D deficiency which may lead to Looser zones, a type of insufficiency fracture (described in answer E).

The other answers describe Graves disease on a nuclear medicine thyroid scan and liver metastases on a CT abdomen and pelvis, which are not associated with hyperparathyroidism.

(The Final FRCR Complete Revision Notes Page 80)

75. (a) Abdominal radiograph in 24 hours

The case demonstrates typical imaging findings of ulcerative colitis with the submucosal low attenuation consistent with fat deposition seen in chronic cases. The patient is at risk of toxic megacolon. This condition also affects patient with colitis of other causes but accounts for the majority of deaths related to ulcerative colitis and should therefore should be kept in mind when reporting acute imaging. Toxic megacolon does not always cause bowel dilatation; however, if the colon is dilated >5 cm, particularly the transverse colon, where gas tends to collect, it should be considered. Colonoscopy and barium studies are contraindicated due to the risk of perforation. Frequent (often daily) abdominal radiographs are suggested to monitor bowel dilatation. Repeat CT may be warranted during admission; however, this patient is relatively young and abdominal radiographs should be considered in the first instance if he is clinically stable. Urgent surgical referral is not indicated at this point.

(The Final FRCR Complete Revision Notes Page 187)

76. (a) Above the urogenital diaphragm

Signs of urethral injury include inability to void, haematuria and blood at the urethral meatus. The urethra is split into anterior and posterior sections, with anterior being penile and bulbous portions, and posterior being prostatic and membranous. The anterior urethra is more commonly injured in straddle type injuries and the posterior urethra in blunt trauma, sometimes with pelvic fractures. Iatrogenic causes are also important to consider.

The Goldman classification helps to distinguish between the different types of injury. The important landmark is the urogenital diaphragm. If the contrast extravasates into the retropubic space it suggests injury above the urogenital diaphragm. Conversely, if the contrast leaks into the perineum it suggests injury below the urogenital diaphragm. Above the urogenital diaphragm relates to the posterior urethra.

Incomplete urethral injuries, such as in this case, are often treated conservatively with catheterization; however complete transection may require surgery. Urethral stricture is the most common long-term complication of urethral injury, with post-traumatic strictures tending

to be short. Post-infectious strictures are more likely to be long.
(The Final FRCR Complete Revision Notes Page 266)

77. (a) Aberrant left pulmonary artery
An aberrant or anomalous left pulmonary artery (also known as a pulmonary sling) is when the artery arises from the right pulmonary artery. Its path takes it between the trachea and oesophagus to reach the left lung, which causes an indentation on the anterior oesophageal wall. It can present in infancy with respiratory distress secondary to right main bronchus compression.
The right subclavian artery usually arises from the brachiocephalic trunk. An aberrant right subclavian artery arises directly from the aortic arch after the left subclavian artery and then passes back towards the right side, frequently posterior to the oesophagus and hence can cause an indentation.
A double aortic arch also indents the oesophagus posteriorly on a lateral view during a barium swallow; however, on the AP view it creates a 'reverse S' appearance.
Evidence of a right-sided aortic arch and significantly enlarged left atrium would be present on plain film rather than barium swallow.
(The Final FRCR Complete Revision Notes Page 311)

78. (e) T2
Pleomorphic adenomas are the most common parotid gland tumours. They can occur elsewhere, for example in the submandibular glands; however they most frequently affect the parotid gland. Although the lesion in this case is in the deep lobe, they are more likely to be located superficially. Pleomorphic adenomas are well-demarcated and appear as hypoechoic masses on ultrasound. On MRI they are T1 hypointense with marked T2 hyperintensity, which helps to differentiate them from other lesions. They tend to have homogenous enhancement.
Another important differential for parotid gland tumours is a Warthin tumour. These tend to be more heterogenous, with both cystic and solid components. The solid components may enhance. Warthin tumours can be bilateral and are associated with smoking.
(The Final FRCR Complete Revision Notes Page 429)

79. (e) Perform a ventilation-perfusion (VQ) scan
The acute concern is whether there is a pulmonary embolus, and the patient has not yet had this diagnosis confirmed or excluded. It is possible that suboptimal opacification could occur again; a VQ scan is a sensible alternative. If a VQ scan is not readily available in your hospital, or if the patient is clinically unstable, repeat attempt at CT pulmonary angiogram would be required (although this is not presented as an option in this question).
The imaging features described on the CT raise the possibility of pulmonary artery hypertension. An echocardiogram would be very useful in this patient, to look for an underlying chronic left to right shunt (such as an atrial septal defect) as well as mitral valve stenosis. Mosaicism can be assessed further using an expiratory phase CT chest where appropriate. In the case of pulmonary hypertension, the central vessel dilatation is indicative of a vascular cause of mosaicism. Furthermore, the low attenuation foci in the lung associated with small peripheral vessels are abnormal and represent oligaema; on expiratory CT the low attenuation foci will demonstrate an increase in attenuation.
CT abdomen and pelvis may be performed in the case of known pulmonary embolus if there is a high clinical suspicion of underlying malignancy. Respiratory referral may be required following further workup, as there are a number of respiratory conditions which cause pulmonary artery hypertension; however in the acute setting it is not considered the most appropriate next step.
(The Final FRCR Complete Revision Notes Page 51)

80. (c) Melorheostosis
The description of dripping candle wax centred on the diaphysis is typical of melorheostosis. In this condition there is progressive cortical hyperostosis along one side of the affected bone in a 'sclerotome', which is a zone supplied by an individual spinal nerve. It is of unknown aetiology and usually asymptomatic initially. It has a slow course in adults and can affect one or more bones of the upper and lower limbs. It may be associated with genu varus, genu valgus and leg length discrepancy.

Caffey disease presents in infancy. Focal scleroderma may demonstrate subcutaneous and periarticular calcification. Osteopoikilosis is a condition of multiple enostoses, a benign condition in which the bone islands align parallel to the trabeculae and tend to cluster around joints. Pyknodysostosis is a condition diagnosed early in childhood in which there is dwarfism with associated with multiple skeletal abnormalities as well as learning disability.

(The Final FRCR Complete Revision Notes Page 82)

81. (c) Hepatopetal portal venous flow

The patient has the clinical signs and symptoms of portal hypertension with bleeding secondary to oesophageal varices. Portal hypertension is defined as an increase in portal venous pressure >10 mmHg.

Sonographic features of portal hypertension include loss of the normal triphasic portal vein Doppler waveform, reduced portal vein flow (<10 cm/sec) and reversal of flow. Normal portal vein flow should be hepatopetal (towards the liver); however, in portal hypertension this can eventually reverse causing hepatofugal flow, and collaterals form, such as oesophageal and splenic varices.

Other common ultrasound findings in portal hypertension include splenomegaly, ascites and gallbladder oedema.

(The Final FRCR Complete Revision Notes Page 218)

82. (b) H-shaped vertebrae

The patient has features consistent with sickle cell disease. Young patients may have splenomegaly but over time the spleen becomes small and calcified. The kidneys are often enlarged in children but over the patient's lifetime may become small due to renal failure. The previous consolidation which has now resolved may represent acute chest syndrome. An associated musculoskeletal finding is H-shaped vertebrae due to endplate infarction.

Anterior inferior vertebral body beaking is a feature of conditions such as Hurler syndrome and achondroplasia.

Posterior vertebral body scalloping is caused by a variety of pathologies including achondroplasia, mucopolysaccharidoses and dural ectasia.

Ribbon ribs are classically associated with neurofibromatosis.

A narrowed interpedicular distance is encountered in achrondroplasia and thanatophoric dysplasia.

(The Final FRCR Complete Revision Notes Page 348)

83. (c) Pineal germinoma

As is the case with other pineal masses, germinomas tend to present with obstructive hydrocephalus and Parinaud syndrome (paralysis of upward gaze). Pineal germinomas are the most common cause of a mass in this region. They usually present in young adults and have a male predilection. The description in this case is typical for a pineal germinoma. Iso or hyperdense on CT with central calcification and isointense to grey matter on T1 and T2 weighted imaging with enhancement post contrast and no haemorrhage. Five to ten percent of patients will have synchronous tumours within the midline at the time of diagnosis.

Pineoblastomas are aggressive lesions and therefore more infiltrative, less well-defined and any calcification is peripheral, causing an 'exploded calcification' appearance.

As well as calcification, teratomas are also likely to contain fat and haemorrhage, both of which are not features of pineal germinomas.

Pineocytomas have quite non-specific imaging findings; however, familiarity with the common features of the other pineal region tumours helps to exclude other causes.

Pineal yolk sac tumours also have no specific imaging findings, but these tumours are unusual and therefore a pineal germinoma is much more likely.

(The Final FRCR Complete Revision Notes Page 403)

84. (e) Porencephaly

The characteristics of the lesion are consistent with it containing cerebrospinal fluid (CSF). The connection with the ventricular system, the lack of septations and the white matter lining are all consistent with porencephaly.

Schizencephaly is a connection between the pial and ependymal surfaces, often communicating with the ventricular system and lacking septations; however, the key differentiating factor is the lining. Schizencephaly is lined with grey matter. In the closed-lip subtype there is no CSF in the cleft, whereas in the open-lipped variety there is CSF in the cleft.

Hydrancephaly is thought to occur secondary to bilateral carotid artery occlusion in-utero and therefore causes significant bilateral forebrain abnormality.

Neuroglial cysts are located in the white matter; however, they do not have a connection with the ventricular system.

(The Final FRCR Complete Revision Notes Page 303)

85. (e) Obliterative bronchiolitis

Obliterative bronchiolitis causes bronchiolar inflammation and fibrosis leading to bronchiectasis and bronchial wall thickening with subsequent air flow obstruction. This causes the CT finding of mosaic perfusion, which is lucency created by trapped air during expiration. The vessels are decreased in calibre in the low attenuation lucent lung and comparatively increased calibre in the normal lung. Causes are varied and can be post-infective, following inhalation of toxic substances and due to aspiration.

The changes associated with acute interstitial pneumonia are non-specific and include ground glass opacification and often dependent consolidation and fibrosis, which can lead to traction bronchiectasis.

Alveolar proteinosis typically causes a 'crazy paving' appearance with ground glass opacification and thickened interlobular septa

CT findings in chronic eosinophilic pneumonia are often described as the photographic negative of pulmonary oedema, with predominantly peripheral consolidation, and pleural effusions are not typical.

The chronic form of hypersensitivity pneumonitis commonly causes mid and upper lobe fibrosis, subsequent traction bronchiectasis and honeycombing. It is often described as sparing the costophrenic angles.

(The Final FRCR Complete Revision Notes Page 24)

86. (a) Haemophilia

The features described are typical for haemophilia. Repeated episodes of bleeding into the joint causes pannus formation which leads to erosion of cartilage and other degenerative features. There may also be proliferation of the synovium and periarticular osteopenia.

In homocysteinuria there is frequently generalised osteoporosis and widespread skeletal abnormalities, rather than the quite focal abnormality described in this case. Lens dislocation is a typical feature. There may be sternal abnormalities and the epiphyses and metaphyses are frequently affected. Imaging of the spine may reveal biconcave vertebrae and scoliosis.

Juvenile rheumatoid arthritis occurs in patients less than 16 years old. The imaging features may also include a squared patella and widened intercondylar notch.

Pigmented villonodular synovitis is a proliferative condition of the synovium with haemosiderin deposition. The radiographic features may include marginal erosions.

In primary synovial chondromatosis there is proliferation of the synovium which can cause intra-articular loose bodies; these may or may not calcify. Imaging features in this condition can include soft tissue swelling around the joint and widening of the joint space as well as erosion of the adjacent bone. Multiple calcific densities may be present in the joint space, which are uniform in size.

(The Final FRCR Complete Revision Notes Page 110)

87. (b) CT chest abdomen pelvis with arterial and portal venous phase contrast

Multiple endocrine neoplasia (MEN) 1 is associated with proliferative lesions in the pancreas, pituitary and parathyroid glands. MEN 2 is associated with medullary thyroid cancer, parathyroid hyperplasia and phaeochromocytomas.

The patient likely has MEN 1, as he has symptoms of Zollinger-Ellison syndrome secondary to a gastrinoma. These commonly occur in the pancreas but are also seen elsewhere, for example in the duodenum.

The most appropriate test is a CT, including arterial phase contrast, as the tumours are hypervascular and are most likely to be seen on this phase of imaging. A barium meal would likely reveal features of Zollinger-Ellison syndrome, such as thickened gastric folds and erosions/ulcers, but would likely not identify the gastrin-secreting lesion. An MRCP would be more helpful than an MRI small bowel, as the gastrinomas commonly occur in the pancreas. 18F-FDG PET/CT may be helpful in poorly differentiated metastatic disease with neuroendocrine tumours but would not be indicated in this case.

A 111In-Octrotide scan may be more helpful in localising the gastrinoma and any metastatic spread. Patients with MEN 1 may also have pituitary lesions which an MRI brain would help to characterise, but in the first instance, the CT would be most helpful.
(The Final FRCR Complete Revision Notes Pages 189, 230)

88. (c) Pyeloureteritis cystica
Horseshoe kidneys are often asymptomatic and discovered incidentally. They are positioned lower than normal and their ascent into the upper abdomen is halted by the inferior mesenteric artery, usually around the level of L3. On ultrasound it may sometimes not be recognised, especially if the lower poles are not well seen and the fusion not appreciated. These abnormally positioned kidneys are more prone to trauma, calculi, pyelouretitis cystica, transitional cell carcinoma (TCC) and pelviureteric junction obstruction due to poor drainage.
TCC is a concern in patients with horseshoe kidneys and potentially in patients with pyelouretitis cystica due to the chronic inflammation associated with the condition. However, with TCC the lesions would be expected to have a soft tissue density and enhance, although compared to the adjacent renal parenchyma this can be difficult to appreciate.
Pyelouretitis cystica causes multiple small cysts and is often associated with diabetes and recurrent infection. This, along with the impeded drainage that can occur in a horseshoe kidney, further predispose patients to the condition.
Multiple calculi are unlikely in the clinical setting of painless haematuria, and the density of these small lesions is not typical for calculi. Leukoplakia is also associated with recurrent infection but is more common in the urinary bladder than the upper tracts. Tuberculous urethritis causes intermittent stricturing and dilatation, as well as urinary tract calcification.
(The Final FRCR Complete Revision Notes Pages 252, 265)

89. (b) Duodenojejunal flexure is at the level of the duodenal bulb
Ultrasound and fluoroscopy can be helpful in assessing for midgut volvulus. Ultrasound findings include the 'whirlpool' sign caused by a twisting of the mesenteric vessels. The superior mesenteric vein usually lies to the right of the superior mesenteric artery; in malrotation it lies to the left. The retro-mesenteric D3 part of the duodenum may not be visible between the aorta and superior mesenteric vessels.
On fluoroscopy establishing the position of the duodenojejunal (DJ) flexure is key. It should cross the midline to lie to the left of the left vertebral body pedicle at, or above, the level of the duodenal bulb. The caecum may have a normal position even in malrotation; however, a cephalad position of the caecum would be suspicious given the other findings. The 'corkscrew' appearance is an additional finding that may be seen due to twisting of the duodenum and proximal jejunum.
(The Final FRCR Complete Revision Notes Page 343)

90. (e) Precuneus, posterior cingulate cortex, posterior temporoparietal lobes
Nuclear medicine studies can be a helpful tool in neurodegenerative conditions but clinical history and correlation is vital because radiological findings often overlap. Alzheimer disease typically has reduced activity in the precuneus, posterior cingulate cortex and the posterior temporal and parietal lobes.
Lewy body dementia tends to also have reduced visual cortex and cerebellar uptake. Reduced uptake in vascular dementia is associated with defects in the basal ganglia and cortex. Focal, and sometimes asymmetrical changes, can be seen in Pick disease with a more anterior temporal and frontal lobe distribution. Progressive supranuclear palsy is associated with reduced uptake in the corpus striatum. Tracer activity in Huntington disease is classically reduced in the caudate nuclei but the basal ganglia and frontal lobes more generally can also demonstrate reduced metabolism.
(The Final FRCR Complete Revision Notes Pages 423–434)

91. (b) Cryptogenic organising pneumonia
The ground glass opacification surrounded by dense crescentic opacification in the left mid zone is a description of the 'atoll sign' or 'reverse halo sign', which is a feature characteristic of organising pneumonia. The migratory consolidation is also typical. Consolidation is often bilateral and predominantly subpleural, affecting the mid and lower zones.
'Halo sign' is associated with invasive fungal infection; in contrast to this case, the

description of this is a solid nodule or opacification with surrounding ground glass change. Pulmonary infarct tends to be found at the lung periphery but is less likely to be migratory. Lung adenocarcinoma in situ was previously known as bronchoalveolar cell carcinoma; it can appear as a ground glass opacification or more dense consolidation. It can be multifocal; however it persists on serial imaging.

(The Final FRCR Complete Revision Notes Page 38)

92. (a) Type I

A slip injury is a type I injury. Table 3.5 describes the Salter-Harris classification of growth plate fractures.

(The Final FRCR Complete Revision Notes Page 124)

TABLE 3.5: The Salter-Harris Classification of Growth Plate Fractures

Type	Frequency	Description
I	6–8%	Slip along the growth plate
II	75%	Fracture line extends proximally into the metaphysis from the physis
III	6–8%	Fracture line extending distally into the epiphysis from the physis (involving the articular surface)
IV	10–12%	Fracture line extending from the metaphysis, across the physis and epiphysis
V	1%	Crush injury

Source: Modified from and reprinted with permission from V Helyar and A Shaw. *The Final FRCR: Complete Revision Notes.* CRC Press, Taylor & Francis Group, 2018, p. 124.

93. (c) Biliary strictures are an uncommon early complication

Biliary strictures, mostly secondary to ischaemia, can occur in up to 30% of patients and it is a late complication of transplant. Hepatic artery thrombosis is the most common and serious early vascular complication post transplant. A tardus parvus wave form is not normal and indicates hepatic artery stenosis.

The gallbladder is removed from the recipient and the donor allograft prior to transplant. A small perihepatic haematoma, small volume ascites, periportal oedema and a right pleural effusion are within normal limits for several weeks following transplant.

(The Final FRCR Complete Revision Notes Page 215)

94. (c) MR venogram

The history and CT findings are suggestive of venous sinus thrombosis. This most commonly affects the superior sagittal sinus, leading to bilateral parasagittal infarcts. Thrombus in the straight sinus or vein of Galen may lead to basal ganglia infarcts. Infarct affecting the temporal lobe could be secondary to a transverse or sigmoid sinus thrombus or thrombus in the vein of Labbe. CT or MR venogram is the next best investigation, depending on availability. MRI will show loss of normal flow venous voids in the area of thrombosis. MRV sequences (either time-of-flight or post gadolinium) will show filling defects in the affected vein. Asymmetrical hypoplastic transverse and sigmoid sinuses can be misleading. Remember to look at the jugular foramen; if it is also small it can help to distinguish between the two.

(The Final FRCR Complete Revision Notes Pages 379–380)

95. (b) Ebstein anomaly

It can be helpful to categorise congenital heart disease into cyanotic versus acyanotic. Within the cyanotic group another important consideration is whether the lungs are oligaemic or congested. The use of categorisation helps to narrow the differentials. For this child, the presence of cyanosis and oligaemia suggests conditions such as tetralogy of Fallot, Ebstein anomaly or pulmonary atresia with an intact ventricular septum. The presence of a very enlarged heart excludes tetralogy of Fallot, when the heart is usually normal in size but classically described as boot shaped with an elevated apex. Pulmonary atresia with an intact ventricular septum is not an option for this question but can have very similar appearances to Ebstein anomaly.

Total anomalous pulmonary venous return causes cyanosis and plethoric lungs. Transposition of the great arteries (the D-transposition subtype) is also a cause of cyanosis, but lung appearance can be variable. It typically cases an 'egg-on-a-string' appearance of the mediastinum due to narrowing of the superior mediastinum.

Aortic coarctation is an acyanotic congenital cardiac disease with normal pulmonary flow.

(The Final FRCR Complete Revision Notes Pages 310, 313)

96. (d) Medullary thyroid carcinoma

Nodules containing medullary thyroid carcinoma, along with their metastases frequently contain microcalcification. The age group it affects tends to be around 30–50 years of age and it is associated with multiple endocrine neoplasia 2 syndrome.

The most common thyroid malignancy is papillary thyroid carcinoma, appearing as a hypoechoic nodule with ill-defined margins, and microcalcifications may be present. Regional lymph node metastases can occur early and may have a cystic component.

Follicular thyroid carcinoma is more likely to have haematogenous metastases compared to regional lymph node involvement, and 20% of patients may have distant disease at presentation.

Anaplastic thyroid carcinoma may contain microcalcification; however, it is usually associated with an older age group and has a poor prognosis, with nodal disease common at presentation.

Thyroid lymphoma is usually the non-Hodgkins type. Microcalcification is uncommon and lymphoma would not usually be treated with total thyroidectomy.

(The Final FRCR Complete Revision Notes Pages 434–435)

97. (c) Pleural thickening and calcification

This is a typical description of round atelectasis associated with asbestos exposure. Although many men who have worked in the construction and manufacturing industries are at risk, their family members would have also potentially been exposed to asbestos fibres on their clothing. Round atelectasis can look mass-like – it is caused by collapsed infolded lung adjacent to calcified or non-calcified pleural thickening. Enhancement is a feature because of the presence of lung parenchyma. The bronchovascular crowding and distortion described is known as the 'comet tail' sign. Round atelectasis tends to be relatively stable over time but can sometimes demonstrate interval growth. Asbestos exposure can also lead to asbestosis – an interstitial lung disease typically associated with lower zone fibrosis.

The other features listed in the question are not associated with round atelectasis. Causes of cavitating pulmonary nodules include tuberculosis, primary or metastatic squamous cell carcinoma, abscesses and septic emboli.

Intralesional fat and popcorn calcification is typical for a pulmonary hamartoma. The water-lily sign is associated with pulmonary hydatid disease.

Right hilum lymph node enlargement in the presence of a solitary lung lesion would be more indicative of a primary lung malignancy.

(The Final FRCR Complete Revision Notes Page 19)

98. (a) An Insall-Salvati ratio of 0.6

Patella baja describes an abnormally low lying patella, compared to patella alta which is a high riding patella – this can be remembered as 'baja – below' and 'alta – above'. The typical presentation is described in the question. The condition has various associations including pathology causing quadriceps dysfunction. For example poliomyelitis and following trauma, whether from fractures or secondary to surgery, including post anterior cruciate ligament repair or knee replacement. Patella baja is usually symptomatic in post-traumatic conditions. Chondromalacia patellae is associated with patella alta.

Patella baja or alta can be assessed on lateral knee radiograph or sagittal MRI with the knee flexed to 30 degrees. The Insall-Salvati ratio calculates the patella tendon length (TL) versus the patella length (PL) and patella baja is when this ratio is <0.8 and patella alta is diagnosed when it is >1.2, although some variation to the quoted figures exists. The Blackburne-Peel ratio is often also described and measures patella height.

(The Final FRCR Complete Revision Notes Page 90)

99. (d) The minor papilla drains the pancreatic body and tail

Pancreas divisum is the most common congenital pancreatic anomaly and is secondary to a failure in fusion of the dorsal and ventral pancreatic ducts. The ventral duct (duct of Wirsung) drains the head of the pancreas via the ampulla of Vater and a minor papilla drains the dorsal duct (duct of Santorini) which drains the pancreatic body and tail. Pancreas divisum is often an incidental finding but it may cause pancreatitis and is associated with an increased risk of pancreatic cancer. There are three subtypes, and type 1, where there is no communication between the ducts, is the most common. It can result in a santorinicoele which is a cystic dilatation of the distal dorsal duct immediately proximal to the minor papilla. Pancreas divisum is not associated with choledochal cysts.

(The Final FRCR Complete Revision Notes Page 229)

100. (c) Magnification views

Following a screening recall for microcalcification, magnification views are obtained to further assess its characteristics. Clustered or branching pleomorphic microcalcification is suspicious for ductal carcinoma in situ. A true lateral view can also be helpful, along with the standard mediolateral oblique (MLO) and craniocaudal (CC) views, to aid localisation of the microcalcification in the breast.

Ecklund technique is used for breast implants to displace the implants more posteriorly and make the breast tissue easier to assess. Paddle views apply focal compression to an area in an effort to assess if apparent distortion or spiculation may be real or caused by overlapping structures. Increasingly paddle views are superseded by tomosynthesis. Contrast-enhanced mammography is available at some breast units and can help detect abnormal areas of enhancement.

(The Final FRCR Complete Revision Notes Pages 282, 284)

101. (a) Brachycephaly

Craniosynostosis presents with abnormal head shape and is due to premature fusion of the cranial sutures. The resulting head shape depends on which suture/s have fused.

Brachycephaly is when the head appears short and wide, and is secondary to fusion of the lambdoid or coronal sutures.

Oxycephaly affects the sagittal, lambdoid and coronal sutures causing a tower-like or conical appearance to the head.

Plagiocephaly is a unilateral abnormality and can be anterior or posterior depending on whether the coronal or lambdoid suture has fused.

Scaphocephaly causes the head to appear long and thin and is caused by fusion of the sagittal suture.

Trigonocephaly is fusion of the metopic sutures and causes a triangular appearance to the front of the skull.

(The Final FRCR Complete Revision Notes Pages 292–293)

102. (a) Craniopharyngioma

The mass in the question is typical for a craniopharyngioma. They are most commonly suprasellar tumours containing solid and cystic components with calcification, but they can be partially intrasellar. They are benign, WHO grade I tumours and they have two peaks of incidence: 5–10 years and around 50–60 years. They often present with hydrocephalus due to obstruction of the foramen of Munro. They often have a mixed solid and cystic appearance. The solid components demonstrate contrast enhancement. Variable signal is seen on T1 weighted MRI due to proteinaceous material.

Rathke cleft cysts will not have a solid enhancing component. Pituitary macroadenoma can look very similar but will tend to have an intrasellar epicentre rather than a suprasellar location and calcification is very rare. Although meningiomas can calcify and enhance following contrast, they are unlikely to have cystic components. Intracranial teratomas tend to be of lower density due to fat.

(The Final FRCR Complete Revision Notes Page 397)

103. (b) Bronchiolitis obliterans

Bronchiolitis obliterans is a manifestation of chronic rejection. It usually occurs 6–18 months after transplant, but can occur as early as 3 months. It occurs in approximately 50% of patients and is a major cause of mortality in these patients. Repeated episodes of acute transplant and cytomegalovirus infection are predisposing factors. The radiological features in this condition are that of bronchiectasis: mildly hyperinflated lungs, airway wall thickening and mosaicism

(representing air trapping). Post-transplant lymphoproliferative disease can occur from 1 month to several years after lung transplantation. It represents lymphoid proliferation (B- or T-cell proliferation) on a spectrum of benign proliferation to high grade lymphoma. It usually occurs after Epstein-Barr viral infection. Radiographically it manifests as single or multiple nodules, less commonly consolidation and hilar or mediastinal lymph nodes. These do not match the description provided in the main stem. The description in the main stem is also not consistent with acute transplant rejection or reperfusion syndrome, as these complications occur in the acute setting. Infection can occur at any time following transplant, however the radiological features described, and the time frame provided is typical for bronchiolitis obliterans.
(The Final FRCR Complete Revision Notes Pages 41, 24)

104. (e) Schmorl nodes are one of the most common features
Scheuermann's disease is also known as adolescent kyphosis, the second most common paediatric spinal deformity. The most common findings are Schmorl nodes and anterior vertebral body wedging and disc space narrowing. The thoracic spine is most commonly affected. Usually three to five vertebral bodies are affected and the kyphosis must be >35°.
(The Final FRCR Complete Revision Notes Page 124)

105. (c) T1: Spleen < liver, T2: Spleen > liver, No change between in- and out-of-phase
Liver MRI is frequently employed to help clarify either CT or ultrasound appearances, especially for challenging cases such as in hepatitis B surveillance or in patients with a high body mass index, which can make ultrasound challenging. Normal liver parenchymal signal is hyperintense compared to the spleen on T1 and hypointense compared to the spleen on T2 and there should be no reduction of signal on out-of-phase imaging. Liver signal is also frequently compared to muscle – it should be a similar signal except on inversion recovery sequences. Diffuse signal reduction on out-of-phase imaging can be suggestive of a fatty liver and similarly the T1 signal may be increased in these patients.
(The Final FRCR Complete Revision Notes Page 193)

106. (d) Osteopetrosis
This is a rare disease of abnormal osteoclast activity leading to thickened sclerotic bones which are weak and brittle. Increased bone density and Erlenmeyer flask deformity are very suggestive for this condition. Other features on appendicular plain film include 'bone-in-bone' appearance and alternative sclerotic and lucent bands in the metaphysis.
Melorheostosis is a bone dysplasia with sclerotic foci, typically described as flowing candle wax. Fibrous dysplasia has varied manifestations and can affect a single bone or multiple bones. It can demonstrate ground glass appearance, lucency or sclerosis. Lead poisoning may demonstrate metaphyseal bands as well as the bone-in-bone appearance. In pyknodysostosis there is generalised increased density of the long bones; however the medullary cavity is spared, unlike in osteopetrosis.
(The Final FRCR Complete Revision Notes Page 117)

107. (d) Corpus callosum agenesis
Partial dysgenesis of the corpus callosum usually manifests as the posterior portion being absent and is frequently asymptomatic. However, this is not the case in complete agenesis. The description of the brain in agenesis is of a 'racing car' appearance due to widely separated lateral ventricles. The third ventricle is elevated, often located between the lateral ventricles; it is dilated and may communicate with the interhemispheric cistern. The interhemispheric fissure is widened and the splenium is absent.
Cavum septum pellucidum, cavum vergae and cavum velum interpositum are all normal variants of an additional cerebrospinal fluid space in the midline.
An interhemispheric arachnoid cyst is possible and associated with corpus callosum abnormality; however, the description in the question is typical for corpus callosum agenesis.
(The Final FRCR Complete Revision Notes Page 290)

108. (a) Enhancement present, Low choline level, Low relative cerebral blood flow (rCBF)
Radiation necrosis can occur in the years following treatment with radiotherapy. The lesions can look very similar to tumour recurrence with rim enhancement; however, there are features which can help to differentiate between them. Whereas tumour recurrence would have a choline peak on MRI spectroscopy, radiation necrosis does not. Similarly, tumour recurrence causes an increase in relative cerebral blood flow, whereas radiation necrosis

causes a reduction. 18F-FDG PET/CT can also be employed; in tumour recurrence there would be increased tracer uptake compared to radiation necrosis. Pseudoprogression also has the same features as radiation necrosis on MRI spectroscopy and perfusion studies.
(The Final FRCR Complete Revision Notes Pages 421, 386)

109. (c) Gallium 68 PET/CT
The question describes a typical carcinoid tumour. These are often centrally located, centred on an airway and therefore can cause peripheral atelectasis and recurrent infection. They often enhance avidly and 30% can calcify. Some carcinoids secrete hormones which can lead to additional symptoms. Although generally considered benign, they can invade locally and metastasise to cause sclerotic bone deposits, enlarged local nodes and liver metastases.
Gallium 68 PET/CT is used to stage carcinoid. Carcinoids can be negative on both 18F FDG PET/CT and 18F DOPA PET/CT. Although carcinoids can metastasise to the liver, the most appropriate test would be the Gallium 68 PET/CT rather than liver MRI as it would help to exclude disease elsewhere, for example in the enlarged right hilar and mediastinal nodes. However, these nodes may also be enlarged due to concurrent infection. Follow-up CT in this symptomatic young patient would not be appropriate.
(The Final FRCR Complete Revision Notes Pages 25–27)

110. (d) Short radius with a triangularised distal epiphysis
The patient has a known Madelung deformity, which is a dysplasia of the radius. Features on plain film include lateral and dorsal curvature and short radius with a triangularised distal epiphysis. The articular surface of the distal radius will be angled in an ulnar and volar direction, and dorsal dislocation of the ulnar head is possible. The proximal carpal row is sometimes described as having a 'V'-shape due to the deformity. The condition can be idiopathic, post-traumatic, dysplastic or genetic.
Madelung deformity may be seen in Turner syndrome. Shortening of the third and fourth metacarpals may be seen in this condition, as well as shortening of the second and fifth middle phalanges (which can also be seen in Down syndrome). Ulnar impingement is seen in negative ulnar variance. Madelung deformity is associated with positive ulnar variance.
(The Final FRCR Complete Revision Notes Page 82)

111. (a) Invasion of the duodenum
Pancreatic cancer is associated with a poor prognosis, and 5-year survival is only around 3%. The most common type (approximately 90% of cases) is ductal adenocarcinoma. Only a minority can be resected at diagnosis with a Whipple procedure.
Factors which make a tumour resectable include involving <25% of the circumference of the superior mesenteric vein, invasion of the duodenum (because it will be removed during a Whipple procedure) and the tumour extending to no more than 25–50% of the circumference of the superior mesenteric artery (SMA).
Irresectability is confirmed when the tumour starts to invade adjacent organs (except the duodenum), there are enlarged regional lymph nodes beyond the planned resection margin and the tumour is contacting >50% of the SMA.
(The Final FRCR Complete Revision Notes Pages 230–231)

112. (c) Renal arterial anatomy with CT angiogram
Horseshoe kidneys are prone to having multiple ectopic renal arteries and therefore a CT angiogram prior to any surgery would be helpful, especially because this patient was diagnosed incidentally on a CT cologram, which is a portal venous phase study.
18F-FDG PET/CT is not routinely indicated in renal cell carcinoma due to limited tracer uptake in renal tumours. Furthermore, the tumour is small with no locoregional nodes so occult metastatic disease is unlikely.
Horseshoe kidneys are associated with conditions that can cause urinary tract filling defects such as pyelouretitis cystica and transitional cell carcinoma; however CT urogram is not part of the imaging workup in a renal cell carcinoma diagnosis.
Nuclear medicine studies can be very helpful for management planning in the Urology multidisciplinary team meeting, especially if there is concern regarding renal function, because the results of these studies may lead to more conservative surgery being considered. However, this kidney is unobstructed with otherwise normal appearances and normal serum renal function tests. Therefore, there are no indications that partial nephrectomy should

significantly impact renal function.

Micturating cystourethrogram is not indicated in this patient. There are no features of urinary reflux with no hydronephrosis or other features of long term reflux.

(The Final FRCR Complete Revision Notes Page 252)

113. (a) Diastematomyelia

This is a congenital cord malformation causing a sagittal division of the spinal cord splitting it into two hemicords which usually join together again more caudally. Each hemicord has its own central canal, dorsal horn and ventral horn. This is in contrast to diplomyelia which is complete cord duplication. In diastematomyelia the lower thoracic and upper lumbar levels are most commonly affected. The condition is almost always symptomatic. Patients frequently have scoliosis and can present secondary to its association with a tethered cord with lower limb neurology and bowel and bladder dysfunction. Radiological signs include a widened interpedicular distance and vertebral anomalies. On MRI the cord can be seen splitting and there is sometimes a fibrous or bony spur between the two hemicords.

Myelomeningocele is a type of spina bifida; not only are the meninges and cerebrospinal fluid present in the neural tube defect, but neural tissue too. This does not involve any splitting of the spinal cord. Syringomyelia, or syrinx, is a collection of fluid centrally in the cord and often occurs secondary to other conditions such as myelomeningocele, Chiari or Dandy-Walker malformations.

(The Final FRCR Complete Revision Notes Page 295)

114. (d) Isointense T1 signal with low T2 signal

It is helpful to know the appearance of haemorrhage on MRI both for exams and everyday reporting. One mnemonic is **I-Be**, **Id-De**, **Bi**D**y**, **Ba**B**y**, **D**o**D**o. Once you can remember the signal intensities and relevant time periods, these questions are quite straightforward. This patient's symptoms suggest she is in the acute period and therefore the haematoma would be isointense on T1 weighted imaging and low signal on T2 weighted imaging.

Hyperacute (up to 6 hours): T1 Isointense, T2 Bright
Acute (8–72 hours): T1 Isointense, T2 Dark
Early subacute (3–7 days): T1 Bright, T2 Dark
Late subacute (Weeks to months): T1 Bright, T2 Bright
Chronic (Months +): T1 Dark, T2 Dark

(The Final FRCR Complete Revision Notes Page 371)

115. (b) In- and out-of-phase imaging

Thymic hyperplasia can be divided into true hyperplasia (secondary to chemotherapy, radiotherapy or steroids) and lymphoid hyperplasia (associated with systemic lupus erythematosus/rheumatoid arthritis/Addison disease/Graves disease). Both types demonstrate diffuse symmetric enlargement of the thymus. Rebound hyperplasia can occur after the stressor has been removed, where the thymus grows even larger. On CT, the diffuse symmetric appearance of the thymus is the key feature in differentiating thymic hyperplasia from neoplasm; the latter is usually a focal mass. In addition to the morphologic features, MRI imaging with in- and out-of-phase sequences may be of use. On the out-of-phase sequences, thymic hyperplasia will demonstrate signal dropout due to chemical shift artefact, this is not seen in thymic neoplasms.

(The Final FRCR Complete Revision Notes Page 59)

Nishino M, Ashiku SK, Kocher ON et al. The thymus: a comprehensive review. RadioGraphics. 2006;26(2):335–348.

116. (b) Expansion of the internal acoustic canal (IAC)

Vestibular schwannomas account for the majority of cerebellopontine angle masses, with meningiomas being the second most common, followed by epidermoid cysts. They are usually isodense masses on CT which enhance and widen the IAC, and can resemble an ice cream cone. They can sometimes contain cystic areas but do not contain calcification. On MRI they are usually low T1 signal or isointense to the brain and have T2 high signal without restricted diffusion. There is an acute angle with the dura.

In contrast to vestibular schwannomas, meningiomas are durally based and have an obtuse angle with the dura. Apart from calcification, they can be more homogenous in appearance. They do not usually widen the IAC.

Epidermoid cysts do not widen the IAC and do not enhance. Unlike a schwannoma, they demonstrate restricted diffusion.
(The Final FRCR Complete Revision Notes Pages 405–406)

117. (c) Grade III
The presence of a parenchymal laceration >3 cm in depth and the absence of active bleeding makes this grade III.
(The Final FRCR Complete Revision Notes Page 240)

TABLE 3.6: The American Association for the Surgery of Trauma (AAST) Spleen Injury Scale (2018 Revision)

Grade	
I	Subcapsular haematoma <10% surface area, parenchymal laceration <1 cm depth, capsular tear
II	Subcapsular haematoma 10–50% surface area, intraparenchymal haematoma <5 cm, parenchymal laceration 1–3 cm
III	Subcapsular haematoma >50% surface area, ruptured subcapsular or intraparenchymal haematoma ≥5 cm, parenchymal laceration >3 cm in depth
IV	Any injury in the presence of a splenic vascular injury or active bleeding confined within splenic capsule parenchymal laceration involving segmental or hilar vessels producing >25% devascularisation
V	Shattered spleen any injury in the presence of splenic vascular injury with active bleeding extending beyond the spleen into the peritoneum

Source: The American Association for the Surgery of Trauma. 2018 revision. AAST Spleen Injury Scale. Table 7. https://www.aast.org/library/traumatools/injuryscoringscales.aspx#spleen.

118. (b) Intraparenchymal haemorrhage
Germinal matrix haemorrhage occurs in premature infants; after around 36 weeks gestation the germinal matrix is no longer present. It is frequently detected on neonatal cranial ultrasound as hyperechoic areas in the caudothalamic groove adjacent to the ventricles. Germinal matrix haemorrhage is graded I to IV in severity. Grade I is limited to the caudothalamic groove, grade II is intraventricular extension without hydrocephalus, grade III is intraventricular extension with ventricular dilatation and grade IV is parenchymal involvement, which is associated with high mortality.
(The Final FRCR Complete Revision Notes Pages 295–296)

119. (a) Elevated serum IgG4
The imaging features are consistent with autoimmune pancreatitis. CT imaging findings include diffuse enlargement of the pancreas with loss of the normal contour. There is usually limited peripancreatic fat stranding but there is commonly a peripancreatic halo of low density. It is not associated with pseudocysts. Focal forms of the condition can mimic pancreatic malignancy. Unsurprisingly, other autoimmune conditions are linked to the condition, including Sjögren syndrome and rheumatoid arthritis. It is associated with high serum IgG4 levels.
Ca19-9 is linked to pancreatic ductal adenocarcinoma. Chromogranin A and B are used as biomarkers for neuroendocrine tumours. Alpha-fetoprotein is elevated in a variety of conditions including some tumours such as hepatocellular carcinoma and germ cell tumours.
(The Final FRCR Complete Revision Notes Page 235)

120. (e) T2 spin echo MRI is one of the tools that can help in the diagnosis and monitoring of multiple sclerosis. Lesions in the brain are typically T2 and FLAIR hyperintense and T1 hypointense. There can be a characteristic 'Dawson's finger' pattern of lesions arranged

perpendicular to the lateral ventricles; this is best appreciated on sagittal FLAIR images. An important feature is multiple white matter lesions separated in time and place, and the use of gadolinium can delineate active plaques versus inactive lesions. FLAIR is the best sequence for supratentorial assessment. T2 spin echo/STIR/proton echo/STIR/proton density sequences are best for imaging the posterior fossa. Active disease may have either increased or decreased diffusion.

(The Final FRCR Complete Revision Notes Page 419)

PAPER 4

1. An 81 year old retired ship builder with a pacemaker has a CT pulmonary angiogram for pleuritic chest pain and shortness of breath. There is no evidence of pulmonary embolus; however you notice that he has small bilateral pleural effusions and widespread bilateral pleural thickening involving the hemidiaphragms. There are a couple of prominent, but not frankly enlarged, hila nodes. Ultrasound guided pleural biopsy is inconclusive. The clinical team call you asking for advice regarding further imaging to help distinguish malignant from benign pleural thickening.

   What is the most appropriate test?

   a. Contrast enhanced ultrasound
   b. CT abdomen and pelvis
   c. MRI
   d. 18F-FDG PET/CT scan
   e. Portal venous phase contrast CT chest

2. A 47 year old female patient is reviewed in the rheumatology clinic with joint pains in her hands. Radiographs are requested which demonstrate a bilateral symmetrical arthropathy with osteopenia, reduction in joint space, osteophytosis and flattening of the index and middle finger metacarpal heads. There are subchondral cysts and irregularity of the articular surface which is particularly affecting the metacarpal phalangeal joints and the carpal bones.

   What other imaging appearance would correspond with these findings?

   a. Dilated oesophagus on chest radiograph
   b. Hyperdensity in the sagittal sinus on CT head
   c. Pancreatic low signal on T1, T2 and T2* sequences on MRI of the upper abdomen
   d. Multiple small foci of subcortical T2* low signal on MRI head
   e. Symmetrical hilar and mediastinal lymph node enlargement on CT chest

3. An adult male patient with abdominal pain undergoes a CT scan of the abdomen and pelvis under the surgical team. The bowel loops are unremarkable and there is no free gas. However, there is a 5.5-cm bulky tumour centred on the right adrenal gland which has an irregular margin, foci of low attenuation and demonstrates heterogeneous enhancement. The tumour does not contain calcification or haemorrhage, and abuts but does not invade the inferior vena cava. There are multiple low attenuation, ill-defined lesions seen within the liver and several lucent foci within the lumbar spine, which are suspicious for metastases. The lungs have not been included on the scan.

   What is the most likely cause of the appearances of the right adrenal gland?

   a. Adrenocortical carcinoma
   b. Collision tumour
   c. Metastasis from adenocarcinoma
   d. Myelolipoma
   e. Phaeochromocytoma

4. A usually fit and well 73 year old man is investigated for weight loss and anaemia. There is a history of left nephrectomy for organ donation 5 years previously. Contrast enhanced CT chest, abdomen, pelvis is performed as part of this workup and demonstrates multiple endophytic, homogenous right renal lesions. The renal lesions appear mildly hypodense to the surrounding parenchyma. There are several enlarged, rounded retroperitoneal and pelvic lymph nodes. The renal vessels opacify normally. There are homogenous appearances of the other solid upper abdominal viscera. The chest is clear. The spleen measures 15.2 cm in craniocaudal extent. Renal MRI is performed to help characterise further and the renal lesions exhibit intermediate T1 and intermediate T2 signal.

   What is the most likely diagnosis?

   a. Leiomyosarcoma
   b. Metastases
   c. Primary lymphoma of the kidney
   d. Renal cell carcinoma
   e. Secondary lymphoma of the kidney

5. A young child has been diagnosed with an infantile haemangioendothelioma on imaging after presenting with a right upper quadrant mass and cardiac failure. An ultrasound confirmed a vascular heterogenous mass which was confirmed as a haemangioendothelioma following an MRI abdomen.

   Which of the following post contrast MRI findings correlates most closely with this diagnosis?

   a. Contrast washout on delayed phase imaging
   b. Early peripheral enhancement with delayed central enhancement
   c. Heterogenous arterial phase enhancement
   d. Heterogenous delayed phase enhancement
   e. Minimal enhancement on all phases

6. A 30 year old male who has multiple cutaneous nodules presents with recurrent episodes of right sided weakness. An intracranial CT angiogram shows bilateral occlusion of the intracranial portion of the internal carotid arteries. There are extensive leptomeningeal and dural arterial vessel collaterals.

   What is the most likely diagnosis?

   a. Radiation vasculitis
   b. Moyamoya syndrome
   c. Sickle cell disease
   d. Cerebral atherosclerosis
   e. Systemic lupus erythematous

7. A 33 year old female undergoes a lung transplant for cystic fibrosis. She has an uneventful recovery from theatre; however her mobile chest radiograph on ITU performed at 24 hours demonstrates bilateral perihilar airspace opacification. This finding continues to worsen over the next 48–72 hours. Echocardiogram excludes left ventricular failure and there is low clinical suspicion of infection. She receives supportive care and after 5 days the opacities improve. They have resolved by day 10.

   What is the most likely aetiology?

   a. Acute transplant rejection
   b. Bronchiolitis obliterans
   c. Infection
   d. Post-transplant lymphoproliferative disease
   e. Reperfusion syndrome

8. A 13 year old boy with a known chromosomal abnormality has a chest radiograph for investigation of fever and general malaise, looking for an infective source. This shows a hypersegmented manubrium as well as 11 pairs of ribs and scoliosis.

   What is the most likely chromosomal abnormality?

   a. Monosomy X
   b. Triploidy
   c. Trisomy 13
   d. Trisomy 18
   e. Trisomy 21

9. A junior radiology colleague asks you to review an upper gastrointestinal barium study that they have performed on a 57 year old male patient referred by his GP for difficulty swallowing and non-specific abdominal discomfort. The oesophagus and stomach outline normally with prompt gastric emptying. In the D2 part of the duodenum there is a posterior well-defined nodular protrusion into the duodenal lumen. Barium collects centrally within this protrusion. Transit through the duodenum is swift and the duodenojejunal flexure is positioned to the left of the vertebral column at the level of the duodenal bulb.

   What is the most likely diagnosis?

   a. Adenocarcinoma of the papilla of Vater
   b. Benign lymphoid hyperplasia
   c. Duodenal ulceration

d. Ectopic pancreatic tissue
e. Malrotation

10. A 10 year old girl has a radiograph of her distal left arm following a fall at school. The radiographer shows you the film. There is no acute fracture but there is shortening and bowing of the radius with positive ulnar variance and distal dislocation of the distal ulnar with a 'V'-shaped appearance of the proximal carpal row.

    What condition is NOT associated with these appearances?

    a. Diaphyseal aclasia
    b. Morquio syndrome
    c. Nail patella syndrome
    d. Ollier disease
    e. Turner syndrome

11. An MRI brain is acquired for an 8 month old child with developmental delay. This shows a thickened, smooth cortex within both cerebral hemispheres. Both occipital horns of the lateral ventricles are dilated. The cerebellum appears spared.

    Which of the following cortical malformation disorders is described?

    a. Hemimegalencephaly
    b. Holoprosencephaly
    c. Lissencephaly
    d. Porencephaly
    e. Schizencephaly

12. A 42 year old patient is referred for imaging by his GP with a painless lump on his jaw. A radiograph demonstrates a lucent lesion at the mandibular ramus. This has a multilocular honeycomb-like appearance. It is well defined and corticated. There is evidence of root resorption affecting the adjacent teeth. An MRI reveals a lesion containing cystic and soft tissue signal elements. There are no fluid-fluid levels. The septations and solid components enhance avidly following contrast injection.

    What is the most likely diagnosis?

    a. Ameloblastoma
    b. Dentigerous cyst
    c. Metastases
    d. Odontogenic keratocyst
    e. Radicular cyst

13. A 64 year old male ex-smoker with a cough is provisionally diagnosed with a T2a N0 M0 primary lung cancer on CT. CT guided biopsy confirms the diagnosis of primary lung adenocarcinoma. Following multidisciplinary team discussion and surgical planning he is admitted for a right lower lobe lobectomy. Several chest radiographs in the week following surgery have shown an appropriately sited right chest drain but with a persistent moderate right pneumothorax. The clinical team report the chest drain continues to bubble. CT chest demonstrates similar findings to the chest radiographs.

    Which of the following could help to confirm the suspected diagnosis?

    a. CT pulmonary angiogram
    b. Insert a larger bore chest drain
    c. Remove the chest drain and repeat chest radiograph after 4 hours
    d. Ventilation-perfusion (VQ) scan
    e. Xenon ventilation study

14. A 10 year old female has a plain film of the thoracic spine which demonstrates vertebral plana of the T4 vertebral body. Further imaging of the skull and appendicular skeleton does not reveal any other site of bone abnormality.

    What is the most likely diagnosis?

    a. Hand-Schüller-Christian disease

b. Langerhans cell histiocytosis
c. Letterer-Siwe disease
d. Leukaemia
e. Vertebral metastases

15. A 25 year old female presents to her GP with right upper quadrant pain. They refer her for an abdominal ultrasound. This shows a 10-cm mass in the right lobe of the liver which has a hyperechoic central scar. A MRI of the liver is arranged. The lesion is isointense relative to the liver on T1 and slightly T2 hyperintense. The central scar is hypointense on both T1 and T2. Following gadolinium administration, the lesion shows heterogeneous enhancement on arterial phase and is isointense on delayed phase. There is no loss of signal on out-of-phase imaging. The central scar does not show any significant enhancement.

    What is the most likely diagnosis?

    a. Focal nodular hyperplasia
    b. Hepatocellular carcinoma
    c. Haemangioma
    d. Fibrolamellar hepatocellular carcinoma
    e. Hepatic adenoma

16. The consultant looking after a 41 year old female outpatient with normal renal function and urine dip comes to ask you for advice. The patient had an ultrasound abdomen for query gallstones due to intermittent epigastric and right upper quadrant pain. The ultrasound confirmed gallstones but the report also mentioned bilateral echogenic renal pyramids with otherwise normal kidneys. A CT urinary tract from an emergency department attendance 1 month previously also demonstrated hyperdense medullary pyramids with no hydronephrosis. A CT urogram confirmed a striated nephrogram.

    What is the most appropriate next step in management?

    a. Antinuclear antibody serum levels
    b. Blood culture and antibiotics
    c. No further investigation required
    d. Review patient medication
    e. Ultrasound renal Doppler

17. A neonate with vomiting has an abdominal radiograph which demonstrates a distended stomach and duodenum causing a 'double bubble' appearance. There is no convincing small or large bowel gas and no free peritoneal gas. Duodenal atresia is suspected. An upper gastrointestinal contrast study is performed.

    Where is the level of obstruction most likely to lie?

    a. At D4 just proximal to the duodenojejunal flexure
    b. At the midpoint of D3
    c. Just distal to the ampulla of Vater in D2
    d. Just distal to the gastric antrum in D1
    e. Just proximal to the ampulla of Vater in D2

18. A 74 year old man presents with a several month history of cognitive impairment. Following a neurology review, a CT brain is performed which demonstrates generalised cerebral atrophy. He goes on to have an MRI brain. This shows high T2 signal within the caudate, putamen and thalami bilaterally. There is also high DWI and T2 signal within the cerebral cortex bilaterally.

    What is the most likely diagnosis?

    a. Alzheimer dementia
    b. Carbon monoxide poisoning
    c. Creutzfeldt-Jakob disease
    d. Lewy body dementia
    e. Manganese poisoning

19. A 67 year old retired patient presents to the GP with increasing shortness of breath. He has a plain film which shows a moderate left sided pleural effusion. The GP goes on to organise a

high resolution CT chest and referral to the respiratory team. The CT scan shows a left sided pleural effusion and extensive, irregular nodular pleural thickening with suspected involvement of the mediastinal surface.

What is the most likely diagnosis?

a. Fibrothorax
b. Liposarcoma of the pleura
c. Metastatic adenocarcinoma
d. Pleural mesothelioma
e. Primary pleural lymphoma

20. An active 61 year old patient has an MRI spine requested by his GP for a 7 month history of lumbar back pain which is stopping him from playing tennis and has not responded to physiotherapy. This is reported as a moderate disc bulge at L3/4, generalised facet joint hypertrophy and Modic type II endplate changes at L4/5.

Which of the options below correlate with the finding of Modic type II endplate changes?

Table 4.1:

	T1 Endplate Signal	T2 Endplate Signal	T2 Disc Signal
a	Low	High	High
b	High	High	Low
c	Low	High	Low
d	Low	Low	Low
e	High	High	High

21. A female patient is discussed at the cancer of unknown primary multidisciplinary team meeting. An MRI lumbar spine incidentally detected multiple liver lesions and several paraaortic lymph nodes measuring up to 15 mm in short axis. A malignant looking gastric lesion was subsequently identified on endoscopy.

Regarding malignant metastatic gastric lesions, what is the most common primary site?

a. Breast
b. Colon
c. Endometrium
d. Pancreas
e. Skin

22. A 6 month old child is referred for an MRI brain due to developmental delay and macrocephaly. This shows an enlarged posterior fossa with elevated torcular herophili. There is cystic enlargement of the fourth ventricle. The cerebellum is hypoplastic and the lateral and third ventricles are dilated.

What is the most likely diagnosis?

a. Chiari I malformation
b. Chiari II malformation
c. Dandy-Walker malformation
d. Dandy-Walker variant
e. Mega cisterna magna

23. A 36 year old woman who is 19 weeks pregnant undergoes an abdominal ultrasound. This demonstrates an echogenic 2-cm mass in the right lobe of the liver. It is well defined and has a lobulated contour.

What is the most appropriate next step?

a. Contrast enhanced low dose CT abdomen
b. Contrast enhanced MRI

c. Non-contrast enhanced MRI
d. Repeat ultrasound following completion of the pregnancy
e. Technetium 99-m red blood cell scan

24. A 30 year old man describes a several month history of bilateral facial weakness. An MRI brain is performed. This shows diffuse, nodular thickening of the leptomeningeal layers predominantly within the basal cisterns. These enhance avidly following gadolinium administration. Further areas of high T2/FLAIR signal are seen involving the facial nerves bilaterally.

What is the most likely diagnosis?

a. Leptomeningeal metastases
b. Lymphoma
c. Multiple myeloma
d. Neurosarcoidosis
e. Tuberculous meningitis

25. A 39 year old female patient with no significant past medical history presents to the emergency department having felt unwell for the past week. She has a raised temperature and is markedly hypoxic. The chest radiograph is abnormal. Full blood count and renal function are normal. The patient proceeds to have a CT chest which demonstrates bilateral patches of consolidation and ground glass opacity with small bilateral pleural effusions and interlobular septal thickening. There are no radiological size significant hila or mediastinal lymph nodes.

What is the most likely diagnosis?

a. Acute eosinophilic pneumonia
b. Eosinophilic granulomatosis with polyangiitis (Churg-Strauss syndrome)
c. Sarcoidosis
d. *Staphylococcus aureus* bronchopneumonia
e. Subacute hypersensitivity pneumonitis

26. A 14 year old boy presents with abdominal pain and vomiting. He is assessed by the paediatric team and found to be anaemic. He is considered to be short for his age and the paediatric team suspect a systemic aetiology, and amongst other investigations he has a plain film of the wrist. The radiograph demonstrates bands of increased density at the distal metaphysis of the radius. There is a 'bone-in-bone' appearance of the bones.

What is the most likely underlying diagnosis?

a. Rickets
b. Lead poisoning
c. Physiological
d. Scurvy
e. Trauma

27. A 61 year old male patient attends hospital with a history of haematemesis. His observations are stable. During admission a contrast enhanced CT abdomen and pelvis reveals a 45-mm soft tissue and cystic density mass centred on the stomach with peripheral enhancement. There is no size-significant lymph node enlargement. Biopsy reveals that the mass expresses c-KIT (CD117) antigen. Apart from some mild lower lobe atelectasis, a CT chest is normal. An MRI head from 5 years ago demonstrated an abnormal left sphenoid wing and several areas of bilateral high T2 weighted signal in the basal ganglia and deep white matter.

What is the most likely diagnosis affecting the stomach?

a. Gastric hamartoma
b. Gastrointestinal stromal tumour
c. Lymphoma
d. Metastatic small cell lung malignancy
e. Gastric scirrhous adenocarcinoma

28. A 65 year old male patient with haematuria is sent by his GP for an ultrasound abdomen which describes a 5-cm isoechoic left renal mass. CT chest abdomen pelvis shows a heterogenous left renal lesion with coarse calcific foci and heterogenous enhancement. There

is no enhancement centrally and no vascular invasion; however there is left perinephric stranding. The adrenal glands are normal, there is no size significant lymph node enlargement and the lungs are clear. Ultrasound guided biopsy was challenging due to the position of the lesion, and the patient did not tolerate it well. Limited tissue was acquired which could not differentiate between oncocytoma and renal cell carcinoma. The patient is referred to the urology multidisciplinary team meeting.

From the following options, what is the most appropriate next step in management?

a. MRI kidneys
b. Referral to a sarcoma centre
c. Surgical resection
d. Repeat US guided biopsy
e. Ultrasound guided ablation

29. A child presents with jaundice and a right upper quadrant mass. Sonographic appearances and MRCP is consistent with Caroli disease.

Which choledochal cyst distribution is consistent with this diagnosis?

a. Dilatation of distal extrahepatic duct within the duodenal wall
b. Dilatation of the intrahepatic ducts
c. Diverticulum of the extrahepatic duct
d. Extrahepatic duct dilatation
e. Intra- and extrahepatic duct dilatation

30. You are reviewing an unenhanced CT head for a 47 year old patient referred by their GP for intermittent headaches. The appearances of the brain are within normal limits; however, you notice a unilateral hyperdensity at the posterior aspect of the right globe. It is well defined and has a lenticular shape which is elevated and minimally protruding into the vitreous. The extraocular structures have normal appearances. Subsequent MRI showed that this was T1 hyperintense, T2 hypointense and enhanced following contrast.

What does this lesion most likely represent?

a. Choroidal osteoma
b. Drusen
c. Melanoma
d. Retinoblastoma
e. Retinal detachment

31. A 29 year old patient with a known genetic condition has a chest radiograph for a new cough productive of sputum. You review the plain film with several previous films that are available. There is a large, well circumscribed opacity in the posterior mediastinum with associated focal thoracic scoliosis. There are also multiple nodules projected over the lungs with evidence of cutaneous soft tissue nodules. These findings are unchanged from the previous imaging. There is also new consolidation in the left lower lobe.

Which of these findings are you LEAST likely to see on subsequent high resolution CT chest?

a. Basal symmetrical lung fibrosis
b. Pectus excavatum
c. Posterior vertebral scalloping
d. Ribbon ribs
e. Tracheobronchomegaly

32. A 50 year old man with a history of sickle cell anaemia is diagnosed with locally advanced prostate cancer. At his outpatient oncology appointment he reports he has been experiencing some lumbar back pain and therefore a lumbar spine MRI is requested. There is no canal stenosis, no evidence of significant intervertebral disc disease but there is multilevel central end plate depression. The marrow is mildly hyperintense on T2 weighted sequences and comparatively lower on T1 weighted imaging. T1 in- and out-of-phase imaging is performed which demonstrates signal reduction on the T1 out-of-phase sequence.

What is the most likely diagnosis?

a. Haemosiderosis
b. Metastatic infiltration
c. Myelofibrosis
d. Red marrow reconversion
e. Yellow marrow reconversion

33. A 26 year old man is a passenger in a road traffic collision. On clinical examination he has a tender right upper quadrant and is noted to be tachycardic and hypotensive. He undergoes a split bolus trauma protocol CT of his chest, abdomen and pelvis. This demonstrates a subcapsular haematoma extending more than 50% around the border of the liver. There is also a linear area of hypodensity in segment VI of the liver extending to the capsule consistent with a laceration. This measures 4 cm in depth. No contrast extravasation or blush is identified to indicate active bleeding.

    Using The American Association of Surgery for Trauma (AAST) grading scale, what is the grade of liver laceration?

    a. Grade I
    b. Grade II
    c. Grade III
    d. Grade IV
    e. Grade V

34. A 3 year old boy is referred to the paediatric neurology team with increasing clumsiness, headache and vomiting over a period of a few weeks. An MRI brain finds a posterior fossa mass. This is poorly defined and in the midline, filling the fourth ventricle. Signal characteristics are low T1 and high T2 compared to the grey matter. There is adjacent oedema causing mass effect and evidence of early hydrocephalus. It enhances homogenously following contrast and demonstrates restricted diffusion.

    What is the most likely diagnosis?

    a. Astrocytoma
    b. Brainstem glioma
    c. Choroid plexus papilloma
    d. Ependymoma
    e. Medulloblastoma

35. A 10 year old girl is referred for an MRI spine due to lower limb sensory and motor deficit. This shows a single cord with termination at the L3 level. There is an intradural, extramedullary mass adjacent to the conus which is T1 and T2 hyperintense. There is no post-contrast enhancement or restricted diffusion. The mass does not extend into the dorsal subcutaneous tissues. Appearances of the vertebrae are within normal limits.

    What is the most likely diagnosis?

    a. Diastematomyelia
    b. Ependymoma
    c. Lipomyelomeningocele
    d. Paraganglioma
    e. Tethered cord syndrome

36. A neonate is born at 35 weeks' gestation following premature rupture of membranes and emergency caesarean section. The child develops tachypnoea and nasal flaring within the first 24 hours. The clinical team are concerned about infant respiratory distress syndrome due to surfactant deficiency. A chest radiograph is requested.

    Which of the following radiographic features would be most likely to be associated with respiratory distress syndrome caused by surfactant deficiency?

    a. Interstitial oedema
    b. Lack of air bronchograms
    c. Normal chest radiograph at 6 hours
    d. Perihilar streaky opacities
    e. Reduced lung volumes

37. A 44 year old male patient has had repeated GP attendances for mild fever, cough and breathlessness over the past 3 months. Several chest radiographs over this time have demonstrated patchy air space opacification varying in distribution with intervening normal chest films.

    Which investigation could confirm the diagnosis?

    a. Anti-basement membrane antibody
    b. Bronchoalveolar lavage
    c. cANCA
    d. Serum eosinophil count
    e. Urine 5-HIAA levels

38. A 15 year old male with pectus excavatum has a plain film of the thoracolumbar spine which demonstrates scoliosis and scalloping of the posterior lumbosacral vertebral bodies. A pelvic radiograph demonstrates acetabular protrusion. He also has several cardiac investigations to assess the mitral valve and aortic root. Of note, he performs well at school academically.

    What is the most likely cause of pectus excavatum in this patient?

    a. Down syndrome
    b. Foetal alcohol syndrome
    c. Homocysteinuria
    d. Marfan syndrome
    e. Prematurity

39. A barium swallow is performed for symptoms of regurgitation and dysphagia in a 42 year old female patient. There is a smooth, wide-based filling defect projecting into the lumen in the lower third of the oesophagus causing slow transit of barium. There is no evidence of mucosal ulceration. On review of the control images there is calcification in this region.

    What is the most appropriate next step?

    a. Breast triple assessment
    b. Endoscopic ultrasound and 18F-FDG PET/CT
    c. Follow-up in 1 year
    d. MRI head, physical assessment and family history
    e. Surgical referral

40. A CT abdomen pelvis requested to assess for diverticulitis as a cause of upper abdominal discomfort in a 63 year old woman identifies a cystic right ovarian lesion. A subsequent MRI pelvis helps to evaluate this lesion further. It is predominantly high signal on T2 weighted imaging with a thin septation and a small amount of enhancing, nodular, peripheral, intermediate T1 and T2 signal. The lesion otherwise demonstrates low T1 signal. There are no size-significant lymph nodes within the pelvis. There is a trace of free fluid in the pouch of Douglas. The left ovary has normal post-menopausal appearances.

    What is the most likely diagnosis?

    a. Kruckenberg tumour
    b. Mucinous cystadenoma
    c. Mucinous cystadenocarcinoma
    d. Serous cystadenoma
    e. Serous cystadenocarcinoma

41. A 3 year old boy is referred for an MRI brain. The request form says he has a facial cleavage abnormality and therefore a diagnosis of holoprosencephaly is suspected by the paediatric team.

    If holoprosencephaly is confirmed on the MRI, which structure will be absent?

    a. Corpus callosum
    b. Falx cerebri
    c. Olfactory tracts
    d. Septum pellucidum
    e. Third ventricle

42. An 8 month old patient under the care of ophthalmology has an MRI orbits following clinical review for right proptosis. This demonstrates a unilateral right orbital mass. The mass spans both intra- and extraconal compartments. It is lobulated and septated with signal which is T1 hypointense to fat and T2 isointense to fat but hyperintense to muscle. The mass enhances intensely following contrast injection. There are thin, curvilinear, very low signal foci within the mass.

    What does this mass most likely represent?

    a. Capillary haemangioma
    b. Cavernous haemangioma
    c. Lymphangioma
    d. Retinoblastoma
    e. Venous varix

43. A 45 year old female with a past medical history of well-controlled diabetes mellitus attends her GP with a productive cough and fever. She has a chest radiograph which shows dense opacification in the right lower zone with the presence of air bronchograms.

    What is the most likely organism?

    a. *Haemophilus influenzae*
    b. *Klebsiella pneumoniae*
    c. *Legionella pneumophila*
    d. *Staphylococcus aureus*
    e. *Streptococcus pneumoniae*

44. A 10 year old boy presents with a couple of months history of intermittent left knee pain and is reviewed by the paediatric team. Radiograph demonstrates soft tissue swelling adjacent to his distal left femur. Within the bone, adjacent to the distal femoral metaphysis, there is a longitudinally orientated, ill-defined lytic lesion with surrounding sclerosis. Emanating from this is a linear lytic area extending towards the physis.

    What is the most likely diagnosis?

    a. Eosinophilic granuloma
    b. Giant cell tumour
    c. Osteomyelitis
    d. Osteoid osteoma
    e. Osteosarcoma

45. A 62 year old male with known liver cirrhosis secondary to hepatitis C presents with an acute upper gastrointestinal bleed. The patient is fluid resuscitated and transfused. Endoscopy is performed which identifies large oesophageal varices. Unfortunately thrombin injection does not stop the bleeding. An emergency transjugular intrahepatic portosystemic shunt (TIPSS) procedure is planned.

    Regarding TIPSS, an iatrogenic communication is made between the portal vein and which vessel?

    a. Inferior vena cava
    b. Aorta
    c. Hepatic vein
    d. Hepatic artery
    e. Splenic vein

46. A 45 year old man of no fixed abode, with a background of alcoholism, is admitted via the emergency department. He appears confused with a fluctuating GCS and is noted to have a spastic quadriparesis. CT brain shows a focal area of low attenuation crossing the midline in the lower pons. The same area on MRI brain demonstrates high T2/FLAIR and low T1 signal. The lesion also shows high DWI/low ADC signal. There is no enhancement of the affected area after intravenous gadolinium administration.

    What is the most likely diagnosis?

    a. Brainstem metastasis

b. Osmotic demyelination syndrome
c. Pontine infarct
d. Pontine astrocytoma
e. Wernicke encephalopathy

47. A 20 year old man is referred for an ultrasound as he has a palpable neck mass. The ear, nose and throat team suspect a type II branchial cleft cyst.

Which of these statements correctly describes the location of a type II branchial cleft cyst?

a. Above the angle of the mandible, close to the external auditory canal
b. Anterior to sternocleidomastoid, below the angle of the mandible
c. In the midline, above the level of the hyoid cartilage
d. Paramidline, infrahyoid adjacent to the thyroid gland
e. Posterior to sternocleidomastoid at the level of the carotid bifurcation

48. A patient with a 30-mm hypoechoic left parotid gland lesion has an ultrasound guided biopsy and is diagnosed with mucoepidermoid carcinoma. The case is discussed at the head and neck multidisciplinary team meeting.

What further MRI head/neck sequence would be most helpful to stage this lesion?

a. Axial DWI/ADC
b. Axial post contrast fat supressed T1
c. Axial small field of view T2
d. Axial T2* GRE
e. Sagittal post contrast T1

49. A 26 year old male cyclist is involved in a serious road traffic collision and intubated at the scene prior to hospital transfer. A trauma CT of the head, neck, chest, abdomen and pelvis and targeted radiographs at the time of hospital admission identified a small right subdural haemorrhage, Malgaigne pelvic fracture, fracture of the right proximal femur, a stable L1 fracture and fracture dislocation of the right ankle joint. No neck or thoracic injuries were identified. The ITU team report increasing oxygen requirements 2 days following admission and difficulty ventilating the patient. CT chest demonstrates bilateral consolidation and ground glass opacity.

What is the most likely diagnosis?

a. Aspiration pneumonia
b. Fat embolism
c. Infective bronchopneumonia
d. Lung contusion
e. Pulmonary laceration

50. A 6 year old male presents with right sided hip pain. He has a pelvic radiograph with frog lateral views. In the right hip, there is widening of the medial joint space. The right epiphysis looks reduced in size, flattened and sclerotic.

What is the most likely diagnosis?

a. Haemophilia
b. Osteomyelitis
c. Perthes disease
d. Slipped upper femoral epiphysis
e. Transient synovitis of the hip

51. A 58 year old woman with dysphagia has a barium swallow following GP referral. This demonstrates a thin transverse filling defect in the upper third of the anterior oesophagus. A diagnosis of Plummer-Vinson syndrome is made.

Which other clinical feature is commonly associated with this diagnosis?

a. Microcytic anaemia
b. Low serum CD4 count
c. Positive serum *Helicobacter pylori* test

d. Raised serum gamma-glutamyl transferase
e. Vitamin B_{12} deficiency

52. Following an ultrasound abdomen of a 32 year old patient which identified multiple hyperechoic bilateral renal lesions, the patient has a CT abdomen pelvis which confirms multiple bilateral exophytic renal masses. The largest measures up to 60 mm. All the lesions have similar appearances, with a soft tissue component as well as lower density areas measuring around −30HU. There is no calcification. The lung bases are included on the CT and there are a couple of small thin-walled cysts visible.

    What is the most appropriate management for the renal lesions?

    a. MRI kidneys
    b. No further management required
    c. Oncology referral
    d. Referral to urology surgeons
    e. Repeat CT in 6 months

53. A 2 year old girl is brought into the emergency department by her parents with fever, cough and inspiratory stridor. The clinical team request a radiograph of the neck. There is subglottic tracheal narrowing and distension of the hypopharynx. The epiglottis and aryepiglottic folds do not appear thickened. The adenoid tonsils are enlarged. On the lateral view the retropharyngeal soft tissues are equivalent in thickness to approximately half a vertebral body width.

    What is the most likely diagnosis?

    a. Croup
    b. Epiglottitis
    c. Exudative tracheitis
    d. Pharyngitis
    e. Retropharyngeal abscess

54. A 60 year old male presents with acute confusion and right upper limb weakness. An MRI brain demonstrates an enhancing mass in the left frontal lobe. The neuroradiologist interpreting the scan is trying to determine the anatomical location of the lesion.

    Which of the following features is indicative of an intra-axial mass?

    a. Buckling of the grey–white matter interface
    b. Cerebrospinal fluid cleft sign
    c. Medial displacement of the subarachnoid vessels
    d. Pial vessels peripheral to the mass
    e. Hyperostosis

55. A 49 year old smoker goes to the GP with persistent cough. On examination he is noted to have clubbed fingernails. He has a plain film of the chest which reports marked symmetrical perihilar ground glass opacification. He is referred to the respiratory team who request a CT chest, which shows a crazy paving appearance. The team perform a bronchial lavage. The overall findings are highly suggestive for pulmonary alveolar proteinosis.

    What is the most likely aetiology?

    a. Acute silicosis
    b. Congenital pulmonary alveolar proteinosis
    c. Haematological malignancy
    d. Infection with immunosuppression
    e. Primary (autoimmune) pulmonary alveolar proteinosis

56. A 51 year old female patient is seen in the orthopaedic hand clinic with soft tissue swelling at the palmar aspect of the right middle finger which a radiograph confirms. The adjacent bone has normal appearances. Ultrasound identifies a well-defined hypoechoic solid lesion with mild internal vascularity around the flexor tendon, through which the tendon can be seen moving. On MRI this lesion is low signal on T1 and T2 sequences with evidence of susceptibility artefact on gradient echo images.

    What is the most likely diagnosis?

a. Desmoid tumour
b. Fibroma of the tendon sheath
c. Ganglion cyst
d. Glomus tumour
e. Tenosynovial giant cell tumour

57. A 70 year old woman undergoes a CT colonography which identifies an incidental pancreatic head mass. This measures 1.5 cm and has a HU density of 10. It contains multiple tiny cysts with a central area of calcification. The pancreatic duct measures 2 mm in diameter.

What is the most likely diagnosis?

a. Serous cystadenoma
b. Main duct intraductal papillary mucinous neoplasm
c. Mucinous cystadenoma
d. Pancreatic adenocarcinoma
e. Islet cell tumour

58. A 12 year old female has ongoing pain in the lower left leg. The pain is worse at night and settles with aspirin. On plain film, there is a 6 mm lucent lesion within the tibial metaphyseal cortex with thickening of the cortex and surrounding sclerosis. On scintigraphy there is a double density sign, with markedly increased uptake centrally and surrounding more modest activity.

What is the most likely diagnosis?

a. Fibrous cortical defect
b. Osteoblastoma
c. Osteochondroma
d. Osteoid osteoma
e. Osteosarcoma

59. Hydrops fetalis is identified on antenatal scans of a male fetus in the second trimester of pregnancy. Following close observation of the mother into the third trimester, the baby boy is delivered early by emergency caesarean section. The baby suffers with respiratory distress and is transferred immediately to the neonatal intensive care unit where a chest radiograph is obtained. The lungs appear clear; however there are bilateral pleural effusions. Drainage of the pleural fluid reveals chylous effusions.

What is the underlying cause likely to be?

a. Extralobar sequestration
b. Lymphangioleiomyomatosis
c. Pulmonary lymphangiectasia
d. Thoracic duct atresia
e. Turner syndrome

60. A 40 year old man with a background of previous renal cell carcinoma presents with nausea and headaches. On clinical examination he is noted to have papilloedema. An MRI brain shows a large cystic mass in the posterior fossa which is obstructing the fourth ventricle causing hydrocephalus. The mass also demonstrates a small enhancing nodule on the T1 post contrast sequence and serpiginous low T2 signal areas at the periphery.

What is the most likely diagnosis?

a. Cavernoma
b. Ependymoma
c. Haemangioblastoma
d. Metastasis
e. Pilocytic astrocytoma

61. A 63 year old male patient is seen in the vascular clinic with a pulsatile mass posterior to his right knee. Ultrasound confirms a 2-cm right popliteal artery aneurysm. The vascular team request a CT angiogram to help plan management.

Which imaging protocol is most appropriate?

a. Arterial phase CT from aortic bifurcation to toes
b. Arterial phase CT from neck to toes
c. Arterial phase CT from aortic bifurcation to knees
d. Arterial phase CT from diaphragm to toes
e. Arterial phase CT from pubic symphysis to toes

62. A GP calls the radiology hot reporting desk and asks for review of a 62 year old female patient's bilateral hand radiographs. The films demonstrate generalised osteopenia and the terminal phalangeal tufts are no longer clearly visible. There are erosions involving the interphalangeal joints and deformity of the first carpometacarpal joint with radial deviation. There are dense scattered soft tissue opacities which are similar density to the adjacent bone. A chest radiograph from 6 months previously shows bilateral distal clavicle erosion and a prominent gas-filled structure in the inferior mediastinum below the level of the carina.

What is the most likely diagnosis?

a. Hyperparathyroidism
b. Psoriatic arthritis
c. Rheumatoid arthritis
d. Scleroderma
e. Systemic lupus erythematosus

63. A 45 year old male patient is admitted under the gastroenterology team following multiple presentations with worsening abdominal pain and bowel symptoms. A barium follow-through demonstrates large circumferential ulcers and deep fissures affecting the caecum and terminal ileum. There is evidence of early stricturing but no significant hold up to the flow of barium or proximal bowel dilatation. The ileocaecal valve is thickened and patulous. A subsequent MRI small bowel reveals circumferential thickening affecting the terminal ileum and caecum. The affected bowel wall demonstrates increased enhancement. There is adjacent mesenteric lymph node enlargement and a trace of abdominal free fluid.

Which radiological feature is most suggestive of gastrointestinal tuberculosis rather than Crohn's disease?

a. Increased bowel wall enhancement
b. Lymph node enlargement
c. Presence of fissures
d. Small volume of ascites
e. Thickened ileocaecal valve

64. A 57 year old patient presents to hospital with right flank pain and haematuria. The team request an unenhanced CT urinary tract as they are concerned about urinary tract calculi. The CT report describes a 6.2-cm exophytic soft tissue mass arising from the right kidney with perinephric fat stranding and a couple of 10-mm retrocaval and aortocaval nodes at the same level. The adrenal glands and other solid abdominal viscera have normal appearances. There is marked expansion of the right renal vein.

What is the most appropriate test to confirm whether this is tumour thrombus or bland thrombus?

a. Contrast enhanced MRI
b. Digital subtraction angiography
c. 18F-FDG PET/CT
d. Portal venous phase CT abdomen pelvis
e. Ultrasound Doppler right kidney

65. A newborn is reviewed by the paediatric cardiologists. She is noted to be cyanotic and a chest radiograph shows an abnormal upper cardiomediastinal silhouette which is dilated superiorly giving a 'snowman appearance'. The lungs are plethoric.

What is the most likely diagnosis?

a. Pulmonary atresia
b. Tetralogy of Fallot

c. Total anomalous pulmonary venous return
d. Transposition of the great arteries
e. Tricuspid atresia

66. A CT and MRI have been performed for an ear, nose and throat clinic patient with chronic sinus symptoms. The MRI confirms a mass centred on the right maxillary sinus. This is low signal on T1 and high signal on T2 sequences. There is peripheral enhancement. On CT the mass is slightly hyperdense and no air is visible within the sinus. The bony walls of the sinus are thinned. The mass passes through a widened maxillary ostium into the nasopharynx.

What does this mass most likely represent?

a. Antrochoanal polyp
b. Esthesioneuroblastoma
c. Inverting papilloma
d. Mucocele
e. Mucous retention cyst

67. A 34 year old patient suffers a high speed road traffic collision and is taken to the nearest trauma centre. A CT traumogram is performed which demonstrates, amongst other serious findings, the presence of pneumomediastinum, right pneumothorax and sagging of the right lung.

Where is the most likely site of injury to cause these findings?

a. Diaphragmatic rupture
b. Fracture of the right first rib
c. Right main bronchus at the site of bifurcation of the upper lobe bronchus and bronchus intermedius
d. Right main bronchus near the carina
e. Tracheal rupture

68. A 32 year old has plain films of the right wrist to investigate ongoing pain. There is a well-defined lucent lesion in the distal radius, which appears lytic and mildly expansile with no matrix mineralisation, periosteal reaction or soft tissue swelling.

Which of the following lucent bone lesions are most likely to have a non-sclerotic rim?

a. Brown tumour
b. Chondroblastoma
c. Epidermoid cyst
d. Fibrous dysplasia
e. Fibrous cortical defect

69. A 22 year old woman is investigated for recurrent episodes of hypoglycaemia. Blood tests confirm endogenous insulin hypersecretion. A CT pancreas is performed.

Which of the following is the most likely imaging finding on arterial phase imaging?

a. Hypoenhancing 3-cm nodule in the tail of pancreas
b. Hyperenhancing 5-cm nodule in the body of the pancreas
c. Hypoenhancing 2-cm nodule in the head of pancreas
d. Hyperenhancing 1-cm nodule in the tail of pancreas
e. Hypoenhancing 4-cm nodule in the head of pancreas

70. A 10 year old girl is referred for a chest radiograph for a productive cough. The lungs are normal, but a well-defined right hilar mass is present. A CT shows a 3-cm mass arising from the middle mediastinum, inferior to and to the right of the carina. Its density is 15HU.

What is the most likely diagnosis?

a. Anterior meningocele
b. Bronchogenic cyst
c. Inhaled foreign body
d. Lymphoma
e. Pericardial cyst

71. A GP requested a CT chest, abdomen and pelvis for a 58 year old post-menopausal female patient with type 2 diabetes and unintentional weight loss. The CT is performed without contrast due to mildly reduced renal function. There is mediastinal, hilar and upper abdominal lymph node enlargement which is noted to be relatively low attenuation compared to adjacent soft tissues.

    Regarding the causes of low attenuation lymph nodes, which one of these is NOT associated with this radiological finding?

    a. Coeliac disease
    b. Kaposi sarcoma
    c. Systemic lupus erythematosus
    d. Tuberculosis
    e. Whipple disease

72. An 11 year old girl is referred to the paediatric neurologist with refractory temporal lobe epilepsy. An MRI brain is performed. This shows a partially cystic mass in the left temporal lobe. The solid component is intermediate T1 signal and T2 hyperintense with heterogenous enhancement. There is no surrounding oedema and no dural tail sign. The mass demonstrates blooming artefact on T2*.

    What is the most likely diagnosis?

    a. Pilocytic astrocytoma
    b. Dysembryoplastic neuroepithelial tumour
    c. Ganglioglioma
    d. Oligodendroglioma
    e. Pleomorphic xanthoastrocytoma

73. A 35 year old male patient is diagnosed with asymptomatic hypertension following a medical examination at his place of work. Following hospital referral and further investigations he is found to have an aortic coarctation. Chest radiograph reveals unilateral inferior rib notching of the left third to eighth ribs.

    What is the most likely cause of this appearance?

    a. Anomalous origin of the left subclavian artery
    b. Anomalous origin of the right subclavian artery
    c. Right sided aortic arch with anomalous left subclavian artery
    d. Stenosed left subclavian artery
    e. Stenosed left costocervical trunk

74. A 63 year old male patient represents to the emergency department febrile following a recent admission for pneumonia. His respiratory symptoms have improved but he now has acute pain in his left elbow without a history of trauma. Radiographs show the anterior fat pad is elevated and there is soft tissue swelling with subtle periarticular osteopenia. The orthopaedic junior doctor on call overnight asks for advice.

    What would the most appropriate next step be?

    a. Joint aspiration
    b. Oral antibiotics and orthopaedic clinic the following day
    c. MRI left elbow
    d. Triple phase nuclear medicine bone study
    e. Ultrasound left elbow

75. A 38 year old female patient with no significant medical history apart from a high body mass index presents to hospital with abdominal pain. Bloods demonstrate slightly raised inflammatory markers. Urine human chorionic gonadotrophin test is negative. The solid abdominal viscera have normal size and appearances on ultrasound and there is no free fluid in the abdomen or pelvis. At the site of maximal tenderness there is an ovoid hyperechoic mass without increased vascularity. It is not compressible. A CT scan is performed to characterise this further. The mass is adjacent to the colon, peripherally enhances, has a density of –90 HU and there is adjacent fat stranding.

    Where is the most common location for this pathology?

a. Anterior to the ascending colon
b. Right iliac fossa
c. Anterior to the sigmoid colon
d. Adjacent to the transverse colon
e. Adjacent to the umbilicus

76. A 52 year old man taking regular aspirin has noticed a change when examining the right side of his scrotum. He is referred by his GP for a scrotal ultrasound. The testicles are normal in size and homogenous in echotexture apart from a couple of tiny hyperechoic foci in the right testicle. Vascularity is symmetrical. The epididymides have normal appearances with no increased vascularity. The right pampiniform plexus is prominent, measuring up to 4 mm in several locations with flow reversal following Valsalva manoeuvre. The left pampiniform plexus has normal appearances.

Which of the following is most appropriate?

a. Abdominal ultrasound
b. Repeat ultrasound in 12 months
c. Suggest serum alpha-fetoprotein and human chorionic gonadotrophin levels
d. Suggest referral for embolisation
e. Suggest referral for surgical ligation

77. An 8 year old girl is referred to the paediatric respiratory team for recurrent infections and a chronic productive cough. A chest radiograph shows hyperinflation, bronchiectasis and multiple bilateral nodular opacities. A sweat test reveals elevated levels of chloride. A high resolution CT chest is arranged.

Which of the following signs is she most likely to have?

a. Basal atelectasis
b. Cardiomegaly
c. Chylothorax
d. 'Finger-in-glove' opacities
e. Thin-walled pulmonary cysts

78. A 67 year old neurology outpatient with cerebellar ataxia has an MRI brain. This reveals cerebellar atrophy and symmetrical high T2 signal in the pons and cerebellum. There is low T2 signal in the putamen with a rim of peripheral higher signal. The ventricles have normal appearances. There is mild generalised volume loss without lobar predilection.

Which of these conditions are these radiological findings most consistent with?

a. Huntington disease
b. Lewy body dementia
c. Multisystem atrophy
d. Pick disease
e. Progressive supranuclear palsy

79. A 24 year old female is investigated for ongoing malaise, chest pain on exertion and shortness of breath. Chest radiograph is unremarkable. She has a ventilation-perfusion (VQ) nuclear medicine scan which excludes a pulmonary embolus. She is subsequently referred to the cardiology team and on examination they discover that she has an absent left radial pulse. The team organise a CT angiogram of the chest. This shows an abnormal appearance of the aortic arch and proximal descending aorta, which is reduced in calibre and thick walled.

Which of the following are most likely to seen in a patient with a diagnosis of Takayasu arteritis in the healed fibrotic phase?

a. Delayed enhancement of the aortic wall
b. Irregular contour of the descending aorta
c. Linear calcification of the ascending aorta
d. Linear calcification of the descending aorta
e. Narrowing of the peripheral arteries

80. A 44 year old male presents with ongoing knee pain. Plain films are performed which demonstrate an eccentrically based lucent lesion which is well defined in the epiphysis of the distal femur. It has a narrow zone of transition and abuts the articular surface.

What is the most likely diagnosis?

a. Aneurysmal bone cyst
b. Eosinophilic granuloma
c. Fibrous dysplasia
d. Giant cell tumour
e. Non-ossifying fibroma

81. A 65 year old patient has an enhanced CT abdomen pelvis at the request of the urology team to monitor recurrent renal calculi. There are bilateral renal calculi which have not significantly changed in size or position compared to the previous symptomatic study and the kidneys are unobstructed. You notice mildly increased density in the fat around the root of the jejunal mesentery, which has a hazy appearance. This has marginally increased compared to the previous CT. There are a couple of small sub-centimetre lymph nodes in this region. The urology team confirm that the patient is currently asymptomatic.

Which other radiological finding would be consistent with mesenteric panniculitis?

a. Displacement of adjacent vessels and bowel loops
b. Low attenuation halo surrounding vessels
c. Low attenuation lymph nodes
d. Nodular shrunken liver
e. Thickening of the adjacent bowel wall

82. A 49 year old male patient is diagnosed with T2b N0 M0 right renal cell carcinoma of clear cell subtype. Also noted on his staging CT are two small left renal angiomyolipomas and several small pancreatic cysts. The patient reports a history of previous brain tumour although there is no imaging of his head available on your PACs system for review.

What is the most likely underlying hereditary condition?

a. Burt-Hogg-Dubé
b. Gorlin-Goltz
c. Osler-Weber-Rendu
d. Tuberous sclerosis
e. Von Hippel-Lindau

83. A 10 year old girl has a systolic murmur. A chest radiograph is performed which shows pulmonary plethora.

Which of the following radiological signs will help differentiate between a diagnosis of patent ductus arteriosus versus ventricular septal defect?

a. Enlarged aorta
b. Enlarged left atrium
c. Enlarged left ventricle
d. Enlarged pulmonary vasculature
e. Normal right atrium

84. A 30 year old woman has been experiencing vague neurological symptoms including left-sided headaches and facial paraesthesia. An MRI brain reveals subtle loss of grey–white matter differentiation in the left temporal and parietal lobes with minor, diffuse gyral expansion. The affected area is extensive and involves the ipsilateral basal ganglia structures; it is T1 hypointense and T2 hyperintense to grey matter. There is moderate effacement of the left lateral ventricle. There is no enhancement following gadolinium administration and the affected area does not restrict on diffusion weighted imaging.

What is the most likely clinical diagnosis?

a. Encephalitis
b. Gliomatosis cerebri
c. Primary CNS lymphoma

d. Progressive multifocal leukoencephalopathy
e. Tumefactive demyelination

85. A 32 year old female patient has an abdominal ultrasound requested by the GP following several urinary tract infections. The right kidney measures 8.2 cm in length and the left kidney measures 10.4 cm. The right renal artery to aortic velocity ratio is 3.7 and the left is 2.6. The kidneys appear structurally normal with no hydronephrosis and no renal calculi identified. There is a 13-mm simple right renal cyst. The urinary bladder appears thin walled.

    Where is the vascular abnormality causing these changes most likely to be sited?

    a. Proximal third of the left renal artery
    b. Proximal third of the right renal artery
    c. Distal left renal artery
    d. Distal right renal artery
    e. Abdominal aorta proximal to the renal arteries

86. A 55 year old female smoker has an accident at work and comes to the emergency department with wrist pain. A radiograph demonstrates no fracture but there is an abnormality in the visualised hand; therefore formal views of the hands are also obtained. These demonstrate soft tissue swelling, cortical thickening and periosteal reaction at the metacarpals and proximal phalanges bilaterally. Joint spaces are well-preserved and no focal bone lesions are identified. The reviewing doctor reports that there is no pain in the hands.

    What other imaging finding would most appropriately correlate with these appearances?

    a. Evidence of scalp skin fold thickening on CT head
    b. Lung mass on CT chest
    c. Symmetrical enlargement of the inferior rectus muscles on MRI orbits
    d. Symmetrical enlargement of the lateral rectus muscles on MRI orbits
    e. Jejunoileal fold pattern reversal on small bowel follow through

87. A 42 year old patient has an ultrasound abdomen requested by his GP for non-specific lower abdominal discomfort. This partially visualises a hypoechoic mass in the pelvis with increased vascularity. Contrast enhanced CT abdomen and pelvis is performed which identifies the mass in the right side of the pelvis. It measures up to 50 mm, is ill defined and inseparable from the pelvic side wall musculature. There is a clear fat plane between the mass and the urinary bladder and the right external iliac vessels. The mass has areas of enhancing soft tissue as well as cystic components and regions measuring –20HU in density. This is within 20 mm of the anterior abdominal wall. There is no ascites. The kidneys are unobstructed. There are a couple of 8-mm right common iliac lymph nodes.

    What is the most appropriate next step in managing this patient?

    a. CT chest with contrast
    b. CT guided biopsy of pelvic mass
    c. Refer to tertiary sarcoma centre for multidisciplinary team discussion prior to biopsy
    d. Ultrasound guided biopsy of pelvic mass
    e. 18F-FDG PET/CT

88. A paediatric junior doctor calls you for advice over the weekend. They have seen a 5 month old girl who has presented to hospital with her parents. Urine dip confirms urinary tract infection. A urine sample taken at the GP surgery by the practice nurse the previous day has grown *Escherichia coli*. The paediatric team are prescribing a course of oral antibiotics with a plan to send home with a clinic review in 48 hours. The junior doctor enquires about the most appropriate imaging.

    According to NICE guidelines, what would the most appropriate recommendation be?

    a. Dimercaptosuccinic acid test
    b. Immediate ultrasound urinary tract
    c. Micturating cystourethrogram within 4 weeks
    d. No imaging required unless recurrent urinary tract infection
    e. Ultrasound urinary tract within 6 weeks

89. A neonate born at term has respiratory distress. A chest radiograph is performed which shows multiple cystic partially air-filled lucencies in the left lower zone. There is associated mass effect with depression of the left hemidiaphragm and contralateral mediastinal shift. The patient then undergoes a CT thorax which shows the left lower lobe is occupied by multiple large-sized cysts with air-fluid levels causing atelectasis of the remaining left lower lobe and associated contralateral mediastinal shift. This lesion is supplied by a branch of the bronchial artery. The diaphragm is intact.

    What is the most likely diagnosis?

    a. Bronchogenic cyst
    b. Bronchopulmonary sequestration
    c. Congenital diaphragmatic hernia
    d. Congenital lobar over inflation
    e. Congenital pulmonary airway malformation

90. A patient is diagnosed with acute Hashimoto thyroiditis following clinical, serological, ultrasound and nuclear medicine assessment in a one-stop thyroid clinic.

    Which of the following profiles fits this diagnosis most accurately?

Table 4.2:

	Serological Result	Greyscale Ultrasound Appearance	Doppler Ultrasound Appearance	Technetium-99m Pertechnetate Tracer Uptake
a	Euthyroid	Hyperechoic gland	Avascular	Increased
b	Euthyroid	Heterogenous hypoechoic gland	Avascular	Reduced
c	Hypothyroid	Heterogenous hypoechoic gland	Increased vascularity	Reduced
d	Hyperthyroid	Heterogenous, hyperechoic gland	Increased vascularity	Increased
e	Hyperthyroid	Hyperechoic gland	Avascular	Reduced

91. A GP contacts you to ask for your advice regarding a pulmonary nodule which has been reported on a CT pulmonary angiogram, performed after a patient attended the emergency department with chest pain. The patient is a 39 year old female with no previous smoking history. The nodule is 8 mm in the right lower lobe with evidence of central calcification. On review of previous imaging, it was present on a unenhanced CT urinary tract performed 6 months prior and is unchanged in size.

    What is the most important feature when assessing for benignity of a pulmonary nodule?

    a. Presence of calcification
    b. Upper lobe location
    c. Volume doubling time ≤400 days
    d. Volume doubling time 400–600 days
    e. Volume doubling time ≥600 days

92. A 17 year old with a known chromosomal abnormality has an MRI of the whole spine which demonstrates a scoliosis, posterior vertebral body scalloping, enlarged neural foramina and dural ectasia as well as several well-defined dumbbell-shaped extra-axial lesions within the nerve exit foramina at multiple levels. All lesions demonstrate low signal on T1 pre-contrast, intermediate signal on T2 and there is T1 post contrast enhancement. A similar intra-axial lesion is seen within the canal at T12.

    You review the patient's previous imaging. What other musculoskeletal finding is the patient most likely to have?

a. Anterior vertebral body beaking
b. Hypertrophy of the vertebral posterior elements
c. Inferior rib notching
d. Sclerotic bone lesions
e. Superior rib notching

93. A 54 year old patient with chronic hepatitis B infection and a high body mass index has an abdominal ultrasound to monitor her liver. Her previous scan was 12 months previously. The most recent ultrasound shows no sonographic evidence of cirrhosis; however there is an indeterminate hypoechoic area in the left lobe. Therefore further liver imaging is advised.

With regard to liver MRI, which of the below is correct regarding normal liver appearances?

Table 4.3:

	MRI T1 Signal	MRI T2 Signal	MRI In- and Out-of-Phase Sequences
a	Spleen < liver	Spleen < liver	No change between sequences
b	Spleen > liver	Spleen < liver	Reduced on out-of-phase sequence
c	Spleen < liver	Spleen > liver	No change between sequences
d	Spleen < liver	Spleen > liver	Reduced on out-of-phase sequence
e	Spleen > liver	Spleen < spleen	No change between sequences

94. A neonatal chest and abdominal radiograph is reported as having a correctly sited umbilical venous catheter in situ.

Which of the following catheter positions would correlate with this statement?

a. Catheter passes inferiorly from umbilicus into pelvis, turning cephalad with the tip at the level of T8
b. Catheter passes inferiorly from umbilicus into pelvis, turning cephalad with the tip at the level of the diaphragm
c. Catheter passes superiorly from umbilicus with the tip at the junction of the superior vena cava and right atrium
d. Catheter passes superiorly from umbilicus with the tip at the level of T8
e. Catheter passes superiorly from umbilicus with the tip projected over the left upper quadrant

95. A neonate has a contrast enema after not passing meconium at 48 hours following delivery. Contrast passes quickly into the rectum and colon. The proximal large bowel is mildly dilated with a transition point to a narrower calibre in the sigmoid colon. The small bowel is normal calibre. The rectosigmoid ratio is 0.8.

Which of the following would help diagnose the underlying condition causing these findings?

a. Antenatal history of oligohydramnios
b. Confirmed maternal history of diabetes
c. Newborn heel prick test
d. Rectal biopsy
e. Sweat chloride test

96. A newborn undergoes a chest radiograph which shows a right sided aortic arch.

What underlying condition are they most likely to have?

a. Ebstein anomaly
b. Tetralogy of Fallot
c. Transposition of the great arteries
d. Tricuspid atresia
e. Truncus arteriosus

97. A 44 year old patient with a history of excess alcohol intake is admitted with acute severe pancreatitis. Initial chest radiograph shows bibasal atelectasis and a small left pleural effusion. Within 24 hours of admission the patient is transferred to intensive care. Following 48 hours on the intensive care unit the team report increased oxygen demand despite optimal therapy. CT scan demonstrates bilateral posterior consolidation with ground glass opacification more anteriorly. There is a small left pleural effusion. Appearances of the pancreas correlate with the clinical diagnosis of pancreatitis.

    What is the most likely explanation for the CT chest findings?

    a. Adult respiratory distress syndrome
    b. Aspiration pneumonia
    c. Cardiac failure
    d. Fat embolism
    e. Hospital-acquired pneumonia

98. An active 38 year old man has repeated GP visits for right hip pain which is stopping him from playing squash and does not improve despite several weeks of physiotherapy. A pelvic radiograph shows preserved joint space of both hips without significant degenerative change. There is relative reduction in the subchondral cortical thickness on the right and reduced bone density of the right proximal femur compared to the left. There is no periosteal reaction or soft tissue mass. An MRI scan reveals a joint effusion and low T1 and high T2 signal in the right femoral head which is particularly marked in the subchondral region with corresponding early post-contrast enhancement.

    What is the most likely diagnosis?

    a. Avascular necrosis of the proximal femur
    b. Complex regional pain syndrome
    c. Idiopathic transient osteoporosis of the hip
    d. Septic arthritis
    e. Stress fracture of the proximal femur

99. A 37 year old female patient with poorly controlled type 1 diabetes has an MRI liver requested. During an inpatient admission for cholecystitis an ultrasound abdomen identified a 50-mm hyperechoic area in the right hepatic lobe. The MRI confirms a heterogenous lesion which is mildly T1 and T2 hyperintense with signal reduction on out-of-phase imaging. There is heterogenous arterial enhancement following gadolinium administration and the lesion washes out, becoming isointense on portal venous phase sequences. A sequence with a hepatocyte specific agent is also performed which reveals the lesion is hypointense.

    What is the most likely diagnosis?

    a. Adenoma
    b. Fibrolamellar carcinoma
    c. Focal nodular hyperplasia
    d. Haemangioma
    e. Metastatic deposit from breast primary malignancy

100. A 13 week old baby boy is being investigated following in-utero diagnosis of bilateral hydronephrosis. Imaging identifies bilateral hydronephrosis and hydroureters with reflux of contrast from the urinary bladder into the ureters. The anterior abdominal wall is underdeveloped with characteristic 'prune belly' appearance. The paediatric team diagnose Eagle-Barrett syndrome.

    What other imaging should be performed in this patient?

    a. Echocardiogram
    b. MRI head
    c. MRI spine
    d. Neck ultrasound
    e. Testicular ultrasound

101. Regarding the imaging findings of choroid plexus papilloma in children, which of the following statements is most accurate?

a. Calcification is present in the majority of cases
b. Hydrocephalus is an uncommon presentation
c. It is a common cause of a posterior fossa mass
d. MRI signal is usually T1 and T2 isointense with homogenous enhancement
e. They are most common at the temporal horn of the lateral ventricle

102. The MRI brain of a 3 year old boy suffering with seizures and spasticity is reviewed. It demonstrates symmetrical high T2 signal throughout the cerebellar white matter and the basal ganglia, including the caudate nucleus, with a similar pattern of abnormal enhancement. A previous MRI brain had less marked changes with symmetrical T2 hyperintensity and enhancement only affecting the frontotemporal lobes.

Which of the following conditions best matches this radiological pattern?

a. Adrenoleukodystrophy
b. Alexander disease
c. Canavan disease
d. Krabbe disease
e. Leigh syndrome

103. A 45 year old male smoker presents with chest pain and cough. After an abnormal chest radiograph, he has a CT which shows a 2-cm pleurally based soft tissue lesion in the left upper lobe with evidence of rib invasion. There is a further 11-mm pulmonary nodule in the left upper lobe. There are enlarged right hilar and mediastinal nodes including the left lower paratracheal lymph node as well as a left-sided pleural effusion. Biopsy of the pleural based lesion demonstrates primary lung cancer.

What is the most likely type of lung malignancy in this case?

a. Adenocarcinoma in situ
b. Invasive adenocarcinoma
c. Mesothelioma
d. Small cell lung cancer
e. Squamous cell carcinoma

104. A 15 year old with known XO chromosomal abnormality has aortic coarctation and a horseshoe kidney. Plain films of the hand demonstrate several characteristic features.

What is the most likely finding?

a. Absent pisiform
b. Avascular necrosis of the scaphoid
c. Increased carpal angle
d. Shortened third and fourth metacarpals
e. Terminal tuft resorption

105. A concerned patient with a complex medical history asks to speak to a doctor regarding Buscopan administration for an MRI small bowel study. The CT radiographer calls asking for your assistance. You are the senior specialist registrar covering MRI.

Which of the following would be a contraindication for Buscopan administration?

a. Chronic open-angle glaucoma
b. History of prostate cancer
c. Hypothyroidism
d. Poorly controlled left ventricular failure
e. Pacemaker device

106. A 34 year old woman attends the breast one-stop clinic with a right breast lump. She noticed it 1 month ago and she is unsure if it has changed over that time. There is no significant past medical or breast-related history. Her grandmother died from breast cancer at the age of 72 years.

On examination, the lump is in the right upper outer quadrant at the 10 o'clock position, 6 cm from the nipple. It is firm, nontender and relatively mobile. At ultrasound the lesion measures 25 mm. It is horizontally orientated, well defined and slightly hypoechoic with a lobular contour. There are internal cystic spaces and posterior acoustic enhancement. There is vascularity in the solid component of the mass. An ultrasound guided biopsy is performed.

Which of the following is the most likely diagnosis?

a. Breast carcinoma
b. Fat necrosis
c. Fibrocystic change
d. Papilloma
e. Phyllodes tumour

107. A newborn baby is noted to have dextrocardia and bilobed lungs. Left isomerism and polysplenia syndrome are suspected.

Which of the following is associated with polysplenia syndrome?

a. Bilateral right atria
b. Bilateral hyparterial bronchi
c. Cyanotic congenital heart abnormality
d. Cystic hygroma
e. Total anomalous pulmonary venous return

108. A 33 year old patient is admitted with fever, headache and reduced GCS. The patient had been previously well apart from a similar fever 1 week previously. A CT head on admission demonstrated patchy hypodensity. On an MRI the following day there are multifocal FLAIR hyperintense subcortical lesions in the right frontal and left temporal lobes with surrounding oedema and mass effect. There are similar areas in the cerebellum. They all have peripheral restricted diffusion and enhancement. Within these areas there are small foci of very low T2 signal with associated hypointensity on gradient echo sequences.

What is the most likely diagnosis?

a. Acute demyelinating encephalomyelitis
b. Acute haemorrhagic leukoencephalitis
c. Cerebral abscesses
d. Herpes simplex encephalitis
e. Progressive multifocal leukoencephalopathy

109. A 58 year old female patient with a history of asthma presents with 2–3 of months of feeling generally unwell, breathlessness, weight loss and cough. CT chest demonstrates bibasal atelectasis with peripheral upper and middle lobe air space opacification, ill-defined ground glass opacities and mildly increased reticular markings. There are no pleural effusions. The hila nodes are prominent bilaterally but there are no size significant hila or mediastinal lymph nodes.

What is the most likely diagnosis?

a. Chronic eosinophilic pneumonia
b. Cryptogenic organising pneumonia
c. Pulmonary infarct
d. Pulmonary oedema
e. Simple pulmonary eosinophilia

110. A 45 year old male has plain films of the left knee for investigation of ongoing knee pain. There is a 3-cm well-defined lucent lesion seen within the proximal tibia. It abuts the articular surface and has a thin sclerotic rim.

What is the most likely feature of an intraosseous ganglion cyst on MRI?

a. Low signal on protein density sequence
b. Internal septations
c. Most common around the knee
d. T2 low signal
e. Periosteal new bone formation

111. A 31 year old male patient has a long history of symptoms of early satiety, abdominal pain after eating and occasional vomiting. The discomfort is relieved when the patient lies down. The patient had been treated as an adolescent for anorexia nervosa and still has a low body mass index. An arterial and portal venous phase CT abdomen and pelvis helps establish the diagnosis and demonstrates an angle of 15° between the superior mesenteric artery (SMA) and aorta.

Which other radiological findings correlate with this diagnosis?

a. Aortomesenteric distance of 15 mm
b. Dilatation of the proximal duodenum and stomach
c. Reduced contrast enhancement of the small bowel in the distribution of the superior mesenteric artery
d. Small bowel wall thickening
e. SMA mural thickening and enhancement

112. A 4-cm right upper pole renal mass is found incidentally on an MRI lumbar spine of a 61 year old female patient performed for lower back pain caused by a protruding L3 disc. She is otherwise fit and well. The renal lesion has multiple well-defined components of variable signal ranging from T2 bright and T1 low signal to intermediate T2 signal and T1 hyperintensity. CT chest abdomen pelvis reveals there is peripheral and septal enhancement between the locules and extension of the mass into the renal pelvis, although no hydronephrosis and no vascular invasion. There is no evidence of distant metastatic disease.

What management is the multidisciplinary team likely to recommend for this patient?

a. Follow-up CT in 6 months
b. Partial nephrectomy
c. Radiological guided embolisation
d. Radiofrequency ablation
e. No further management required

113. A neonate, born at 28 weeks, has an ongoing need for ventilation and oxygenation. A chest radiograph performed at 30 days shows hyperinflation, coarse linear densities and focal areas of emphysema.

What is the most likely diagnosis?

a. Bronchopulmonary dysplasia
b. Bronchopulmonary sequestration
c. Congenital lobar emphysema
d. Transient tachypnoea of the newborn
e. Viral pneumonia

114. A 66 year old female presents with a sudden decrease in GCS. A non-contrast CT head is performed which shows multiple bilateral, supratentorial, hyperdense intra-axial lesions (55HU). The lesions are predominantly distributed at the grey–white matter junction of the cerebral hemispheres. There is hypodensity surrounding the lesions consistent with oedema and associated mass effect.

From which of the following primary malignancies are these lesions most likely to be disseminated?

a. Cervical squamous cell carcinoma
b. Colonic adenocarcinoma
c. Endometrial endometroid carcinoma
d. Pancreatic ductal adenocarcinoma
e. Thyroid papillary carcinoma

115. A 3 day old neonate with respiratory distress has a chest radiograph which shows increased lucency in the right middle and lower zones with increased rib interspacing on the right compared to the left. A water-soluble contrast upper gastrointestinal (GI) study and arterial phase CT chest are performed and a vascular cause is identified, confirming the diagnosis of an aberrant left pulmonary artery.

What did the upper GI study most likely show?

a. Anterior oesophageal indentation and posterior tracheal indentation
b. Anterior tracheal indentation
c. Anterior tracheal and posterior oesophageal indentation
d. Normal appearances of the trachea and oesophagus
e. Posterior oesophageal indentation

116. A barium swallow is performed for a 64 year old female patient with a history of recurrent aspiration pneumonia. Recent CT identified left lower lobe consolidation, bilateral peripheral reticulation and enlarged mediastinal lymph nodes with an air-fluid level in the oesophagus. The barium swallow finds a patulous distal oesophagus with poor motility, although tertiary contractions are visualised.

What is the most likely diagnosis?

a. Achalasia
b. Chagas disease
c. Oesophageal carcinoma
d. Presbyoesophagus
e. Progressive systemic sclerosis

117. A 5 year old boy is referred to the paediatric neurologists having presented with visual field defects and diabetes insipidus. A CT head shows a partially calcified suprasellar mass. On MRI the mass is partially cystic and part solid. It demonstrates high signal on both T1 and T2 weighted imaging. There is heterogenous enhancement following gadolinium administration.

What is the most likely diagnosis?

a. Craniopharyngioma
b. Germinoma
c. Meningioma
d. Pituitary macroadenoma
e. Rathke cleft cyst

118. A 42 year old patient with newly diagnosed ascending colon cancer is discussed at the colorectal multidisciplinary team meeting. He has a past medical history of hypertension and left nephroureterectomy for cancer 5 years previously. The patient was recently seen in outpatient clinic and reported a positive family history of colorectal cancer, with his father and two brothers affected. His father was successfully treated for colorectal cancer but later died from glioblastoma. His sister has recently had a hysterectomy following a diagnosis of endometrial cancer.

Which of the following hereditary syndromes does the patient most likely have?

a. Familial adenomatous polyposis
b. Lynch syndrome
c. Peutz-Jeghers syndrome
d. Tuberous sclerosis
e. Turcot syndrome

119. Following an MRI of the auditory canal, an ear, nose and throat clinic patient with conductive hearing loss is diagnosed with a cholesteatoma located in the attic.

Which of the following imaging characteristics is most consistent with this diagnosis?

Table 4.4:

	T1 Signal	T2 Signal	Restricted Diffusion	Ossicular Displacement
a	High	High	Present	Medial
b	Low	High	Absent	Lateral
c	Low	High	Absent	Medial
d	Low	High	Present	Lateral
e	Low	High	Present	Medial

120. A 17 year old male has a CT of the spine for ongoing mid-thoracic back pain. There is a lytic, expansile lesion within the posterior elements of the T5 vertebral body, with extension into the vertebral body. On MRI the lesion is multicystic of different signal intensities, there are fluid-fluid levels within the multiple thin-walled cysts. Heterogeneous enhancement of the septae is seen post-contrast.

What is the most likely diagnosis?

a. Aneurysmal bone cyst
b. Fibrous dysplasia
c. Giant cell tumour
d. Simple bone cyst

ANSWERS 4

1. (d) 18F-FDG PET/CT scan

18F-FDG PET/CT scan is used to help differentiate benign from malignant pleural thickening and can also help to assess for nodal metastases in malignant mesothelioma.

Contrast-enhanced ultrasound is not typically used for this indication.

CT abdomen and pelvis would be more appropriate once malignancy was confirmed to exclude peritoneal involvement.

On MRI, high T2 signal intensity when compared to muscle, and contrast enhancement of the pleural thickening is suggestive of malignancy; however, this patient has a pacemaker which would likely contraindicate MRI. MRI is sometimes used in the staging of malignant mesothelioma, particularly where there is a question regarding surgical resection and the extent of chest wall or diaphragmatic involvement.

Portal venous phase contrast CT chest is better at demonstrating pleural enhancement than an arterial phase CT; however, 18F-FDG PET/CT is more sensitive for distinguishing between malignant and benign disease. CT features that favour a malignant process include pleural thickness >1 cm, nodularity and mediastinal pleural involvement.

(The Final FRCR Complete Revision Notes Page 44)

2. (c) Pancreatic low signal on T1, T2 and T2* sequences on MRI of the upper abdomen

Haemochromatosis causes a symmetrical arthropathy typically affecting the second and third metacarpal phalangeal joints causing osteopenia, reduction in joint space, subchondral cysts, flattening of the metacarpal heads and 'hook-like' osteophytes. Chondrocalcification is common and overlaps with calcium pyrophosphate dihydrate crystal deposition disease. Haemochromatosis is associated with iron deposition in the liver, spleen, heart, pancreas and central nervous system, causing low signal on T1, T2 and T2* MRI sequences.

A dilated oesophagus would be associated with scleroderma – acro-osteolysis causing 'pencil-in-cup' deformities; soft tissue atrophy and calcification and contractures are also features. There is often marked ulnar deviation of the phalanges.

Systemic lupus erythematosus (SLE) causes symmetrical muscle wasting, periarticular osteopenia and reversible deformities such as 'swan-neck' deformities and ulnar deviation. SLE is associated with hypercoagulability, and patients are at risk of venous thrombosis which could manifest as intracranial venous sinus hyperdensity.

Multiple small foci of subcortical T2* low signal on MRI head are typical of microhaemorrhages in amyloidosis. Larger joints tend to be affected rather than the hands, and features include subchondral cysts, erosions and osteoporosis without joint space narrowing. Soft tissue deposition of amyloid can lead to periarticular nodularity.

Sarcoidosis causes symmetrical hilar and mediastinal lymphadenopathy. The musculoskeletal manifestations include a typical 'lace-like' appearance along with soft tissue swelling, cyst formation and resorption of the terminal tufts.

(The Final FRCR Complete Revision Notes Page 78)

3. (c) Metastasis from adenocarcinoma

The most likely diagnosis is metastatic adenocarcinoma. Metastases to the adrenal gland can be large with a heterogeneous appearance, central necrosis, haemorrhage and irregular borders. The most common sites of primary malignancy are lung, breast, melanoma, gastrointestinal tract and renal.

The main differential diagnosis is adrenocortical carcinoma. This has peak incidences in early childhood and in the fourth and fifth decade of life. This tumour is usually large at diagnosis and typically has central necrosis or haemorrhage. There is calcification in 30% and it can invade the inferior vena cava or the renal vein. However, adrenocortical carcinoma is relatively rare compared to metastatic adenocarcinoma.

A collision tumour is a rare occurrence of two different pathologies in the same place and can be benign or malignant.

There are no specific features described to indicate that lesion could be a myelolipoma, such as fat density or punctate calcification.

A phaechromocytoma would usually demonstrate homogeneous enhancement. They are prone to haemorrhage and then can appear heterogeneous. Most are benign but some may be malignant and demonstrate metastases; however, this occurs less commonly than adenocarcinoma metastases.

(The Final FRCR Complete Revision Notes Page 268)

4. (e) Secondary lymphoma of the kidney

   The imaging characteristics of the lesions, along with abdominopelvic lymphadenopathy and mild splenomegaly, make lymphoma most likely.

   Lymphoma of the kidney can be split into primary and secondary forms. The primary form is uncommon because the kidneys do not contain lymphoid tissue. The secondary form occurs because of haematogenous spread and is most likely to be non-Hodgkin's lymphoma.

   Unlike renal cell carcinoma (RCC), typically lymphoma does not significantly affect the renal contour. Lymphomas often look slightly denser compared to adjacent normal renal tissue prior to contrast and are comparatively hypodense to the rest of the kidney following contrast. The MRI appearances are usually intermediate T1 and intermediate to low T2 signal. Lymphoma is typically more homogenous in appearance compared to RCC.

   Vascular invasion is an important feature when evaluating renal masses; RCC and leiomyosarcoma are more likely to invade the vessels, whereas lymphoma can encase them. Metastases do not typically invade the vessels either and are usually small lesions and cortically based. The most common primaries which metastasise to the kidneys are melanoma, lung, colorectal and breast. No other primary site is identified on the CT, although a melanoma primary is unlikely to be radiologically visible. The patient is male, making breast malignancy unlikely. CT cannot exclude gastrointestinal malignancy, and endoscopy could be considered, although if there was disseminated colorectal cancer, liver and lung metastases would also be expected.

   Leiomyosarcomas spread haematogenously; therefore lymphadenopathy is uncommon and the lesions are often positioned close to the renal pelvis and vessels.

   (The Final FRCR Complete Revision Notes Page 253)

5. (b) Early peripheral enhancement with delayed central enhancement

   Infantile hepatic haemangioendothelioma are vascular lesions causing arteriovenous shunting which can lead to high-output cardiac failure. These lesions are also associated with thrombocytopaenia due to consumptive coagulopathy. They are heterogenous vascular masses which can contain calcification. The aorta above the level of the coeliac trunk may be enlarged compared to the aorta below this level. Enhancement of these lesions is similar to a hepatic haemangioma with peripheral early enhancement and central filling in on delayed phases.

   (The Final FRCR Complete Revision Notes Pages 340–341)

6. (b) Moyamoya syndrome

   The description of multiple cutaneous nodules and the finding of bilateral internal cerebral artery (ICA) occlusion is suggestive of Moyamoya syndrome in the setting of neurofibromatosis (NF) 1.

   Two conditions containing the name Moyamoya exist – a disease and a syndrome. Moyamoya disease translates as 'puff of smoke' from Japanese and is a vasculo-occlusive angiopathy. The puff-of-smoke description arises from the appearance of the intracranial collateralisation that occurs secondary to congenital stenosis and occlusion of the distal ICAs; however, it can affect other vessels within the circle of Willis too. On imaging there are commonly watershed infarcts and it may present with intraventricular haemorrhage.

   Moyamoya syndrome gives the same appearance on angiography but is not the result of a congenital ICA occlusion. It is associated with NF1, sickle cell, radiation, chronic infection,

tuberculosis and atherosclerosis.
(The Final FRCR Complete Revision Notes Page 375)

7. (e) Reperfusion syndrome
The imaging features described are typical for reperfusion syndrome. This occurs in 95% of transplant patients within 48 hours of the procedure. It is non-cardiogenic oedema and is seen radiographically as bilateral perihilar airspace opacification and can occur alongside bibasal effusions. It resolves by day 10; persistence after this time is suggestive of infection or acute rejection.
Acute transplant rejection usually occurs 10 days after transplant. Chest radiographs are normal in 50% of patients but there may be heterogeneous perihilar opacification, septal thickening and a pleural effusion. Diagnosis can be made by transbronchial biopsy.
The imaging appearances of bronchiolitis obliterans are of bronchiectasis and air trapping, and this condition usually occurs 6–18 months after transplant.
Post-transplant lymphoproliferative disease represents a proliferative disorder occurring from 1 month onwards. It manifests as lung nodules and adenopathy. The clinical scenario and imaging findings in this case are not in keeping with this.
Infection can occur at any time and is the most common complication after transplantation; however reperfusion syndrome is the most common immediate complication and the imaging features described in the stem are in keeping with this condition.
(The Final FRCR Complete Revision Notes Page 41)

8. (e) Trisomy 21
The description is one of Down syndrome. The hypersegmented manubrium occurs in 90% of patients with trisomy 21, and 11 pairs of ribs are seen in 25%. A bell-shaped thorax and scoliosis can also be seen on plain films in this condition.
Monosomy X is Turner syndrome. Chest radiograph may demonstrate thinning of the lateral aspect of the clavicles as well thinned and narrow ribs with pseudo notching. Triploidy is the third commonest fatal chromosomal anomaly, with most associated with spontaneous abortions. Trisomy 13 is Patau syndrome. Most infants do not live more than a few days. Trisomy 18 is Edwards syndrome. The mean infant survival in this condition is 48 days.
(The Final FRCR Complete Revision Notes Page 109)

9. (d) Ectopic pancreatic tissue
The finding of a smooth nodular protrusion into the duodenum with a central depressed duct remnant is diagnostic for ectopic pancreatic tissue. Benign lymphoid hyperplasia typically demonstrates multiple filling defects and can be a normal variant in children but is indicative of hypogammaglobulinaemia in adults. Duodenal ulcers are most commonly more proximally in the bulbar part of the duodenum and are also more commonly anteriorly rather than posteriorly positioned. An adenocarcinoma of the papilla of Vater would be positioned laterally, expected to have ill-defined edges and may lead to obstruction. The duodenojejunal flexure is normally positioned in this patient and so malrotation would not be a concern.
(The Final FRCR Complete Revision Notes Page 166)

10. (b) Morquio syndrome
Madelung deformity is a condition where the radius is bowed and shortened with subsequent positive ulnar variance causing a 'V'-shaped appearance of the proximal carpal row. This can potentially lead to distal ulna dislocation. Reverse Madelung deformity has similar appearances but affects the ulna, causing negative ulnar variation.
Causes include diaphyseal aclasia, nail-patella syndrome, Ollier disease and Turner syndrome. Morquio syndrome is not associated with it; however Hurler syndrome is. Some causes can be remembered with the mnemonic **HIT DOC**:
Hurler syndrome
Infection
Trauma
Dyschondrosteosis, for example Leri-Weill syndrome
Osteochondromatosis (also known as diaphyseal aclasia)
Congenital, for example Turner syndrome, nail-patella syndrome, achondroplasia

(The Final FRCR Complete Revision Notes Page 82)

11. (c) Lissencephaly

Lissencephaly is an abnormally smooth brain surface. The cortex is thickened and the lateral ventricles may be dilated, especially posteriorly. The cerebellum is usually not affected. Pachygyria (broad gyri) and agyria (no gyri) also exist as subtypes within this spectrum of disorders.

Schizencephaly is a cleft lined by grey matter extending between the pia mater and ependymal surface and often connecting the surface of the brain to the lateral ventricles. The open-lipped subtype has cerebrospinal fluid in the cleft and the closed lip subtype does not.

Porencephaly occurs secondary to an in-utero insult, usually before the second trimester. It leaves a fluid-filled space communicating with the ventricles lined by white matter.

Holoprosencephaly is incomplete septation of the two cerebral hemispheres. Hemimegalencephaly is when part of the brain is enlarged due to hamartomatous overgrowth; this can be an entire hemisphere or more limited.

(The Final FRCR Complete Revision Notes Page 291)

12. (a) Ameloblastoma

Ameloblastoma typically affect patients >40 years of age and presents as a painless hard lump. They are multilocular and characteristically have a 'bubbly' or 'honeycomb' appearance. On MRI they have both cystic and soft tissue components which enhance avidly. In contrast to this, odontogenic keratocysts often enhance poorly. Ameloblastomas are commonly expansile and can cause root resorption.

Metastases are an important differential in this age group; however they usually have more ill-defined margins.

Dentigerous and radicular cysts are more commonly unilocular lucencies related to dentition, the former related to the crown of an unerupted tooth and the latter related to the roots.

(The Final FRCR Complete Revision Notes Page 441)

13. (e) Xenon ventilation study

The ongoing pneumothorax and bubbling chest drain are suspicious for a bronchopleural fistula. They can occur following surgery or as a sequelae of chemo- or radiotherapy and also sometimes with infections, such as tuberculosis. CT can often be used to diagnose this condition; however, in this case when further clarification is required, a Xenon ventilation study can confirm the diagnosis by demonstrating tracer activity in the pleural space.

A CT pulmonary angiogram and a ventilation perfusion (VQ) study would not add anything further to the existing CT chest for this indication and would be more appropriate if pulmonary embolus was suspected.

Inserting a larger bore chest drain is unlikely to clinically improve the situation and would not aid diagnosis. Larger bore chest drains can be indicated in the context of pleural effusions with thick fluid, for example empyema or haemothorax.

Removing the chest drain when there is suspicion of a bronchopleural fistula could potentially lead to tension pneumothorax and therefore this is not an appropriate management plan.

(The Final FRCR Complete Revision Notes Page 25)

14. (b) Langerhans cell histiocytosis

Langerhans cell histiocytosis is the most common cause of vertebral plana in children. Other imaging features include lucent bone lesions, occurring most commonly in the skull, mandible, ribs and pelvis. Bone lesions are associated with periostitis. Lesions may resolve or become sclerotic.

Hand-Schüller-Christian disease is a variant which typically affects children 1–5 years old. Multiple bones are involved, with evidence of extraskeletal involvement (classic triad of diabetes insipidus, proptosis, and lytic bone lesions). Letterer-Siwe disease is a multisystem variant which affects children less than 2 years old and is often fatal.

(The Final FRCR Complete Revision Notes Page 113)

15. (d) Fibrolamellar hepatocellular carcinoma (HCC)

Fibrolamellar HCC is an uncommon variant of HCC affecting young patients with no risk factors. The tumour is typically large at diagnosis. The central scar is usually hyperechoic on ultrasound and hypointense on MRI sequences, which helps to differentiate it from the T2 hyperintense central scar in focal nodular hyperplasia (FNH). The central scar generally does not enhance in fibrolamellar HCC but does in FNH.

The age of the patient in this case is highly suggestive of fibrolamellar HCC over standard HCC. Fibrolamellar HCC can calcify; however this is less likely in HCC. Furthermore, fibrolamellar HCC is commonly isointense on venous phase imaging, whereas HCC shows early washout.

Hepatic adenoma can occur in a similar age group; however they do not contain a central scar. They frequently contain fat and haemorrhage. The former leads to a drop of signal on out-of-phase imaging.

Haemangiomas can appear hyperechoic on ultrasound but their enhancement is quite characteristic with peripheral enhancement that progresses centrally with time. They do not contain a central scar.

(The Final FRCR Complete Revision Notes Pages 205–206)

16. (c) No further investigation required

The imaging appearances are consistent with medullary sponge kidney. On intravenous urograms the appearance used to be likened to a paintbrush; otherwise known as a 'striated nephrogram'. Other causes for this appearance bilaterally include acute pyelonephritis, acute tubular necrosis, hypotension and autosomal recessive polycystic kidney disease. The latter is associated with paediatric patients. The history does not fit with hypotension, acute pyelonephritis or acute tubular necrosis. Urine dip would typically be abnormal in pyelonephritis and acute tubular necrosis, either showing signs of nitrites, blood or protein. If these conditions were suspected clinically, then answers B and D may be appropriate.

If systemic lupus erythematous is suspected then an antinuclear antibody test would be helpful; however, this tends to be associated with glomerulonephritis, which causes swollen kidneys.

Renal vein thrombosis would cause a unilateral striated nephrogram and is also unlikely in a patient without risk factors; therefore an ultrasound Doppler is unlikely to provide any additional information.

Medullary sponge kidney does not progress to renal failure, and for most patients the condition is asymptomatic. It is often picked up incidentally and further follow-up is not required.

(The Final FRCR Complete Revision Notes Page 253)

17. (c) Just distal to the ampulla of Vater in D2

The case describes a classic case of duodenal atresia. This may be suspected antenatally if there is polyhydramnios and postnatally within the first week when infants experience vomiting. The radiographic appearance in the case is called the 'double bubble' sign. The majority of cases have an obstructive level which is just distal to the ampulla of Vater and hence the vomiting is bilious. Non-bilious vomiting would suggest a more proximal obstruction. The finding that there is no gas more distally in the bowel excludes other differentials such as duodenal stenosis or a duodenal web. Duodenal atresia is associated with an annular pancreas, VACTERL anomalies and Down syndrome.

(The Final FRCR Complete Revision Notes Page 336)

18. (c) Creutzfeldt-Jakob disease (CJD)

CJD is a spongiform encephalopathy which causes abnormal signal in the thalamus, basal ganglia (particularly the caudate and putamen) and cortex with T2 hyperintensity and restricted diffusion. The condition causes myoclonus and dementia. The sporadic type is most common and tends to affect older age groups. CT findings are frequently of atrophy.

The history may fit with manganese poisoning, which causes parkinsonism; however the area of the brain affected is different, with T1 hyperintensity in the globus palladi. Similarly the globus pallidi are affected in carbon monoxide poisoning; however, the history is not consistent.

Imaging findings in Alzheimer's and Lewy body dementia can be non-specific and they require clinical correlation. The typical description in Alzheimer's disease is mesial temporal lobe volume loss and volume loss in the parietal-occipital region. Similarly Lewy body dementia also leads to volume loss, usually in the frontal, parietal and temporal regions.

(The Final FRCR Complete Revision Notes Page 381)

19. (c) Metastatic adenocarcinoma

The imaging features described are suspicious for a malignant process, with secondary metastases to the pleura being the most common pleural malignancy. Lung, breast, ovarian and lymphoma are the most common malignancies to metastasise to the pleura.

Pleural mesothelioma is the second most common pleural malignancy (after metastases), strongly associated with exposure to asbestos and a latency period of up to 40 years.

Primary pleural lymphoma is extremely rare. When it occurs, it tends to be associated with immunodeficiency and chronic pyothorax. Secondary pleural lymphoma is more common than primary pleural lymphoma.

Liposarcoma of the pleura is demonstrated as a mixed attenuation mass with some areas of fat tissue (this is a different entity to liposarcomatous differentiation of malignant mesothelioma).

Fibrothorax is a benign entity that can occur as a sequelae to inflammation, tuberculosis or haemothorax. In this condition, pleural thickening is smooth, it may be calcified and does not usually involve the mediastinal surface.

(The Final FRCR Complete Revision Notes Page 44)

Jaramillo FA, Gutierrez F, Bhalla S. Pleural tumours and tumour-like lesions. Clinical Radiology. 2018;73(12):1014–1024.

20. (b) High T1 and T2 endplate changes with low T2 disc signal

Modic endplate changes are associated with degenerative disease of the lumbar spine. Type II changes are most common.

The difference between Modic type I changes and discitis is the disc signal. Normally discs are intermediate signal or, if there is disc dehydration, they may demonstrate low T2 signal, whereas in discitis they would be high on T2 and low signal on T1 sequences, due to inflammation. Answer A would be consistent with discitis.

Modic type I is associated with pain and due to bone marrow oedema, and inflammation there is increased fluid in the region, hence T1 endplate signal is low and T2 endplate signal is high. Answer C would be consistent with Modic type I change.

Modic type II changes are due to red marrow replacement, which is fatty; hence T1 endplate signal is high, as is T2 signal.

Modic type III changes are due to subsequent sclerosis and so both T1 and T2 endplate signals are low. Answer D would be consistent with Modic type III change.

(The Final FRCR Complete Revision Notes Page 83)

21. (e) Skin

The most common metastatic lesion in the stomach is malignant melanoma. Other common primary sites of metastatic malignancy include breast, lung, cervix, prostate and renal. Spread can be contiguous from adjacent structures, for example via the gastrocolic ligament, or haematogenous. The latter is more common. On a barium meal haematogenous metastases can produce multiple nodules and a characteristic 'bull's-eye' appearance, which is so called due to the central ulceration the lesions demonstrate. Metastases often affect the proximal and middle part of the stomach and can present with weight loss, melaena and haematemesis.

(The Final FRCR Complete Revision Notes Page 170)

22. (c) Dandy-Walker malformation

Dandy-Walker malformation is a constellation of congenital anomalies including absent or hypoplastic cerebellar vermis, a posterior fossa cyst connected to the fourth ventricle and a resulting enlarged posterior fossa. The torcular herophili (the confluence of the intracranial venous sinuses) is abnormally elevated. The variant condition is when not all of the findings are present and often the posterior fossa is not enlarged.

If there is a posterior fossa cerebrospinal fluid cyst and the cerebellar vermis are normal in appearance, then the differential lies between arachnoid cyst and mega cisterna magna. The latter is a normal variant. An arachnoid cyst is suspected if there is adjacent mass effect.

Chiari malformations do not cause an enlarged posterior fossa. Chiari I is when the cerebellar tonsils descend >5 mm through the foramen magnum. Chiari II is more severe and can cause a small posterior fossa and descent of the torcular herophili. There is caudal descent of the medulla, cerebellar vermis and fourth ventricle with a myelomeningocele.

(The Final FRCR Complete Revision Notes Pages 293–294)

23. (c) Non-contrast enhanced MRI

The most likely cause of a hyperechoic liver lesion in a young patient is an incidental haemangioma and if the patient was not pregnant than a contrast enhanced MRI would be the most appropriate investigation. However, gadolinium-based contrast agent is avoided in pregnancy unless essential for diagnosis and management. An unenhanced MRI may still be helpful and is worth pursuing in the first instance. MRI should be avoided in the first trimester, and then in the second and third trimesters it is worth considering whether acoustic noise and specific absorption rate (SAR) can be reduced by amending the protocol.

A contrast-enhanced CT would not be suitable in a pregnant patient for this indication due to the risks of ionising radiation. Similarly, Technetium 99-m red blood cell scan, although very helpful in diagnosing haemangioma, would also be contraindicated.

Imaging could be performed following completion of the pregnancy; however this is >4 months away. A repeat ultrasound is unlikely to add more information.

(The Final FRCR Complete Revision Notes Page 209)

24. (d) Neurosarcoidosis

Central nervous system involvement of sarcoidosis can cause symptoms including bilateral facial nerve palsy, seizures and diabetes insipidus. It characteristically causes basal leptomeningeal thickening which can lead to hydrocephalus. Appearances can be similar to tuberculous meningitis; however, bilateral cranial nerve involvement, most commonly the facial or optic nerves, is suggestive of sarcoidosis.

Leptomeningeal carcinomatosis can be due to a primary intracranial tumour however there would be evidence of this on the MRI. Lymphoma, leukaemia and metastatic disease, for example from a breast or lung primary, are possible; however this tends to cause diffuse thickening affecting all parts of the brain rather than having a basal predilection.

(The Final FRCR Complete Revision Notes Page 382)

25. (a) Acute eosinophilic pneumonia

Acute eosinophilic pneumonia often presents with a short febrile illness and marked hypoxia. CT changes include bilateral consolidation and ground glass opacification with pleural effusions and interlobular septal thickening. In contrast to the chronic and simple subtypes of eosinophilic lung disease, the acute form is not associated with serum eosinophilia and instead there are elevated eosinophil levels in the bronchoalveolar fluid.

Eosinophilic granulomatosis with polyangiitis (previously known as Churg-Strauss) can have ground glass opacification and consolidation but you may also expect centrilobular nodularity and serum eosinophilia.

Sarcoidosis is also associated with nodularity, and mediastinal and hilar lymphadenopathy is also common. Pleural effusions are not typical.

Bronchopneumonia can cause bilateral scattered consolidation with *Staphylococcus aureus* infection potentially leading to cavitating pneumonia and empyema; however, in a young patient the full blood count would usually be abnormal.

Subacute hypersensitivity pneumonitis is usually associated with centrilobular nodularity as well as air trapping and mosaicism.

(The Final FRCR Complete Revision Notes Page 29)

26. (b) Lead poisoning

Lead poisoning may present with loss of appetite, abdominal pain, constipation and vomiting; patients may also be anaemic. The presence of high-density bands within the metaphysis represents lead deposition. Patients may be short for their age, with skeletal immaturity present on imaging, and a 'bone-in-bone' appearance may also be seen.

Metaphyseal bands can also be seen in healed rickets; however 'bone-in-bone' appearance is not a typically described feature of this condition.

The presence of dense metaphyseal bands may be physiological in children aged less than 3 years old.

Dense metaphyseal bands can be seen in scurvy, which is relatively uncommon. It is caused by dietary lack of vitamin C. Other imaging features include generalised osteopenia, cortical thinning, periosteal reaction, Wimberger ring sign, Frankel line and Trümmerfeld zone.

Fracture at the distal radius may cause increased density at the metaphysis; however it does not account for the other clinical and radiographic features described.

(The Final FRCR Complete Revision Notes Page 113)

27. (b) Gastrointestinal stromal tumour

The gastric soft tissue mass has imaging features in keeping with a gastrointestinal stromal tumour (GIST). They can be very large and have necrotic, haemorrhagic and cystic components. They may be asymptomatic or present with vague abdominal symptoms. Sometimes, similar to this case, they can present with haemorrhage. The most common site is the stomach, followed by the small intestine. They are usually benign but larger tumours, greater than 5 cm, are more likely to have malignant potential. Ninety percent of GISTs express c-KIT (CD117) antigen, a tyrosine kinase growth factor receptor.

GISTs can be associated with several syndromes, including neurofibromatosis type I. The intracranial appearances are consistent with this – sphenoid wing dysplasia and focal areas of signal intensity (FASIs). Carney triad is also associated with GISTs. The lack of lymph node enlargement makes malignancy such as gastric adenocarcinoma, metastatic malignancy or lymphoma less likely. Gastric hamartomas can be seen in several polyposis syndromes such as Cowden and Peutz-Jegher syndrome.

(The Final FRCR Complete Revision Notes Page 172)

28. (c) Surgical resection

The imaging description is of a heterogenous renal lesion with coarse calcification and a central scar. The differential lies between renal cell carcinoma and oncocytoma. Classical imaging characteristics for an oncocytoma include an isoechoic renal mass with a hypoechoic centre on ultrasound. CT of larger lesions such as this one can demonstrate a heterogenous mass and there can be perinephric fat stranding. Both CT and MRI demonstrate the typical non-enhancing central scar. Other MRI features include T1 hypointensity and T2 hyperintensity compared to the renal cortex. In this case an MRI is unlikely to add more information.

Oncocytomas are benign but they are difficult to differentiate from renal cell carcinoma on imaging alone, and even a biopsy of a carcinoma can contain oncocytic components.

Renal sarcomas are aggressive lesions. Often at this size there may be vascular invasion, and early haematogenous metastases are common. The CT scan on this patient does not demonstrate evidence of metastatic infiltration.

Therefore, the most appropriate answer is surgical resection to help confirm what the lesion is and plan for the most appropriate management. Repeat ultrasound guided biopsy may not be successful given the issues during the first attempt. Ablation would not help with histological diagnosis and is therefore not indicated.

(The Final FRCR Complete Revision Notes Pages 255–256)

29. (b) Dilatation of the intrahepatic ducts

The Todani classification helps differentiate between choledochal cysts, and ranges from I to V. Caroli disease is the cystic dilatation of intrahepatic ducts and consistent with Todani type V.

Type I is fusiform cystic dilatation of the extrahepatic duct.

Type II is an extrahepatic bile duct diverticulum.

Type III is dilatation of the extrahepatic bile duct within the duodenal wall.

Type IV is the presence of intra- and extrahepatic cysts.

(The Final FRCR Complete Revision Notes Page 335)

30. (c) Melanoma

Uveal melanoma is the most common primary eye tumour in adults, and when they affect the choroid at the posterior aspect of the globe, they can be detected incidentally or following visual loss caused by retinal detachment. Cutaneous melanoma can also metastasise to the eye, along with other primary tumours such as breast and lung. Typically ocular melanoma is hyperdense on CT with a lenticular, well-defined shape. The mass enhances and demonstrates high T1 and low T2 signal due to melanin content. There may be haemorrhage associated with it.

Drusen are usually small areas of bilateral calcification overlying the optic nerve and are not a unilateral finding, such as in this case. Choroidal osteomas do occur unilaterally and manifest as curvilinear calcification which are usually larger than drusen and normally spare the optic disc.

Retinoblastoma affects a younger age group than this patient and are the most common paediatric eye tumour. On imaging they manifest as a heterogenous soft tissue mass containing areas of necrosis and calcification.

Retinal detachment can sometimes be incidentally identified on imaging as a 'V' shape

emanating from the optic disc.
(The Final FRCR Complete Revision Notes Page 440)

31. (e) Tracheobronchomegaly
Basal lung fibrosis, pectus excavatum, posterior vertebral scalloping and ribbon ribs are all thoracic manifestations of neurofibromatosis (NF) type 1 (von Recklinghausen disease). This is the genetic condition described in the main stem. The cutaneous nodules seen on the plain film represent cutaneous neurofibromas. The posterior mediastinal mass described could represent a meningocele or neurofibroma (fluid content would favour meningocele). Posterior scalloping of the vertebral bodies and ribbon ribs can occur secondary to adjacent neurofibroma. Pectus excavatum is sometimes associated with other conditions including Marfan syndrome and Ehlers-Danlos syndrome. It can be seen on plain film as blurring of the right heart border and displacement to the left, mimicking middle lobe consolidation. The posterior ribs are also more horizontal and the anterior ribs are more vertical. Tracheobronchomegaly is not a feature of NF 1.
(The Final FRCR Complete Revision Notes Page 44)

32. (d) Red marrow reconversion
In childhood red (haematopoietic) marrow predominates in the skeleton but as we age this is converted, distally to proximally, to yellow (fatty) marrow. In adulthood only the axial skeleton continues to contain red marrow.
Some conditions promote the reconversion of yellow to red marrow, including conditions associated with anaemia, long distance running and altitude. Signal characteristics of yellow marrow follow subcutaneous fat on all sequences, demonstrating high signal on T1 and T2 sequences. Red marrow is mildly hyperintense on T2 sequences but although on T1 imaging will be hyperintense to disc and muscle, it can be comparatively lower than the T2 signal and can be difficult to differentiate from metastatic marrow infiltration. In- and out-of-phase imaging can be helpful as the fat in yellow marrow will cause a drop in signal on the out-of-phase sequence which will not occur in metastatic infiltration.
Haemosiderosis may be possible in this case due to episodes of haemolysis or potentially repeated transfusion but it would be expected to cause reduced T1 and T2 signal.
Myelofibrosis is unlikely in this case but causes low signal on T1 and T2 sequences.
(The Final FRCR Complete Revision Notes Page 85)

33. (c) Grade III
(The Final FRCR Complete Revision Notes Page 221)

Table 4.5: American Association for the Surgery of Trauma (AAST) Grading of Liver Laceration (2018 Revision)

I	Subcapsular haematoma <10% surface area, laceration <1 cm deep
II	Subcapsular haematoma 10–50% surface area, intraparenchymal haematoma <10 cm, laceration <3 cm deep/10 cm long
III	Subcapsular haematoma >50%, intraparenchymal haematoma >10 cm, laceration >3 cm deep and >10 cm long, active bleeding contained within liver parenchyma
IV	Active bleeding beyond liver parenchyma into peritoneum, parenchymal disruption of 25–75% of liver lobe
V	Parenchymal disruption of >75% of lobe, juxtahepatic venous injuries – IVC, major hepatic vein, etc.

Source: The American Association for the Surgery of Trauma. 2018 revision. *AAST grading of liver laceration. Table 8.* https://www.aast.org/library/traumatools/injuryscoringscales.aspx#liver.

34. (e) Medulloblastoma
An astrocytoma is the most common posterior fossa mass, but the radiological features of this mass favour medulloblastoma, which is the second most common.

Medulloblastomas are solid masses which can grow quickly causing a relatively rapid onset of symptoms. They typically have low T1 signal and are T2 iso/hyperintense to grey matter. They are commonly more homogenous than other posterior fossa masses and demonstrate both enhancement and restricted diffusion. They arise from the roof of the fourth ventricle. It is important to image the rest of the neuroaxis to exclude drop metastases.

Astrocytomas typically have a large cystic component with an enhancing mural nodule. The fourth ventricle is often displaced anteriorly.

Ependymomas are frequently also in the fourth ventricle; however, they arise from the floor of the fourth ventricle and can extend out of the foramen of Magendie and Luschka. They are more heterogenous and commonly calcify.

Brainstem glioma tend to occur in the pons causing diffuse enlargement, although they can sometimes cause an exophytic masses. Like medulloblastoma, they can return low T1 and high T2 signal; however, their enhancement and restricted diffusion is minimal in comparison.

Paediatric choroid plexus papilloma are more common in the lateral ventricles and are usually well-defined cauliflower-like masses rather than the ill-defined mass described in this child.

(The Final FRCR Complete Revision Notes Page 300)

35. (e) Tethered cord syndrome

The cord usually terminates around the level of L1/2; below this level it is low and is associated with a tethered cord. There are various associations with tethered cord including spinal lipoma, diastematomyelia, thickened filum terminale, Chiari malformation, myelomeningocele and dermal sinus. In this case, the cord is tethered due to a lipoma; it follows fat on all sequences and does not enhance.

Ependymoma and paraganglioma are other causes of filum terminale masses. Ependymomas are the most common but they are often more heterogenous than the mass described in this question with haemorrhage, cystic change and calcification. Paragangliomas are also usually more heterogenous and they also intensely enhance.

Lipomyelomeningocele is a form of spina bifida. Although they do contain fat, it extends within the subcutaneous tissues and there are other important features such as neural arch defects. The bones in this case are normal.

Diastematomyelia is a split cord malformation however the question states that there is a single cord.

(The Final FRCR Complete Revision Notes Pages 305, 451)

36. (e) Reduced lung volumes

Respiratory distress syndrome in neonates is due to surfactant deficiency. It affects premature infants (<37 weeks) and is associated with low lung volumes, air bronchograms and granular opacities. If a chest radiograph is normal at 6 hours it excludes the diagnosis.

Interstitial oedema is more commonly associated with transient tachypnoea of the newborn, which also affects babies relatively quickly following delivery and is more commonly associated with term infants delivered by caesarean section. It usually resolves within days.

Meconium aspiration is typically associated with increased lung volumes, streaky perihilar opacities and lack of air bronchograms. Perihilar opacities may also be seen in neonatal pneumonia.

(The Final FRCR Complete Revision Notes Page 328)

37. (d) Serum eosinophil count

Simple pulmonary eosinophilia, or Löffler syndrome, is associated with elevated serum eosinophil levels and presents with transient air space opacification.

Anti-basement membrane antibody is associated with Goodpasture syndrome. This tends to cause pulmonary haemorrhage which may have similar appearances on chest radiograph but would be associated with more constitutional symptoms and haemoptysis.

Bronchoalveolar lavage demonstrating eosinophils would help to diagnose acute or chronic eosinophilic pneumonia. Both are associated with raised eosinophils in bronchoalveolar fluid, and the latter also with serum eosinophilia.

Serum cANCA positivity is found in vasculitic conditions such as eosinophilic granulomatosis with polyangiitis (Churg-Strauss) and microscopic polyangiitis.

The presence of 5-HIAA in urine suggests increased serotonin metabolism, which may be a feature of a carcinoid tumour.

(The Final FRCR Complete Revision Notes Page 29)

38. (d) Marfan syndrome
All of the options provided are possible causes of pectus excavatum. The imaging features described are consistent with underlying diagnosis of Marfan syndrome, which is a connective tissue disorder. Skeletal features in this condition include posterior vertebral body scalloping due to dural ectasia, scoliosis, spondylolisthesis, acetabular protrusion and arachnodactyly. Cardiac complications in this condition include aortic root dilatation, mitral valve regurgitation and aortic dissection. Cardiac disease is the cause of death in 90% of patients. Homocystinuria is rare. Patients can have Marfanoid features, and mortality in these patients is also mostly due to cardiovascular complications. Screening for this condition is performed in the neonate with the heel-prick test. Patients often have developmental delay.
(The Final FRCR Complete Revision Notes Page 114)

39. (e) Surgical referral
The appearances of a single, broad-based intraluminal filling defect without mucosal irregularity is suggestive of a benign lesion. The calcification is typical of a leiomyoma – they are the only oesophageal masses that calcify. If these are asymptomatic, then they do not need treatment; however, this patient does have symptoms and therefore surgical referral would be indicated.
Breast carcinoma is the most common metastatic lesion to affect the oesophagus and often causes multiple submucosal nodules.
The appearance of this lesion is also not typical for an oesophageal carcinoma, which frequently causes shouldered stricturing, often with mucosal irregularity. Staging for this would include endoscopic ultrasound and 18F-FDG PET/CT.
Neurofibromas can affect the oesophagus and can be difficult to differentiate from a leiomyoma; however they do not typically calcify and they are much rarer. If neurofibromatosis is suspected, then physical and family history assessment would be indicated along with neurological imaging.
(The Final FRCR Complete Revision Notes Page 179)

40. (e) Serous cystadenocarcinoma
The ovarian lesion has features concerning for malignancy due to the enhancing, peripheral, intermediate T1 and T2 signal area. The most common malignant ovarian tumour is a serous cystadenocarcinoma. These often have a large cystic component and enhancing soft tissue which may be papillary in appearance and demonstrate restricted diffusion. In contrast to this, serous cystadenomas should be simple and cystic with no soft tissue component.
Mucinous cystadenomas often have multiple septations, and due to their mucin content may have more varied signal than a serous cystadenoma. The lesion is frequently described as having a 'stained glass' appearance on MRI. A mucinous cystadenocarcinoma would have these features but also suspicious findings such as mural thickening or solid components.
Kruckenberg tumours are metastatic ovarian lesions, commonly from the gastrointestinal tract, breast or lung. They are frequently bilateral and have complex appearances containing enhancing solid components and mucin.
(The Final FRCR Complete Revision Notes Page 275)

41. (d) Septum pellucidum
There are differing severities of holoprosencephaly, ranging from alobar to lobar depending on the degree of cleavage that has occurred. The unifying characteristic of all forms is the absence of the septum pellucidum.
With the alobar subtype there is no cleavage of the cerebral hemispheres. There is no corpus callosum or falx cerebri, just one anterior cerebral artery and the thalami are fused. There is commonly an associated facial abnormality.
In semilobar holoprosencephaly there is partial cleavage posteriorly and the thalami are partially separated, but anteriorly there is still no hemispheric cleavage. The corpus callosum may be absent or hypoplastic.
In lobar forms of the condition it is just the frontal lobes and the frontal horns of the lateral ventricles which remain fused. There is either complete or partial cleavage of the thalami and the falx and interhemispheric fissure is formed. The corpus callosum may be hypoplastic.
(The Final FRCR Complete Revision Notes Page 296)

42. (a) Capillary haemangioma

Capillary haemangiomas often affect the periorbital region and are also called strawberry haemangiomas when they are external on the skin surface. However, they can cause intraorbital masses presenting with proptosis. They usually increase in size over the first few months of life and then slowly regress. On imaging they appear as lobulated, septated masses which can span both the intra and extraconal compartments. They have curvilinear flow voids and enhance intensely.

Cavernous haemangioma are more common in the adult population and are usually intraconal. They are rounded and well defined with the appearance of a capsule. Their enhancement tends to be slower and more patchy than a capillary haemangioma.

Lymphangioma are usually extraconal and are more heterogenous with solid and cystic components and fluid-fluid levels. They can cause sudden proptosis due to haemorrhage. Due to their proteinaceous cystic components they are commonly high on T1 and T2 with minimal enhancement.

Retinoblastomas are related to the globe and are heterogenous solid masses containing necrosis and calcification.

On imaging, a venous varix appears as a dilated intraconal vessel and can be congenital or acquired, following trauma for example. It presents with intermittent proptosis on coughing or straining, and therefore imaging before and after Valsalva manoeuvre can be helpful.

(The Final FRCR Complete Revision Notes Page 437)

43. (e) *Streptococcus pneumoniae*

The chest radiograph is describing lobar consolidation. Opacification usually appears rapidly on a chest radiograph and resolves slowly after treatment. The most common causative organism is *Streptococcus pneumoniae* (pneumococcal pneumonia). This accounts for more than 50% of bacterial pneumonia. It can be multi-lobar or bilateral, and pleural effusions are also common. In children, consolidation can appear mass-like, referred to as 'round pneumonia'.

Haemophilus influenzae is a Gram-negative pneumonia, usually found in debilitated patients. This usually affects the lower lobes.

Klebsiella produces consolidation similar to streptococcus. It may be associated with bulging fissures and it can cavitate.

Legionella pneumophila (Legionnaires' disease) can produce consolidation similar to *Streptococcus pneumoniae*. There is often rapid progression to other lobes and cavitation may be present.

Staphylococcus aureus usually occurs in debilitated inpatients. It is commonly associated with cavitation and pleural effusion, sometimes empyema.

(The Final FRCR Complete Revision Notes Page 47)

44. (c) Osteomyelitis

The case describes a Brodie abscess, which is a form of chronic osteomyelitis and represents an intraosseous abscess. Typical radiographic appearances are described in the question, in particular the orientation along the long axis of the bone. They usually occur in the metaphysis, and the pathognomic sign is the lucent channel extending towards the physis in a patient with an unfused skeleton. They can have similar appearances to osteoid osteoma, although the latter are usually cortically based, but this can vary.

Eosinophilic granulomas do occur in children and can affect the metadiaphysis; however they would not typically have a sclerotic rim.

Osteosarcomas are more aggressive lesions and would usually cause more adjacent periosteal reaction and soft tissue extension without the sclerosis

Giant cell tumours typically involve the metaphysis but tend to occur in an older age group with fused skeletons.

(The Final FRCR Complete Revision Notes Pages 87, 106)

45. (c) Hepatic vein

A transjugular intrahepatic portosystemic shunt (TIPSS) is performed to treat portal hypertension and can be utilised for bleeding oesophageal or gastric varices when endoscopic therapy has failed. Vascular access is usually via the right jugular vein and a shunt is created between the portal vein and a hepatic vein with a stent to allow blood to bypass the liver. Contraindications include severe right heart failure, severe encephalopathy, sepsis and severe chronic liver disease. Complications include haemorrhage, infection and specifically

arteriovenous fistula, unintentional gallbladder puncture and hepatic infarct.
(The Final FRCR Complete Revision Notes Page 221)

46. (b) Osmotic demyelination syndrome
Osmotic demyelination syndrome (formally known as central pontine myelinolysis) refers to an acute demyelination in the setting of rapid osmotic changes, classically due to rapid correction of hyponatraemia. There are usually initial symptoms secondary to the hyponatraemia and then within days of correction of the electrolyte imbalance, symptoms of demyelination ensue with quadriparesis and reduced consciousness.
Typical CT findings are of pontine hypodensity crossing the midline. On MRI this is T2 and FLAIR hyperintense with T1 hypointensity and restricted diffusion. It can also affect the basal ganglia and subcortical white matter.
A pontine infarct could have similar signal characteristics but would typically be a unilateral abnormality that does not cross the midline.
Wernicke encephalopathy is associated with chronic alcohol abuse but does not typically affect the pons, instead favouring the thalami, periaqueductal grey matter and mamillary bodies with T2 hyperintensity, contrast enhancement and restricted diffusion.
A metastatic lesion and pontine astrocytoma would cause a mass-like lesion with enhancement and causing mass effect, potentially leading to hydrocephalus. Evidence of disease elsewhere within the brain may also be expected in metastatic disease.
(The Final FRCR Complete Revision Notes Pages 417–418)

47. (b) Anterior to sternocleidomastoid, below the angle of the mandible
Branchial cleft cysts are within the differential for a non-midline, anterior triangle cystic neck mass. The most common type is a second branchial cleft cyst. The Bailey classification has traditionally been used to differentiate between them, although other helpful anatomical landmarks are worth knowing. Type II cysts are commonly described as anterior to sternocleidomastoid, between the angle of the mandible and carotid bifurcation, deep to the level of platysma. The sternocleidomastoid muscles help divide the neck into anterior and posterior triangles.
The other types of branchial cleft cysts are much less common; however answer A describes a type I cyst and answer D describes a type IV cyst.
(The Final FRCR Complete Revision Notes Page 307)

48. (b) Axial post contrast fat supressed T1
Mucoepidermoid carcinoma is the most common cancer to affect the parotid glands, followed by adenoid cystic carcinoma. Both of these primaries have a predisposition to perineural spread. A post contrast fat supressed T1 sequence is the best way to assess the base of skull and cranial nerves. Lymph node metastases are also possible.
Classically on ultrasound mucoepidermoid carcinoma appears as a hypoechoic lesion containing cystic areas. When high grade, they can be more ill defined and infiltrative. MRI demonstrates low T1 signal and heterogenous T2 signal due to the solid and cystic nature of the lesion. The solid components usually enhance.
(The Final FRCR Complete Revision Notes Page 428)

49. (b) Fat embolism
Fat embolism can be encountered following trauma or other significant insults such as pancreatitis, burns, liposuction and severe sepsis. In the setting of trauma, long bone fractures are often the underlying cause due to fat from bone marrow entering the circulation. Initial imaging is normal, followed by delayed development at around 24–48 hours of consolidation, and ground glass opacity within the lungs, with fat density pulmonary artery filling defects also possible.
In contrast to this, lung contusions and pulmonary lacerations would usually be present at the time of the initial trauma imaging. Lung contusions are often seen in the form of consolidation which is frequently peripherally sited at an interface between the lung and a firmer structure, for example the ribs or mediastinum. Pulmonary lacerations cause a defect in the lung which can fill with blood or air, in which case it is called a pneumatocele.
Aspiration pneumonia is possible following trauma but the patient was intubated on admission to hospital so if it was not visible on the trauma CT it is unlikely to have developed since then in the presence of an inflated endotracheal tube. The short time interval between admission and the

pulmonary abnormalities developing makes bronchopneumonia less likely.
(The Final FRCR Complete Revision Notes Page 30)

50. (c) Perthes disease
The description in the question is that of Perthes disease, also known as Legg-Calvé-Perthes disease. This is avascular necrosis of the capital femoral epiphysis, more common in boys between 4 and 8 years. Early changes include subchondral lucency, widened medial joint space and a small epiphysis with sclerosis. Later in the disease there may be fragmentation of the femoral head.
Slipped upper femoral epiphysis typically affects adolescents aged 10–16 years. It is best seen on the frog-leg lateral views; the epiphysis is slipped posteriorly and the epiphyseal height reduced.
Whilst osteomyelitis is an important consideration and appearances may include a joint effusion, osteopenia, periosteal reaction and focal bone lysis or cortical destruction, the features described in this case are typical for Perthes.
Transient synovitis is the most common cause of hip pain in children. A joint effusion is common but would not account for the changes seen in the epiphysis.
Haemophilic arthropathy is associated with a joint effusion, periarticular osteoporosis and epiphyseal enlargement.
(The Final FRCR Complete Revision Notes Page 121)

51. (a) Microcytic anaemia
Plummer-Vinson syndrome is characterised by an oesophageal web, iron deficiency anaemia and dysphagia. The web is often anteriorly located in the upper third of the oesophagus, but it can be circumferential. Other causes of oesophageal webs include graft-versus-host disease, gastroesophageal reflux disease and pemphigoid.
A low CD4 count is associated with an impaired immune system, most commonly secondary to HIV infection. On a barium swallow this may manifest with signs of herpes simplex infection causing small superficial ulcers, candidiasis causing large plaque-like abnormalities with pseudomembrane formation, or cytomegalovirus oesophagitis causing giant ulcers.
Raised gamma-glutamyl transferase suggests excess alcohol intake. This may be associated with variceal formation in chronic abuse which cause serpiginous luminal filling defects.
Helicobacter pylori is associated with gastro-oesophageal reflux disease and peptic and duodenal ulcers.
Vitamin B_{12} deficiency can be secondary to gastric causes such as atrophic gastritis and following gastrectomy or due to ileal malabsorption, for example in Crohn's disease.
(The Final FRCR Complete Revision Notes Page 181)

52. (d) Referral to urology surgeons
The multiple fat-containing renal lesions along with lung cysts are consistent with a diagnosis of tuberous sclerosis; therefore these lesions are likely angiomyolipomas. The main risk for angiomyolipoma is retroperitoneal haemorrhage and lesions that are >40 mm should be considered for embolisation or surgical removal. Lesions that are <20 mm generally do not require follow-up due to slow growth, and angiomyolipoma between these measurements can be followed up with interval imaging. A patient may require MRI kidneys if there is any doubt about the lesions, for example if they are fat poor. Fat-saturated and in- and out-of-phase MRI sequences can be helpful.
Patients with tuberous sclerosis are more likely to have renal cysts and can develop renal cell carcinoma at a younger age than the general population.
(The Final FRCR Complete Revision Notes Pages 246, 263)

53. (a) Croup
Croup or laryngotracheobronchitis is a viral upper respiratory tract infection usually affecting children up to the age of 3 years. It causes a characteristic barking cough and can cause inspiratory stridor. The findings on radiograph include subglottic narrowing, referred to as the 'steeple' sign, and hypopharyngeal distension.
Epiglottitis is an important and potentially life-threatening differential to exclude. This causes epiglottic and aryepiglottic fold swelling which can cause the epiglottis to resemble a thumb. Epiglottitis is less common now due to infant *Haemophilus influenzae* type B vaccination; however, *Streptococcus* A can also cause it. These patients should not be laid flat for imaging as this could lead to complete airway obstruction.

Exudative tracheitis is less likely in this age group as it usually affects older children. Radiographic findings would include membranous tracheal filling defects and irregularity.

Retropharyngeal abscess is suspected if the retropharyngeal soft tissues are thickened; however, they are normal in this case.

The subglottic narrowing and hypopharyngeal distension in this case is below the pharynx and therefore not consistent with pharyngitis.

(The Final FRCR Complete Revision Notes Page 322)

54. (d) Pial vessels peripheral to the mass

Differentiating intra- from extra-axial masses helps to narrow the imaging differential. Extra-axial masses can have various characteristics that may aid this task. An extra-axial mass will displace the subarachnoid and pial vessels medially towards the brain. If the pial vessels are peripheral to the mass it suggests it is a parenchymal, intra-axial mass.

Extra-axial masses can cause adjacent skull changes such as hyperostosis with meningiomas; however, this is unlikely with an intra-axial lesion. Buckling of the grey–white matter interface is caused by the pressure exerted by an extra-axial mass on the adjacent brain. In contrast, an intra-axial mass will usually cause swelling and expansion of the white matter and cortex. The cerebrospinal fluid (CSF) cleft sign is described as a thin rim of CSF or FLAIR hyperintensity between the mass and the brain parenchyma.

(The Final FRCR Complete Revision Notes Page 386)

55. (e) Primary (autoimmune) pulmonary alveolar proteinosis

Pulmonary alveolar proteinosis (PAP) usually affects middle-aged men. It is strongly associated with smoking. It represents filling of airspaces with proteinaceous fluid with preservation of the interstitium. Imaging features are often more severe than the clinical symptoms. The 'crazy paving' description is typical for PAP but not pathognomonic. It refers to ground glass opacification in combination with smooth interlobular septal thickening. It is usually of primary (or autoimmune) origin (approximately 90%).

Secondary PAP is less common. It can be precipitated by silica dust inhalation or haematological malignancy as well as immunodeficiency with infection, for example *Cryptococcus*, *Nocardia* or *Aspergillus*. The information provided in the main stem is most likely in keeping with primary PAP, as this is most common, and no information that could account for a secondary cause has been provided. Congenital PAP presents in the neonatal period and so is not considered a possible aetiology in this case.

(The Final FRCR Complete Revision Notes Page 49)

56. (e) Tenosynovial giant cell tumour

These tumours are pigmented villonodular synovitis affecting the tendon sheath and have similar imaging characteristics on MRI with low T1 and T2 signal and evidence of blooming on gradient echo sequences due to haemosiderin deposition.

Although desmoid tumours are most common in the abdomen, they can affect limbs but tend not be in direct contact with the tendon sheath. They can look similar on ultrasound if well defined, and also demonstrate low signal on T1 and T2 sequences; however, they would not demonstrate susceptibility artefact.

Fibromas can look similar but are not associated with susceptibility artefact either.

Ganglion cysts are cystic rather than solid lesions and would not demonstrate internal vascularity.

Glomus tumours are vascular tumours also known as glomangiomas, and present as painful small blue/red nodules under the fingernails. Due to their small size they are difficult to see on radiograph and there may just be mild soft tissue swelling. The lesions will be hypervascular if visible on ultrasound.

(The Final FRCR Complete Revision Notes Pages 90, 142)

57. (a) Serous cystadenoma

The mass fits well with being a serous cystadenoma; it is in the pancreatic head, there are multiple small cysts, calcification is central and the patient is an elderly woman.

A mucinous cystadenoma is more common in middle-aged women and the cysts are less numerous and larger. Calcification is peripheral and the majority of masses are in the pancreatic body or tail.

Main duct intraductal papillary mucinous neoplasms (IPMNs) do occur in a more elderly age group and more commonly in the pancreatic head; however, they usually cause pancreatic duct dilatation (>3 mm). Calcification is not a typical feature.

Islet cell tumours are neuroendocrine tumours, and when small are usually homogenous solid lesions rather than the cystic mass described in this question. The most common islet cell tumour is an insulinoma followed by gastrinoma. They exhibit arterial phase enhancement and so usually appear isodense to the pancreas on portal venous phase CT.

(The Final FRCR Complete Revision Notes Page 229)

58. (d) Osteoid osteoma

The history of night pain relieved by salicylate is typical for an osteoid osteoma. This is a benign bone lesion which has a lucent central nidus (<1.5 cm) with surrounding sclerosis centred on the metaphyseal or diaphyseal cortex. On scintigraphy there is 'double density sign' where the central nidus demonstrates focal intense activity and the surrounding sclerosis demonstrates more modest activity. Treatment options include radiofrequency ablation of the lucent focus.

Fibrous cortical defect are benign, well-defined lytic lesions less than 2 cm. They are intracortical affecting the metaphysis, have a narrow zone of transition with a thin sclerotic rim, and on scintigraphy there is increased uptake.

Osteoblastomas are histologically similar to an osteoid osteoma. The central nidus is larger than 1.5 cm and they are usually seen between 20 and 30 years old.

Osteochondromas are composed of cortical and medullary bone protruding from a bone with the presence of a cartilage cap.

Osteosarcoma is the most common primary bone tumour in children. It is an ill-defined lytic/sclerotic metaphyseal lesion with an internal osteoid matrix.

(The Final FRCR Complete Revision Notes Page 147)

59. (d) Thoracic duct atresia

Chylothorax is most commonly due to an iatrogenic injury of the thoracic duct, for example following thoracic surgery such as oesophagectomy. Chylothoraces can also be caused by traumatic injury or by malignancy. In a neonate these causes are less likely, although birth trauma is a possibility. The most likely causes are thoracic duct atresia, lymphangiectasia and pulmonary abnormalities such as congenital pulmonary airway malformation and extralobar sequestration. Certain congenital conditions such as Turner, Noonan and Down syndrome are also associated with chylothoraces.

In this case, the child is male so this excludes Turner syndrome. The normal appearance of the lungs excludes lymphangiectasia and extralobar sequestration. The former causes dilated lymphatics, which leads to other radiological findings such as interstitial thickening and perihilar infiltrates. Lymphangioleiomyomatosis is not a diagnosis made in this age group, as it usually affects young women. Therefore the most likely cause in this patient is thoracic duct atresia.

(The Final FRCR Complete Revision Notes Page 320)

60. (c) Haemangioblastoma

The most common cause of a posterior fossa mass in adults is a metastasis; however the second most common is a haemangioblastoma, which fits the description in this case. The history of a relatively young man with a history of renal cell carcinoma is also suggestive of possible von Hippel-Lindau syndrome. On imaging, haemangioblastomas are most commonly located in the posterior fossa. They are well-defined cystic masses with an enhancing mural nodule. They may demonstrate flow voids, particularly at the periphery of the lesion.

Pilocytic astrocytomas can have a similar appearance with a cystic mass and enhancing mural nodule; however, they usually occur in a much younger age group.

A cavernoma is not a cystic mass and on MRI can have variable appearances depending on the presence of haemorrhage and haemosiderin. This causes blooming on susceptibility weighted imaging.

Ependymomas often contain cystic components; however they also contain significant solid elements, calcification and haemorrhage.

(The Final FRCR Complete Revision Notes Page 392)

61. (d) Arterial phase CT from diaphragm to toes

Approximately 30–50% of popliteal artery aneurysms are associated with an abdominal aortic aneurysm; therefore the abdominal aorta needs to be included on the study. In lower limb studies, the contralateral lower limb will automatically be included on the study and assessment of the contralateral popliteal artery is also vital, as they can be bilateral. Other important factors to consider when planning interventional radiological management is the tortuosity of the common and external iliac arteries and mural calcification, particularly at the femoral vessels where vascular access will be required for endovascular repair. The CT should extend to the toes to assess the vessel quality peripheral to the aneurysm, as popliteal aneurysms are associated with peripheral thromboembolic complications.

(The Final FRCR Complete Revision Notes Page 2)

62. (d) Scleroderma

The differentials for acro-osteolysis, or terminal tuft resorption, include scleroderma, psoriatic arthritis, hyperparathyroidism, syringomyelia and trauma, such as burns or frostbite.

Clavicle involvement further narrows the differential; it is described in scleroderma and hyperparathyroidism as well as rheumatoid arthritis and other less common congenital conditions such as cleidocranial dysostosis and pyknodysostosis.

Therefore, the acro-osteolysis and clavicle erosions combined with the other findings make scleroderma the most likely answer.

Hyperparathyroidism, particularly secondary hyperparathyroidism, can also cause generalised osteopenia, soft tissue calcification, acro-osteolysis and distal clavicle resorption. However, the described deformity and the dilated oesophagus on chest radiograph make scleroderma more likely.

Scleroderma causes an erosive arthropathy affecting the interphalangeal joints and there is commonly deformity with ulnar deviation of the fingers or radial subluxation at the first carpometacarpal joint. Osteopenia can be either periarticular or generalized, and soft tissue wasting and calcification is also common. Another typical finding on chest radiograph is oesophageal dilatation.

(The Final FRCR Complete Revision Notes Pages 95, 107)

63. (e) Thickened ileocaecal valve

Tuberculosis (TB) affecting the bowel can present with pain, weight loss, bowel symptoms and fever. It most commonly involves the ileocaecal region, and often preferentially affects the caecum. The ileocaecal valve can become thickened, patulous and over time, rigid. Like Crohn's disease, there can be both deep fissures and ulceration. The ulceration in TB is usually circumferential, whereas in Crohn's they are typically longitudinal and typically on the mesenteric border. With chronicity, both conditions can lead to strictures, and in TB the caecum can appear retracted.

Crohn's disease tends to be associated with very little ascites whereas there is often more fluid in cases of TB, which can be relatively high density. Both conditions may cause abdominal lymph node enlargement; however in TB these lymph nodes typically demonstrate low attenuation. TB can also cause peritonitis with nodularity and peritoneal thickening.

(The Final FRCR Complete Revision Notes Pages 183–184)

64. (a) Contrast enhanced MRI

Renal cell carcinoma extending into the renal vein corresponds to at least T3 disease, with proximal extension an important factor in surgical planning. If it extends into the inferior vena cava, then a midline laparotomy is required, and if beyond the level of the hepatic veins, then thoracic surgeons will likely need to be involved.

It can be difficult to assess tumour thrombus versus bland thrombus. Sometimes contrast enhancement is identified on post-contrast CT within the thrombus, consistent with tumour; however, MRI is superior to CT for assessment. Tumour thrombus on MRI would also enhance and on T1 weighted imaging the normal vascular flow voids would be replaced by comparatively high tumour signal.

18F-FDG PET/CT currently has a limited role in the staging of renal cell carcinoma due to renal excretion causing high renal tracer uptake and therefore making assessment difficult. However, there are reports of tracer uptake in tumour thrombi.

Ultrasound Doppler may identify thrombus; however the assessment of bland thrombus versus tumour thrombus would be challenging on ultrasound.

Digital subtraction angiography does not have a role in this case.

(The Final FRCR Complete Revision Notes Page 258)

65. (c) Total anomalous pulmonary venous return (TAVPR)

When assessing congenital heart disease, the best approach is to categorise the conditions into cyanotic and acyanotic and then further divide them using the appearance of the lungs into plethoric and oligemic. Of the options listed, TAPVR and transposition of the great arteries (TGA) are the only ones that cause cyanosis and plethoric lungs. Tetralogy of Fallot and pulmonary atresia cause oligaemic lungs. Tricuspid atresia can cause variable lung appearances, but usually it is associated with oligaemia. TGA classically gives a narrowed upper mediastinal silhouette (egg-on-a-string) whereas the most common form of TAPVR (the supracardiac type I) gives the snowman appearance.

(The Final FRCR Complete Revision Notes Pages 310, 317)

66. (a) Antrochoanal polyp

Antrochoanal polyps are benign lesions occurring in the maxillary sinus which fill the antrum and extend into the nasopharynx via an enlarged ostium. Typically they are low signal on T1 and high signal on T2 sequences with peripheral enhancement.

Mucoceles may have similar MRI signal characteristics but they do not pass into the ipsilateral nasopharynx. Another differential is a mucous retention cyst. These are more likely when there is air visible in the sinus, whereas this finding would exclude a mucocele. Mucous retention cysts are also not associated with bony expansion.

An inverting papilloma originates in the nose but can extend into the ipsilateral paranasal sinuses. The signal tends to be more isointense on T1 and T2 sequences.

An esthesioneuroblastoma also arises from the nose, and these masses are more likely to affect the ethmoid air cells. They can invade the anterior cranial fossa and typically demonstrate marked contrast enhancement rather than the peripheral enhancement described in this case.

(The Final FRCR Complete Revision Notes Page 426)

67. (d) Right main bronchus near the carina

The description of the sagging right lung indicates that there is an underlying tracheobronchial injury. This injury is associated with high mortality. It usually occurs close to the carina which is fixed relative to the bronchi. Imaging features include presence of a pneumothorax which is refractory to drainage, as well as the presence of the 'fallen lung' sign, in which the lung sags towards the floor of the hemithorax, away from the hilum. There may also be a fractured first rib, indicating high impact force; however this is not the cause of pneumothorax in the case vignette. Diaphragm rupture can occur in cases of trauma and may be associated with complications such as herniation of abdominal viscera.

(The Final FRCR Complete Revision Notes Page 59)

68. (a) Brown tumour

(The Final FRCR Complete Revision Notes Pages 132, 149)

Table 4.6: Lucent Bone Lesions with and without Sclerotic Margination

Sclerotic rim	Non-sclerotic Rim
Simple bone cyst	Giant cell tumour
Chondroblastoma	Aneurysmal bone cyst
Chondromyxoid fibroma	Brown tumour
Fibrous dysplasia	
Fibrous cortical defect	
Epidermoid cyst	

Source: Reprinted with permission from V Helyar and A Shaw. *The Final FRCR: Complete Revision Notes.* CRC Press, Taylor & Francis Group, 2018, p. 149.

The features are in keeping with a Brown tumour, also known as an osteoclastoma. These are solitary lesions seen in primary and secondary hyperparathyroidism. They can mimic metastases and myeloma.

69. (d) Hyperenhancing 1-cm nodule in the tail of pancreas
Endocrine tumours of the pancreas, also known as islet cell tumours, are a type of neuroendocrine tumours. The most common type is an insulinoma followed by a gastrinoma, but other types include glucagonoma and VIPoma. Insulinomas tend to present when small due to the episodes of hypoglycaemia they induce. They are usually avidly arterially enhancing solid masses but they can be necrotic when large. They may also contain calcification.
(The Final FRCR Complete Revision Notes Page 232)

70. (b) Bronchogenic cyst
Bronchogenic cysts are congenital malformations causing mediastinal or, less commonly, intrapulmonary masses. They are often incidental findings but when large can impact adjacent structures, causing respiratory symptoms. They are typically in the middle mediastinum, subcarinal and right-sided. They are usually of fluid density with no contrast enhancement.
Meningoceles would be located in the posterior mediastinum.
Pericardial cysts mainly occur at the cardiophrenic angle.
A radiopaque inhaled foreign body may be projected over the hilum or mediastinum; however many foreign bodies are radiolucent.
Lymphoma would be expected to be of soft tissue density.
(The Final FRCR Complete Revision Notes Page 319)

71. (b) Kaposi sarcoma
Low attenuation lymph nodes can be due to cystic or fatty components. Causes of cystic components include metastatic malignancy, typically squamous cell carcinoma, and sometimes lymphoma is associated with this. Tuberculosis and coeliac disease can also cause this appearance. Fat is deposited in lymph nodes in Whipple disease. It has also been described in systemic lupus erythematosus.
High attenuation lymph nodes have been described in conditions such as Kaposi sarcoma, Castleman disease and carcinoid.
(The Final FRCR Complete Revision Notes Pages 189, 214)

72. (c) Ganglioglioma
Gangliogliomas most commonly occur in the temporal lobes causing seizures in children and young adults. They can have variable appearances with both solid and cystic elements. They frequently demonstrate calcification which causes blooming on susceptibility weighted imaging.
Oligodendrogliomas can have similar appearances to ganglioglioma and present with seizures; however they are uncommon in children.
The other options are all likely in the temporal lobes, causing little if any adjacent oedema or seizures as a common presentation. Dysembryoplastic neuroepithelial tumours (DNETs) usually do not enhance much, if at all. Pleomorphic xanthoastrocytomas are rare tumours. Calcification is not a feature and although intra-axial, commonly demonstrate a dural tail sign.
Pilocytic astrocytomas are not common in the temporal lobes and usually affect the cerebellum or optic pathways. They are also largely cystic with an enhancing solid nodule.
(The Final FRCR Complete Revision Notes Page 391)

73. (b) Anomalous origin of the right subclavian artery
Inferior rib notching in aortic coarctation is caused by dilated intercostal vessels which act as collateral supply bypassing blood to the thoracic aorta distal to the coarctation. Unilateral left inferior rib notching is seen in aortic coarctation when there is an anomalous origin of the right subclavian artery distal to the coarctation. Anomalous origin of the left subclavian artery, a right-sided aortic arch with an anomalous left subclavian artery and a stenosed left subclavian artery are all potential causes of unilateral right inferior rib notching. The costocervical trunks are important anatomically as they arise directly from the subclavian arteries on both sides and supply the first and second intercostal arteries. The other intercostal arteries arise directly from the thoracic aorta, hence there is sparing of the first and second ribs from rib notching with aortic coarctation.
(The Final FRCR Complete Revision Notes Pages 3, 94)

74. (a) Joint aspiration
This patient is suffering from septic arthritis until proven otherwise and should therefore not be sent home. Radiographs can be normal initially but can also reveal relatively

non-specific changes such as joint effusion and joint swelling. More advanced manifestations include periarticular osteopenia, joint space narrowing and bone destruction.

The history is key; the patient is febrile and the recent pneumonia suggests this could be caused by haematogenous spread from the recent infection. The most commonly affected joints are hip, knee, elbow or ankle, and the most common pathogen is *Staphylococcus aureus*.

The best way to obtain a diagnosis and target antibiotics appropriately is with joint aspiration followed by microscopy and culture of the synovial fluid. Radiology can offer assistance with ultrasound-guided aspiration if needed, but if clinical suspicion is high, joint washout may be pursued regardless.

MRI in septic arthritis can confirm the joint effusion and demonstrate marrow and soft tissue oedema and synovial enhancement.

There will be increased tracer uptake on all phases of a triple phase nuclear medicine bone scan.
(The Final FRCR Complete Revision Notes Page 96)

75. (c) Anterior to the sigmoid colon

The imaging characteristics are typical for epiploic appendagitis. This usually affects women more than men and is more common in patients with a raised body mass index. Differentials would include appendicitis and diverticulitis; however the patient is young and diverticulitis would be less likely. The imaging appearances are not characteristic for appendicitis.

The epiploic appendages are small fatty appendages sited along the large bowel. When these twist they cause acute abdominal pain which can be difficult to clinically differentiate from other causes of pain. This most commonly occurs anterior to the rectosigmoid colon. On ultrasound the appearance of a hyperechoic mass indicates fat. Sometimes a slightly hypoechoic line can be seen peripherally, and there is no internal vascularity. CT is usually diagnostic and demonstrates a lesion of fat density adjacent to the colon with peripheral enhancement and surrounding fat stranding. Sometimes a hyperechoic dot centrally can be seen representing thrombosed vessels.
(The Final FRCR Complete Revision Notes Page 167)

76. (a) Abdominal ultrasound

The patient has a right-sided varicocele. Varicoceles are more common on the left due to the drainage of the left testicular vein into the left renal vein. The right testicular vein drains directly into the lower pressure inferior vena cava. If a varicocele is just on the right side, then ultrasound of the abdomen, to focus on the retroperitoneal structures, should be performed to ensure there is not an underlying pathology, such as a mass, impeding venous return. If ultrasound cannot be confidently used to assess this, for example in patients with a high body mass index, then other modalities could be considered. Treatment for uncomplicated varicoceles include surgical ligation or embolisation.

There are a couple of tiny hyperechoic foci in the right testicle of unlikely clinical significance; when >5 this is consistent with microlithiasis. Guidance from the European Society of Urogenital Radiology suggests annual follow-up until the age of 55 only if there are other risk factors present, such as a history of orchidopexy or maldescent. The presence of a testicular mass would prompt tumour marking testing but is not indicated in this case.
(The Final FRCR Complete Revision Notes Page 281)
Richenberg J, Brejt N. Microlithiasis: is there a need for surveillance in the absence of other risk factors. European Radiology. 2012:22(11);2540–2546.

77. (d) 'Finger-in-glove' opacities

The child has cystic fibrosis. The first signs on chest radiograph are hyperinflation and bronchial wall thickening. High resolution CT can show cylindrical bronchiectasis, mucous impaction and mosaic attenuation due to air trapping. Although the entire lung can be affected, there is a predilection for the upper lobes, the apices of the lower lobes and a perihilar distribution. The 'finger-in-glove' appearance is due to bronchial obstruction by mucous. The bronchus distal to the obstructing mucous is dilated. This can be observed in other conditions such as allergic bronchopulmonary aspergillosis which can occur in isolation, or in combination with cystic fibrosis.

Atelectasis in cystic fibrosis is more likely to be in the upper lobes. Cardiomegaly may eventually occur secondary to pulmonary hypertension and resulting cardiac failure; however, this is unlikely at diagnosis. Chylothoraces and thin-walled pulmonary cysts are not associated with cystic fibrosis.
(The Final FRCR Complete Revision Notes Page 322)

78. (c) Multisystem atrophy

There can be overlap between the radiological appearances in neurodegenerative disease. Multisystem atrophy is classically associated with the 'hot cross bun' sign due to pontine T2 hyperintensity. Hyperintensity can also be seen in the cerebellum and cerebellar peduncles. Typically there is low signal in the basal ganglia, specifically the putamen, with a peripheral rim of T2 hyperintensity. Atrophy of the pons, cerebellum and midbrain is also reported.

Progressive supranuclear palsy is associated with midbrain atrophy causing flattening of the superior midbrain leading to the characteristic 'hummingbird' appearance. T2 hyperintensities in the pons, midbrain and inferior olivary nucleus, as well as cisternal and ventricular dilatation, may be evident.

Huntington disease is characterised by enlargement of the frontal horns of the lateral ventricles due to atrophy of the caudate nuclei. The basal ganglia may become T2 hypointense due to iron deposition.

Features of Lewy body dementia include generalised volume loss with enlargement of the lateral ventricles. Hippocampal atrophy, which is frequently associated with Alzheimer disease, is not a feature. Pick disease classically has more focal volume loss which can be asymmetrical and affect the temporal and frontal lobes.

(The Final FRCR Complete Revision Notes Page 425)

79. (b) Irregular contour of the descending aorta

Takayasu arteritis is a vasculitis of large arteries, affecting predominantly the aorta and major branches. It can also affect the pulmonary arteries (in approximately 15%). It is divided into two phases, acute inflammatory phase and healed fibrotic phase, which have differing CT appearances. In the acute phase the aorta wall is thickened and demonstrates delayed enhancement (on imaging performed approximately 20 minutes after contrast injection). The most common feature in healed fibrotic phase is an irregular contour of the descending aorta. Absent enhancement of a thickened wall can also be seen as well as calcification of the arch and descending aorta; however these are less frequent. Whilst Takayasu arteritis has a predilection for the aortic arch and descending aorta, calcification of the ascending aorta may be seen as sequelae to syphilitic aortitis.

(The Final FRCR Complete Revision Notes Page 16)

Chung MP, Chin AY, Lee HY et al. Imaging of pulmonary vasculitis. Radiology. 2010;255(2):322–341.

80. (d) Giant cell tumour

The features described are typical of a giant cell tumour, which is an eccentric lesion occurring in a fused skeleton, abutting the articular surface with a well-defined non-sclerotic margin. Aneurysmal bone cysts are lucent lesions occurring in the metaphysis with thinning of the cortex and fine internal trabeculation; however, they usually occur in patients less than 30 years old. Eosinophilic granuloma also occurs in patients less than 30 years old. Fibrous dysplasia can look like anything. It typically has a sclerotic rim. Non-ossifying fibromas are rarely seen in patients over 30 years old. They usually have a thin sclerotic border.

(The Final FRCR Complete Revision Notes Page 141)

81. (b) Low attenuation halo surrounding vessels

Mesenteric panniculitis is a chronic inflammatory condition of the small bowel mesentery, often affecting the jejunal root. It is described as haziness of the mesenteric fat which is not associated with adjacent bowel wall involvement and does not cause displacement of adjacent structures. A low attenuation perivascular halo is frequently described.

Mesenteric oedema causes diffuse hyperdensity of the mesentery which can often make visualisation of the vessels difficult. One cause of this would be liver cirrhosis, which would be associated with a shrunken, nodular liver. Other causes include hypoalbuminaemia and cardiac failure. Low attenuation lymph nodes are not associated with mesenteric panniculitis but are seen in conditions such as tuberculosis, Whipple disease and coeliac disease.

(The Final FRCR Complete Revision Notes Page 190)

82. (e) Von Hippel-Lindau

Von Hippel-Lindau is an autosomal dominant inherited condition which can exhibit multisystem involvement. The intracranial tumour described by the patient in the question likely represents a haemangioblastoma; however, choroid plexus papillomas are also possible. Patients can have cysts in the liver, pancreas and kidneys as well as renal angiomyolipoma, phaechromocytomas and pancreatic neuroendocrine tumours. This group of patients is at increased risk of renal cell carcinoma, which can be bilateral and is typically of clear cell subtype.

Tuberous sclerosis can cause angiomyolipomas. It carries an increased risk of renal cell carcinoma and is associated with intracranial tumours such as subependymal giant cell astrocytomas as well as other parenchymal brain abnormalities. However, the other features in the question are not typical. Pulmonary cysts, sclerotic bone lesions and cardiac rhabdomyomas are also encountered.

Osler-Weber-Rendu is also known as hereditary haemorrhagic telangiectasia and is characterised by multiple arteriovenous malformations.

Birt-Hogg-Dubé is associated with renal tumours such as renal cell carcinomas and oncocytomas as well as pulmonary cysts and cutaneous manifestations; however, the other lesions mentioned in the question are not consistent with this diagnosis.

Gorlin-Goltz is characterised by multiple basal cell carcinomas and musculoskeletal and craniofacial abnormalities. Intracranial tumours are possible but the other features are not described.

(The Final FRCR Complete Revision Notes Pages 266, 306)

83. (a) Enlarged aorta

With a patent ductus arteriosus, a left-to-right shunt occurs as high-pressure blood passes from the aorta to the pulmonary circulation via the patent ductus. The ductus arteriosus usually closes within 48 hours of birth. If this remains open, then eventually the left atrium and ventricle can become enlarged and the aorta dilated; however the right heart is unaffected. With a ventricular septal defect the left atrium and both ventricles may enlarge; however, the aorta remains normal in size.

(The Final FRCR Complete Revision Notes Page 314)

84. (b) Gliomatosis cerebri

Gliomatosis cerebri is a diffuse infiltrative parenchymal process involving two or more lobes of the brain. The peak onset is 30–40 years of age. It affects large portions of the brain with relatively little mass effect considering the extent of involvement. Due to its isodense appearance relative to adjacent brain, it can be difficult to define on CT. On MRI there is often T1 hypointensity and T2 hyperintensity within the white matter and gyral thickening. There is limited enhancement and restricted diffusion.

The history is not suggestive of progressive multifocal leukoencephalopathy (PML) which is encountered in the setting of immunosuppression, for example HIV and AIDS. There is also no mass effect in PML. Primary CNS lymphoma would usually demonstrate avid, uniform enhancement. Tumefactive demyelinating lesions also typically enhance with incomplete ring enhancement. Encephalitis has a different clinical presentation. The most common type is due to herpes simplex infection usually causing bilateral temporal lobe abnormalities.

(The Final FRCR Complete Revision Notes Page 392)

85. (d) Distal right renal artery

The case is describing findings of right renal artery stenosis, which in this patient is an incidental finding identified on an ultrasound performed for another clinical indication. Sonographic findings include a size discrepancy in the kidneys, a renal artery to aortic velocity ratio of >3.5, a renal artery peak systolic velocity >180 cm/sec, increased resistive index (>0.7) and a slow rising parvus and tardus waveform distal to the stenosis. The most common cause for renal artery stenosis is atheroma, which affects the proximal renal artery close to its origin; however this is most common in older patients. In young patients, such as in this case, the most common cause is fibromuscular dysplasia, which causes multiple short stenoses leading to a 'string of beads' appearance. This tends to affect the mid-distal renal artery; however other arteries such as carotid, iliac and mesenteric arteries can also be affected. Treatment is with angioplasty and tends to have good results.

(The Final FRCR Complete Revision Notes Pages 14, 252)

86. (c) Symmetrical enlargement of the inferior rectus muscles on MRI orbits

The appearance of painless symmetrical periosteal reaction in the tubular bones, particularly of the hands and feet, is typical for thyroid acropachy. The thyroid itself does not have to be abnormal, as patients can be euthyroid or post-treatment. The condition is almost always associated with thyroid eye disease, which manifests as an increase in orbital fat and bilateral symmetrical enlargement of the extraocular muscles. There is a characteristic pattern of involvement, with the mnemonic **'I'M SLOW'** being a helpful way to remember it:

Inferior rectus
Medial rectus
Superior rectus
Lateral rectus
Obliques

Another cause for periosteal reaction of the long bones is hypertrophic osteoarthropathy, but this tends to be painful. Secondary causes of hypertrophic osteoarthropathy include lung cancer, bronchiectasis and mesothelioma as well as non-pulmonary causes such as inflammatory bowel disease and coeliac disease. The latter causes reversal of the normal jejunoileal fold pattern with increased ileal folds and reduced jejunal folds.

Primary hypertrophic osteoarthropathy, or pachydermoperiostosis, is most common in young black men and typically has skin changes with skin fold thickening, often on the scalp. The patient demographics do not fit with this diagnosis.

(The Final FRCR Complete Revision Notes Page 99)

87. (a) CT chest with contrast

The imaging features are suspicious for a soft tissue sarcoma. The most appropriate next step is a CT chest to assess for any evidence of disease elsewhere. An MRI pelvis may also be helpful to more accurately delineate the extent of the mass. Discussion at a tertiary sarcoma centre prior to biopsy is important; however imaging should be completed prior to this referral. There are frequently concerns regarding tumour seeding with sarcomatous lesions, and sometimes sarcoma centres will request to biopsy the lesion themselves. Identifying the most appropriate biopsy site may also be aided by completing imaging, as a more superficial lymph node could be more easily accessible than an intrapelvic or abdominal mass. 18F-FDG PET/CT may be helpful but would not be clearly indicated at this point.

(The Final FRCR Complete Revision Notes Page 192)

88. (e) Ultrasound urinary tract within 6 weeks

NICE guidelines state that for children less than 6 months old an ultrasound within 6 weeks of a lower urinary tract infection (LUTI) is appropriate. If there are atypical features, such as raised creatinine, poor urine flow, failure to respond to treatment with 48 hours, sepsis or non-*Escherichia coli* bacteria, this would necessitate an immediate ultrasound. This child is being prescribed oral treatment with close outpatient follow-up and therefore atypical infection is unlikely.

For children older than 6 months the recommendation is for immediate ultrasound if there are features of atypical LUTI and dimercaptosuccinic acid (DMSA) test within 4–6 months. Otherwise, imaging is not routinely indicated for a single episode of LUTI unless infections are recurrent (≥3 LUTI episodes) when an ultrasound within 6 weeks and DMSA test within 4–6 months is indicated.

Micturating cystourethrograms are only advised if there is a family history of vesicoureteral reflux, a non-*E. coli* infection, poor urine flow or urinary tract dilatation on ultrasound.

(National Institute for Health and Care Excellence (NICE) Clinical Guideline 54: Urinary tract infection in under 16s: diagnosis and management, 2007, updated 2018)

89. (e) Congenital pulmonary airway malformation (CPAM)

CPAM was previously known as congenital cystic adenomatoid malformation. It can be diagnosed on antenatal ultrasound scans. It is a condition causing cystic lung lesions arising from abnormal airway development. There are three subtypes; however the most common is as described with multiple large air-filled cysts. Immediately following birth these lesions may predominantly contain fluid and air-fluid levels. They can cause mass effect with atelectasis of adjacent lung and flattening of the diaphragm.

The mass described in the question is unlikely to be a bronchogenic cyst because there is no airway connection and therefore no gas in bronchogenic cysts unless complicated by infection, for example.

The supply of the lesion by the bronchial artery helps exclude pulmonary sequestration, which receives a systemic arterial supply. Similarly, this makes a diaphragmatic hernia, such as a Bochdalek hernia, unlikely. The question also states that the diaphragm is intact.

Congenital lobar over inflation would have a hyperlucent and hyperinflated lung segment and would not have any cystic components.
(The Final FRCR Complete Revision Notes Page 321)

90. (b) Euthyroid, heterogenous hypoechoic gland, avascular, reduced tracer uptake
Hashimoto thyroiditis can have variable ultrasound appearances but there is reduced tracer uptake on pertechnetate scans. The gland is usually enlarged and hypoechoic with reduced vascularity. Patients are commonly euthyroid or hypothyroid. There is an increased risk of non-Hodgkin's lymphoma and therefore follow-up and biopsy of any focal nodularity is recommended. Chronic changes include a shrunken heterogenous gland.
Graves disease is associated with hyperthyroidism and would be consistent with answer D in this case. Patients may present with extrathyroid signs such as ophthalmopathy. Ultrasound appearances are typically of an enlarged hyperechoic gland with hypervascularity and on nuclear medicine studies there is increased tracer activity.
(The Final FRCR Complete Revision Notes Page 433)

91. (a) Presence of calcification
When assessing the incidental pulmonary nodule (nodule found incidentally in a patient without active or previous history of cancer) there are a number of features which should be reported, including whether the nodule is solitary or multiple, the location in the lungs, solid/ground glass/mixed, size, margins and presence of calcification/fat. The presence of calcification is reassuring as this is considered a feature of benignity. The most recent British Thoracic Society guidelines advise not to offer routine follow-up in patients with a nodule containing diffuse, central, laminated or popcorn calcification. Whilst volume doubling time of ≥600 days is reassuring, there are some malignancies which demonstrate slow growth, and so follow-up is required. Volume doubling time of ≤400 days is considered a suspicious feature and may warrant further investigation.
Upper lobe location of pulmonary nodules is also considered more suspicious than lower lobe location.
(The Final FRCR Complete Revision Notes Page 55)
Callister MEJ, Baldwin DR, Akram AR et al. British Thoracic Society Guidelines for the investigation and management of pulmonary nodules. Thorax. 2015;70(2):ii1–ii54.

92. (c) Inferior rib notching
The chromosomal abnormality described is neurofibromatosis type 1. The well-defined intra- and extra-axial lesions are neurofibromas. The description of enlarged neural foramina is secondary to the presence of neurofibromas. Lateral meningocoeles may also be present and can cause this finding. The posterior elements may be hypoplastic, also due to the presence of neurofibromas/meningocoeles. Inferior rib notching is more likely to occur for the same reason; superior rib notching is possible if the neurofibroma is large.
Anterior vertebral beaking is a feature of mucopolysaccharidoses, Down syndrome and other conditions. Multiple non-ossifying fibromas may also be seen in neurofibromatosis type 1, which are typically lucent lesions with sclerotic margins. Other musculoskeletal manifestations include pseudarthrosis of the wrist, tibia, fibula and clavicle as well as other bony dysplasias.
(The Final FRCR Complete Revision Notes Page 116)

93. (c) T1: Spleen < liver, T2: Spleen > liver, No change between in- and out-of-phase
Liver MRI is frequently employed to help clarify either CT or ultrasound appearances, especially for challenging cases such as in hepatitis B surveillance or in patients with a high body mass index, which can make ultrasound challenging. Normal liver parenchymal signal is hyperintense compared to the spleen on T1 and hypointense compared to the spleen on T2, and there should be no reduction of signal on out-of-phase imaging. Liver signal is also frequently compared to muscle – it should be a similar signal except on inversion recovery sequences. Diffuse signal reduction on out-of-phase imaging can be suggestive of a fatty liver, and similarly the T1 signal may be increased in these patients.
(The Final FRCR Complete Revision Notes Page 193)

94. (d) Catheter passes superiorly from umbilicus with the tip at the level of T8
Umbilical venous catheters pass superiorly from the umbilical vein into the portal vein and then through the ductus venosus into the hepatic vein and inferior vena cava. The tip should

ideally lie at the junction of the inferior vena cava and right atrium, which is around the level of the diaphragm at T8/9. It is important that the catheter is sited correctly because if the tip is within the portal venous system it can lead to thrombosis. The catheter may also pass into the superior mesenteric artery or splenic vein (and be projected over the left upper quadrant (as described in answer E). If the catheter is inserted too far, the tip may be within the right ventricle or the superior vena cava.

The path of umbilical arterial catheters should be inferior from the umbilicus going into the pelvis before turning cephalad and passing into the aorta. The aim is for the tip to be within the aorta in either a high or low position but not between the levels of T10-L3, which is where the main aortic branches arise.

(The Final FRCR Complete Revision Notes Page 332)

95. (d) Rectal biopsy

The case describes a patient with Hirschsprung disease. There is a transition point, most commonly at the rectosigmoid colon, where the bowel transitions to a narrowed aganglionic segment. A longer segment can also be affected, with a transition at the splenic flexure, or less commonly the entire colon may be involved. There is frequently dilatation of the bowel proximal to this transition point. There may be a 'sawtooth' appearance of the narrowed segment. The rectosigmoid ratio is an important factor, as normally the rectum is larger than the sigmoid colon and should be >1. A ratio <1 is indicative of Hirschsprung disease and this is confirmed with rectal biopsy.

If Hirschsprung disease was associated with an abnormal antenatal scan, the abnormality would lead to polyhydramnios rather than oligohydramnios. A sweat chloride test and the routine neonatal heel prick test could help in the detection of cystic fibrosis, which is commonly associated with meconium ileus. A maternal history of diabetes is associated with meconium plug syndrome.

(The Final FRCR Complete Revision Notes Page 340)

96. (b) Tetralogy of Fallot

A right-sided aortic arch with mirror imaging branching is the most common subtype of a right-sided aortic arch and is nearly always associated with congenital heart disease. Of these, 90% are associated with tetralogy of Fallot. Therefore other radiological findings to look for are a 'boot-shaped' heart and pulmonary oligaemia.

A right-sided aortic arch with an aberrant left subclavian artery is the second most common subtype, and the persistent ductus ligament can cause tracheal compression. A Kommerell diverticulum is also a feature, which manifests as dilatation of the aberrant left subclavian artery at the right aortic arch origin.

(The Final FRCR Complete Revision Notes Page 315)

97. (a) Acute respiratory distress syndrome

Acute respiratory distress syndrome (ARDS) can be split into pulmonary causes (e.g. toxic inhalation, drowning, lung contusion, pneumonia and fat embolus) and extrapulmonary causes (e.g. burns, sepsis, blood transfusion and pancreatitis). This case describes an extrapulmonary cause. The features of symmetrical consolidation with a gradient from posterior to anterior with more ground glass changes anteriorly is typical. Pulmonary causes tend to lead to asymmetrical changes without a gradient.

A hospital-acquired pneumonia is possible, although the patient has only had a brief admission so far. An aspiration pneumonia is also possible, especially if there has been vomiting with recent alcohol excess, but in an intensive care patient with pancreatitis and such typical features of ARDS, this is less likely.

In cardiac failure, other features such as cardiomegaly, prominent vascular markings, interstitial lines and pleural effusions would be more common. This patient does have a small left pleural effusion but this is likely secondary to the pancreatitis.

One of the causes of fat embolism is pancreatitis, and features can resemble ARDS. Typical appearances of fat embolism include geographic ground glass opacities rather than the gradient seen in ARDS. Interlobular septal thickening and nodularity are also features, which are less common in ARDS.

(The Final FRCR Complete Revision Notes Page 16)

98. (c) Idiopathic transient osteoporosis of the hip

This tends to be unilateral, affecting males more than females, although it is described in late pregnancy. The history of hip pain is long, and the classic radiological description is of osteopenia and subchondral cortical loss. An MRI will demonstrate bone marrow oedema, centred on the subchondral region, and early post-contrast enhancement of the abnormal marrow.

The history and presentation is not characteristic for septic arthritis and there is no indication that the patient is unwell, as this has been managed as an outpatient.

In avascular necrosis the early post-contrast enhancement would not be typical. Although bone marrow oedema is a feature, other signs such as subchondral linear low signal and the 'double line' sign are usually present.

A stress fracture in an active young patient is possible but in the proximal femur this tends to occur at the femoral neck rather than at the femoral head. A cortical breach and a linear low T1 signal fracture line would also be expected.

Complex regional pain syndrome commonly occurs following trauma. Due to sympathetic dysfunction, other symptoms such as alteration to skin blood flow, hyperalgesia and oedema are often described. This condition typically affects the extremities rather than a large joint such as the hip. There is some overlap in radiographic features, with joint space preservation and osteopenia being typical.

(The Final FRCR Complete Revision Notes Page 100)

99. (a) Adenoma

The appearances are typical for a hepatic adenoma. These lesions can be large and heterogenous due to areas of necrosis and haemorrhage. Despite being benign, they are often removed due to the risk of bleeding. They may contain fat, leading to the hyperechoic appearance on ultrasound, T1 hyperintensity and signal drop on out-of-phase imaging. Adenomas can demonstrate washout, and are the only benign lesions which may do so.

The hypointensity following hepatocyte specific contrast helps to differentiate it from focal nodular hyperplasia (FNH) which would be iso to hyperintense due to their hepatocellular origin. Similarly, the absence of a high T2 signal intensity central scar differentiates it from FNH.

A fibrolamellar carcinoma typically has a low signal intensity central scar and many cases demonstrate calcification.

Hepatic metastases are often T1 hypointense and there is not usually fat present.

Haemangiomas commonly cause incidental hyperechoic hepatic lesions on ultrasound but the other features in this case are not typical. They characteristically exhibit centripetal enhancement.

(The Final FRCR Complete Revision Notes Page 195)

100. (e) Testicular ultrasound

Eagle-Barrett, or prune belly syndrome is a congenital condition causing urinary tract abnormalities, a characteristic 'prune belly' appearance of the anterior abdominal wall and cryptorchidism. A testicular ultrasound would be able to confirm whether the testicles have descended into the scrotum, and if not, may be able to locate them in the inguinal canal. Undescended testes at birth may descend by around 3 months of age. Locating an intrapelvic or abdominal testicle with ultrasound can be more challenging, and sometimes MRI would be required. Eagle-Barrett syndrome is associated with cardiac anomalies in approximately 10%.

(The Final FRCR Complete Revision Notes Page 257)

101. (d) MRI signal is usually T1 and T2 isointense with homogenous enhancement

Choroid plexus papilloma are thought to increase cerebrospinal fluid production and impede absorption by the arachnoid granulations, so hydrocephalus is a common presentation. They typically occur at the trigone of the lateral ventricle. In children a supratentorial location is most likely; however in adults they are more common in the posterior fossa. The majority of tumours are benign but in up to 20% of cases they can become malignant. MRI signal is often described as T1 and T2 isointense with avid homogenous enhancement. Calcification occurs in around 20% of cases.

(The Final FRCR Complete Revision Notes Page 289)

102. (b) Alexander disease

Alexander disease is a progressive disease affecting the white matter in infants. It characteristically starts in the frontal lobes and progresses posteriorly, affecting the basal ganglia too. This causes white matter T2 hyperintensity and enhancement. In the late stages of the disease there can be cystic cavitation.

X-linked adrenoleukodystrophy has a more posterior distribution of T2 hyperintensity with changes affecting the periventricular parieto-occipital white matter and splenium of the corpus callosum progressing to affect the visual and auditory pathways, with peripheral enhancement commonly seen.

Canavan disease has a symmetrical, diffuse, bilateral involvement of subcortical white matter. However, there is usually sparing of the caudate nucleus, corpus callosum and internal capsule. In contrast to Alexander disease, there is no contrast enhancement. MR spectroscopy will reveal elevated *N*-acetyl-aspartate, which is a hallmark of the condition.

Krabbe disease affects the white matter with a periventricular predilection but in a more central and posterior distribution with involvement of the centrum semiovale, thalami and basal ganglia. There is no contrast enhancement in these regions and unlike other leukodystrophies there is enlargement of the optic nerves.

Leigh syndrome is a mitochondrial disorder. The changes seen on imaging tend to be symmetrical with T2 hyperintensity in the brainstem, medulla, midbrain and putamen. In contrast to the conditions already discussed above, cerebral white matter involvement is not commonly a feature.

(The Final FRCR Complete Revision Notes Page 421)

103. (b) Invasive adenocarcinoma

The most common type of lung malignancy is non-small cell lung cancer which comprises adenocarcinoma and squamous cell carcinoma, of which adenocarcinoma is the most common. The imaging features are in keeping with lymph node involvement, and the effusion may also be malignant. Adenocarcinoma may also present as consolidation which is resistant to antibiotics, whilst adenocarcinoma in situ usually manifests as persistent predominantly ground glass opacification.

Squamous cell carcinoma tends to cavitate. The common sites of metastasis are the skeleton, brain, adrenal glands, liver and soft tissues.

Small cell lung cancer typically presents when it is systemically disseminated. Imaging commonly demonstrates extensive lymph node enlargement, occasionally without evidence of significant lung parenchymal abnormality.

Mesothelioma is a relatively rare thoracic malignancy; however it is the most common primary pleural malignancy. It is usually nodular, but can be diffuse and is often associated with pleural effusion. It is strongly associated with previous asbestos exposure.

(The Final FRCR Complete Revision Notes Pages 39–41)

104. (d) Shortened third and fourth metacarpals

Turner syndrome is a chromosomal abnormality occurring only in females. It is associated with cardiovascular anomalies including hypoplastic left heart and aortic coarctation and renal anomalies including ectopia and horseshoe kidney. Radiographs of the hand may show shortened third and fourth metacarpals, Madelung deformity, carpal coalition and narrowing of the scapholunate angle. The other findings listed in the question are not seen in Turner syndrome.

Terminal tuft resorption is associated with inflammatory processes rather than congenital conditions such as scleroderma and psoriatic arthritis.

(The Final FRCR Complete Revision Notes Page 130)

105. (d) Poorly controlled left ventricular failure

Buscopan is used as an antispasmodic agent for studies where bowel motion may cause image degradation. A complication of Buscopan is acute angle closure glaucoma; however, the chronic open angle form of the condition is not a contraindication. Patients may not know they are at risk of acute angle closure glaucoma until they develop symptoms of eye pain, altered/reduced vision and nausea and vomiting, and so it is important that patients are warned about this. If a patient develops acute angle closure glaucoma, both eyes are usually treated by laser iridotomy at the first presentation to prevent recurrence.

Unstable cardiac disease such as poorly controlled left ventricular failure, unstable angina, recent admission with acute coronary syndrome and recent arrythmia are all contraindications for Buscopan. Hypothyroidism is not a contraindication. There should be caution exercised with hyperthyroidism due to its potential association with tachycardia.

Buscopan can hypothetically lead to urinary retention; however, due to its short-acting effects and the relatively low dose used in radiology this is considered to be low risk. A history of prostate cancer should not be a contraindication for Buscopan usage.

A conventional pacemaker device is a contraindication for MRI but not for Buscopan administration. Some newer pacemakers are marketed as MRI compatible within certain parameters. A pacemaker will have most likely been inserted due to dysrhythmia and therefore should be able to counteract any Buscopan-induced tachycardia; however, it may be prudent to discuss with cardiology first.

Dyde R, Chapman AH, Gale R et al. Precautions to be taken by radiologists and radiographers when prescribing hyoscine-N-butylbromide. Clinical Radiology. 2008;63(7):739–743.

106. (e) Phyllodes tumour

A phyllodes tumour is difficult to differentiate from other lesions, such as fibroadenoma, without a biopsy. Typical features include a predominantly solid lesion with posterior acoustic enhancement which may contain cystic spaces and vascularity. Rapid growth is also a characteristic.

Breast carcinoma is commonly described as an ill-defined, hypoechoic and spiculate mass with posterior acoustic shadowing. The mass is typically vertically orientated, disrupting tissue planes. High-grade cancers can appear as more focal well-defined masses and hence why biopsy of solid breast lesions is so important. Lobular cancers may be difficult to identify on ultrasound.

Fat necrosis follows trauma to the breast, and eliciting this history is important. Its appearance depends on the age of the lesion. It may initially be a focal hyperechoic area in the fat, then become more cystic manifesting as an oil cyst, and finally it can appear as a spiculate area due to desmoplastic reaction. Eggshell calcification is typically associated with it on mammograms.

Fibrocystic change is common in young women and can be painful. Simple cysts on ultrasound are anechoic and well defined. A cyst with solid components requires biopsy of the solid component. Prominent fibrous glandular tissue may be palpated and visualised at ultrasound.

Papillomas are a cause of nipple discharge and may appear as a solid lesion within a dilated duct or as a solid and cystic mass.

(The Final FRCR Complete Revision Notes Page 286)

107. (b) Bilateral hyparterial bronchi

Polysplenia syndrome is a form of left isomerism and one of the heterotaxy syndromes. Patients with polysplenia have multiple small spleens, bilobed lungs, hyparterial bronchi, bilateral left atria, partial anomalous pulmonary venous return (APVR), a midline liver and absent gallbladder. The superior vena cava continues as the azygous or hemiazygous vein.

Hyparterial bronchi arise inferior to the pulmonary artery, whereas eparterial bronchi arise superior to it.

Right isomerism, or asplenia, is associated with eparterial bronchi, trilobed lungs, bilateral right atria, total APVR, absence of the spleen and cyanotic congenital heart disease.

Cystic hygromas are associated with chromosomal abnormalities and other congenital conditions but not with heterotaxy syndromes.

(The Final FRCR Complete Revision Notes Page 316)

108. (b) Acute haemorrhagic leukoencephalopathy

Acute haemorrhagic leukoencephalopathy, also known as Hurst disease, is a severe haemorrhagic form of acute demyelinating encephalomyelitis (ADEM). The features are similar except that in Hurst disease there is increased oedema, mass effect and microhaemorrhages. It is usually fatal, whereas ADEM frequently responds to steroids.

ADEM is a white matter abnormality favouring the subcortical white matter, but the brainstem and cerebellum can also be affected. The lesions are FLAIR hyperintense and can have peripheral restricted diffusion and enhancement. The history of recent illness or vaccination is key to the diagnosis.

Herpes simplex encephalitis classically involves bilateral temporal lobes and cingulate gyrus. There is commonly both cortical and white matter and cortex T2 hyperintensity rather than the subcortical distribution in this case. There may also be microhaemorrhages.

Cerebral abscesses are a differential for peripherally enhancing lesions; however they would usually have central restricted diffusion rather than just peripherally.

Progressive multifocal leukoencephalopathy is not typical with this history because it is associated with an immunocompromised state. The white matter changes are also asymmetric and frequently parieto-occipital, affecting the periventricular as well as the subcortical white matter.

(The Final FRCR Complete Revision Notes Page 412)

109. (a) Chronic eosinophilic pneumonia

The peripheral air space opacification described in the question is describing the so-called 'reverse bat-wing' appearance, which has a short list of differentials including simple pulmonary eosinophilia, chronic eosinophilic pneumonia, cryptogenic organising pneumonia (COP), pulmonary haemorrhage, vasculitis and contusion. The clinical history is typical for chronic eosinophilic pneumonia, whereas simple pulmonary eosinophilia tends to cause minimal systemic upset.

COP can present similarly but tends to affect all lung zones rather than the upper and middle lobe predominance described in chronic eosinophilic pneumonia. Peribronchial nodules are also a feature of COP.

Pulmonary infarcts can also cause subpleural air space opacification and are secondary to obstructing pulmonary emboli, often leading to wedge shaped areas of abnormality. The history also makes this less likely.

Pulmonary oedema is one of the causes of the 'bat-wing' appearance, where pulmonary changes are perihilar rather than the peripheral changes described in the question. Pleural effusions are commonly encountered with pulmonary oedema but are not typically associated with chronic eosinophilic pneumonia.

(The Final FRCR Complete Revision Notes Pages 29–30)

110. (b) Internal septations

Ganglion cysts are benign bone lesions containing mucous material. They can be intra-articular, extra-articular, intra-osseous and periosteal. They are most common around the wrist and hand. Internal septations may or may not be present. MRI features are T1 low to intermediate signal, T2 high signal and high signal on protein density sequences. Periosteal new bone formation is a feature of periosteal ganglia rather than an intraosseous ganglion cyst.

(The Final FRCR Complete Revision Notes Page 140)

111. (b) Dilatation of the proximal duodenum and stomach

The patient has symptoms and radiological signs of superior mesenteric artery (SMA) syndrome. This frequently affects patients with a low body mass index due to reduced intrabdominal fat; however, conditions such as lumbar lordosis can also predispose patients. The aortomesenteric angle is reduced to between 6 and 22° and the aortomesenteric distance is reduced to 2–8 mm. Sagittal reconstructions usually aid diagnosis. Another radiological sign is dilatation of the proximal duodenum and stomach, which fits with the symptoms of early satiety and vomiting.

Reduced contrast enhancement of the small bowel in the distribution of the SMA and small bowel wall thickening are not features but would be more in keeping with SMA thrombus and ischaemia. SMA mural thickening and enhancement are findings consistent with a large vessel vasculitis such as Takayasu.

(The Final FRCR Complete Revision Notes Page 186)

112. (b) Partial nephrectomy

The lesion described is a well-defined, multiloculated cystic mass with an enhancing periphery and septations. The protrusion of the mass into the renal hilum and imaging description is typical for a cystic nephroma. The component cysts can contain simple fluid or more complex fluid such as haemorrhage. Cystic nephromas have a bimodal distribution often occurring in children or middle-aged females. However, these lesions are difficult to macroscopically differentiate from multilocular cystic renal neoplasm of low malignant potential and are therefore resected. Follow-up is also not appropriate in this patient who is otherwise fit and well.

This patient has no features to suggest that a partial nephrectomy would be contraindicated, and radiological-guided embolisation and radiofrequency ablation are less likely options in the setting of a renal mass of unknown malignant potential.

(The Final FRCR Complete Revision Notes Page 254)

113. (a) Bronchopulmonary dysplasia

The history of a baby born prematurely with long-term oxygen and ventilator requirements (>30 days) is consistent with bronchopulmonary dysplasia. The radiological appearances of hyperinflation, focal emphysema and coarse lung markings are also typical.

Sequestration and congenital lobar overinflation are conditions affecting part of the lung rather than all of the lungs and therefore the radiological findings and history are not consistent with these diagnoses.

Viral pneumonia can cause hyperinflation and perihilar densities but the emphysematous changes in this child are not consistent with this diagnosis.

As the name suggests, transient tachypnoea of the newborn exists for a short time, usually resolving by 2–3 days following delivery.

(The Final FRCR Complete Revision Notes Page 319)

114. (e) Thyroid papillary carcinoma

The lesions described in the question are consistent with haemorrhagic metastases with a density of 55 HU and adjacent mass effect. Malignancies associated with haemorrhagic metastases include melanoma, thyroid (particularly papillary carcinoma), choriocarcinoma and renal cell carcinoma. The other available cancers do not typically cause haemorrhagic metastases.

(The Final FRCR Complete Revision Notes Page 394)

115. (a) Anterior oesophageal indentation and posterior tracheal indentation

The question described typical findings in a pulmonary sling or aberrant left pulmonary artery. Neonates can present with respiratory distress due to narrowing of the trachea and narrowing of the right main bronchus or bronchus intermedius, which can lead to air trapping. The left pulmonary artery arises from the right pulmonary artery and passes between the trachea anteriorly and the oesophagus posteriorly, hence indenting the posterior wall of the trachea and the anterior wall of the oesophagus. It is the only vascular anomaly to pass between the trachea and oesophagus.

A double aortic arch causes anterior tracheal and posterior oesophageal indentation.

Anterior tracheal compression is caused by innominate artery indentation, which tends to occur in infants who have an arterial origin more towards the left than in adults. The mediastinum is more crowded in infants due to the thymus, and the vessel can therefore indent the trachea just inferior to level of the thoracic inlet.

Posterior oesophageal indentation can either be caused with a normal left aortic arch with an aberrant right subclavian artery or with a right aortic arch if there is an aberrant left subclavian artery.

(The Final FRCR Complete Revision Notes Pages 1, 311)

116. (e) Progressive systemic sclerosis

Progressive systemic sclerosis, also known as scleroderma, causes dilatation of the distal two-thirds of the oesophagus due to fibrosis of the smooth muscle in this region. This leads to poor motility, dilatation and places patients at risk of aspiration.

Other causes of oesophageal dysmotility include gastro-oesophageal reflux disease, presbyoesophagus, achalasia and Chagas disease. The patient also has thoracic features of scleroderma with peripheral lung reticulation and lymph node enlargement.

Presbyoesophagus is considered to be age related and affects elderly patients frequently with comorbidities such as dementia and diabetes.

Chagas disease is caused by a protozoal infection and also leads to cardiomyopathy and dilatation elsewhere in the gastrointestinal tract.

Achalasia frequently presents with dysphagia; over time the oesophagus becomes dilated, lacking normal motility with distal tapering rather than dilatation.

Despite the mediastinal lymph node enlargement, the other radiological features described in this case are not typical for oesophageal carcinoma.

(The Final FRCR Complete Revision Notes Page 180)

117. (a) Craniopharyngioma

Craniopharyngiomas are the most common suprasellar mass in children, and the history in this question is typical with visual field defects and diabetes insipidus. Radiologically they are usually part cystic and solid and exhibit T1 and T2 hyperintensity due to proteinaceous content. Calcification is very common.

Germinomas are typically solid and are neither cystic nor calcified. In contrast to this, meningiomas do commonly calcify, but a cystic component is not usually a feature. Pituitary macroadenomas occur in an older age group and calcification is rare. Rathke cleft cysts are thin walled, cystic and generally show no enhancement.

(The Final FRCR Complete Revision Notes Page 292)

118. (b) Lynch syndrome

Along with colorectal cancer, there is a patient history of nephroureterectomy, consistent with previous urothelial malignancy. The family history reveals endometrial cancer and glioblastoma. These all fit with Lynch syndrome, otherwise known as hereditary non-polyposis colorectal cancer. This is the most common cancer syndrome and increases the risk of urinary tract transitional cell carcinoma, endometrioid endometrial cancer and glioblastoma as well as ovarian, small bowel and gastric cancers.

Apart from colorectal cancer, familial adenomatous polyposis is also associated with other conditions such as hepatoblastoma, osteomas, papillary thyroid cancer and desmoid tumours.

Peutz-Jeghers syndrome is a condition which causes non-neoplastic hamartomas. These are not premalignant; however, the syndrome is associated with malignancies such as cervical adenoma malignum, breast, pancreas, ovarian and testicular tumours.

Tuberous sclerosis predisposes patients to multiple gastrointestinal polyps but it is not associated with colorectal cancer. Associations with neurological tumours such as subependymal giant cell astrocytoma and renal angiomyolipoma, oncocytomas and renal cell carcinoma are documented.

Turcot syndrome is characterised by colon cancer as well as primary brain tumours, such as glioblastoma and medulloblastoma. Although the father in this case died from glioblastoma, Turcot syndrome is rare compared to Lynch syndrome.

(The Final FRCR Complete Revision Notes Page 173)

119. (e) T1 hypointense, T2 hyperintense, Restricted diffusion, Medial displacement

Cholesteatoma are middle ear masses, which unlike other masses in this region demonstrate restricted diffusion. They are T1 hypointense and T2 hyperintense and do not typically enhance. They most commonly affect the superior tympanic membrane (pars flaccida) occurring in the attic, otherwise known as Prussak's space. They can erode the scutum and displace the ossicles and in this location displace them medially. When cholesteatomas less commonly involve the pars tensa, the ossicles are displaced laterally.

(The Final FRCR Complete Revision Notes Page 431)

120. (a) Aneurysmal bone cyst

The description is typical for an aneurysmal bone cyst (ABC). This is a benign lesion, more common in patients in the second decade, typically lucent, expansile with multiple thin walled, blood filled cavities (fluid-fluid levels). ABCs are more common in the posterior elements with involvement of the vertebral body.

Giant cell tumour (GCT) is an important differential diagnosis; however this usually affects patients in the third or fourth decades, and usually affects the vertebral body rather than the posterior elements. Fluid-fluid levels may be seen if there is secondary formation of an ABC within the GCT.

A simple bone cyst may be multilocular and can have fluid-fluid levels representing haemorrhage. It usually affects the metaphysis/diaphysis of a long bone, pathological fractures are common and a fallen fragment is seen in 5%.

Fibrous dysplasia has a variety of appearances. It is usually ground glass in appearance with a sclerotic margin, most commonly affecting the ribs, femur, tibia and craniofacial bones. The appearances described are not typical for bone metastasis.

(The Final FRCR Complete Revision Notes Page 130)

Index

Boldface page numbers denote tables.

C

D

E

F

G

H

I

J

K

L

M

U

V

W

X

Z